Resistance to Targeted Anti-Cancer Therapeutics

Volume 2

Series Editor

Benjamin Bonavida

For further volumes:
http://www.springer.com/series/11727

Benjamin Bonavida
Editor

Resistance to Immunotherapeutic Antibodies in Cancer

Strategies to Overcome Resistance

Springer

Editor
Benjamin Bonavida, Ph.D.
Department of Microbiology,
Immunology and Molecular Genetics
University of California
Los Angeles, CA
USA

ISSN 2196-5501 ISSN 2196-551X (electronic)
ISBN 978-1-4614-7653-5 ISBN 978-1-4614-7654-2 (eBook)
DOI 10.1007/978-1-4614-7654-2
Springer New York Heidelberg Dordrecht London

Library of Congress Control Number: 2013943719

Printed on acid-free paper

Springer is part of Springer Science+Business Media (www.springer.com)

Preface

A new era of anti-cancer therapeutics has emerged with significant objective clinical responses, prolongation of survivals, and even cures. These have been the result of the successful introduction of monoclonal antibodies (mAbs) directed against surface-bound membrane antigens on cancer cells. More than 20 mAbs have been approved for human use targeting a range of different cancers. The observed successes achieved by such antibodies against cancers stem from their high levels of specificity, long biological half lives, ability to recruit host effector cells, synergy with conventional drugs, and minimal toxicity. However, a major drawback of mAbs therapeutics, like any other therapeutics, is that a subset of patients does not initially respond and another initially responding subset develops resistance to further treatments. At the present time, there are no effective therapies for these subsets of cancer patients. Clearly, it is imperative that analyses of underlying mechanisms responsible for resistance will be required to develop and generate new targeted therapies that overcome the resistance. In addition, it will be possible to determine a priori whether a patient will be susceptible to response or not and which will allow oncologists to make proper decisions for treatment of the cancer patient at the individual level.

This volume titled, *Resistance to Immunotherapeutic Antibodies in Cancer: Strategies to Overcome Resistance* has been developed with the objective of highlighting up-to-date information on several investigations that deal with various mechanisms of resistance to anti-cancer mAbs therapeutics as well as those that deal with novel approaches to overcome resistance. The reviews in this volume are written by highly qualified, established, and experienced leaders in the field of resistance to anti-cancer mAbs.

This volume consists of 10 reviews that cover a wide range of topics on resistance. A summary highlighting each chapter is briefly presented. Dr. Dumontet's review titled, *Resistance to Anticancer Antibodies: From Mechanism to Solutions* discusses the importance of finding closed links between preclinical observations and the clinic. These links are imperative to unravel various mechanisms of resistance for the benefit of the patients. He raises the important point that not a simple mechanism of resistance will be found in a cancer patient type but multiple mechanisms will work in concert, due primarily to the heterogeneity of the cancer in question. As an example, he discusses HER2^{+} breast cancer response to trastuzumab and how to identify both biomarkers to predict an optimal response and gene products that regulate resistance for novel targeted therapies. Dr. Ferrone's review titled, *Tumor Antigen-Specific Monoclonal Antibody-Based Immunotherapy, Cancer Initiating Cells and Disease Recurrence* discusses an important facet of resistance, namely, the intrinsic resistance of a small subgroup of cancer initiating cells (CICs) that are primarily responsible for mAb resistance, relapse, and metastasis. He presents several examples of mAbs that do not affect CICs, however, the use of combination therapies with drugs/radiation and inhibitors of the CIC signaling pathways resulted in significant killing of CICs but not all. He suggests the development of additional targeted therapies and combination to completely eliminate CICs. Dr. Cragg's review titled, *Overcoming Resistance to Therapeutic Antibodies by Targeting Fc Receptors* discusses the clinical finding demonstrating the important role of Fc gamma receptors (FcγRs) polymorphism and response to mAb therapeutics. Due to the number of various FcRs with activating or inhibitory functions, their biology is very complex indeed. Noteworthy, while the role of FcγRs expression by cytotoxic effector cells was primarily reported for the observed polymorphism, however, new findings show that FcRs on both the cancer cell and the effector cell participate in determining the therapeutic efficacy of the monoclonal antibody in question. Several novel strategies are provided to circumvent the unresponsiveness of resistance with the aim to develop more successful mAb therapeutics. Dr. Hernandez-Ilizaliturri and Dr. Czuczman's review titled, *Understanding the Mechanisms of Resistance to Rituximab: Paving the Road for the Development of Therapeutic Strategies to Overcome Rituximab Resistance* discusses the clinical problem of cancer patients resistance to rituximab (antiCD20 mAb) therapy. They discuss several reported mechanisms of resistance that have been observed in cancer patients, including surface receptors and intracellular hyperactivated survival pathways. Their approach to determine potential underlying mechanisms of rituximab-resistance has been to develop preclinically rituximab-resistance lymphoma cell lines. These have been analyzed for their therapeutic phenotypes and molecular properties compared to the parental wild-type cells. Such approaches are clearly important to identify new biomarkers of resistance for both prognostic and novel therapeutics. Dr. Bonavida's review titled, *Tumor Resistance to Antibody-Mediated Immunotherapy and Reversal of Resistance: Rituximab as Prototype* discusses several studies that investigated cell-mediated signaling by rituximab on B-Non-Hodgkin's lymphoma cell lines and which demonstrated the inhibition of several intracellular pathways (example NFκB, p38 MAPK, Raf/ERK/MEK, and PI3K/Akt) leading to inhibition of cell growth and inhibition of anti-apoptotic gene products. In addition, this review discusses the chemo-immunosensitization-mediated by rituximab when used in combination with chemo-immunotherapeutic drugs and various mechanisms of sensitization. Like the above studies by Dr. Hernandez-Ilizaliturri and Dr. Czuczman, the potential mechanism of rituximab resistance has been analyzed by generating rituximab-resistant clones in vitro and their general molecular profiles were compared to wild-type cells. While the resistant clones were unresponsive to rituximab treatment alone or in combination with drugs, however, intracellular intervention inhibiting the hyper-activated survival pathways by various inhibitors resulted in the reversal resistance to cytotoxic drugs. The analysis with the resistance clones yielded several candidate targets of potential prognostic and therapeutic values. Doctors Saridaki and Souglakos's review titled, *Resistance to the Anti-EGFR Therapy, Beyond KRAS, in Patients with Metastatic Colorectal Cancer* discuss the role of mutation profiles in the treatment decision in patients with metastatic colorectal cancer. They critically reviewed the underlying mechanisms of resistance to anti-EGFR mAbs and their relationship to various mutations. The reported studies are aimed to identify novel biomarkers that may be useful to select cancer patients who will respond favorably to anti-EGFR mAbs. Dr. Hersey and colleagues' review titled, *Overcoming Resistance of Melanoma to Immunotherapy with Monoclonal Antibodies Against Checkpoint Inhibitors* discusses the poor clinical response in melanoma patients following treatment with monoclonal antibodies against checkpoint inhibitors on T cells such as Ipilimumab (anti-CTLA-4) and PD1 (programmed death receptor-1). They discuss various mechanisms of resistance to immunotherapy including changes in the microenvironment, regulation of T-cells infiltration into melanoma tumors and suggest mechanisms to augment T-cell infiltration into the tumors. They also discuss the important role of NF-κB activation as a key regulator of anti-tumor immune resistance. Dr. Fulda's review titled, *Strategies to Overcome TRAIL Resistance in Cancer* discusses the mechanism that underlies the resistance of cancer cells to TRAIL/agonist antibodies directed against TRAIL receptors DR4 or DR5 currently under clinical investigation. She discusses several mechanisms conferring resistance to TRAIL such as the impairment of various members of the TRAIL signaling apoptotic pathways. These include signaling by death and decoy receptors that result in both the activation and the inhibition of apoptosis, the aberrant expression of anti-apoptotic gene products and the regulation of caspases. She implies that a better understanding of the mechanisms that regulate the sensitivity to resistance to TRAIL-apoptosis should lead to the successful application of TRAIL and agonist monoclonal antibodies as new therapeutics in the treatment of cancer.

The above chapters discuss several limitations by the use of therapeutic monoclonal antibodies. The next two chapters discuss the new engineered monoclonal antibody-conjugates as the new generation of antibody therapy. Dr. Smider's review titled, *Unnatural Amino Acid Antibody Conjugates as Next Generation Biologics* discusses the first approved monoclonal antibody against solid tumors, namely, trastuzumab (anti-HERT2$^+$ mAb; herceptin) in 1998 for the treatment of HERT2$^+$ overexpressing metastastatic breast cancer. He reviews several mechanisms of resistance to trastuzumab. He discusses the use of novel antibody-conjugates as novel therapies to overcome resistance. For example, unnatural amino acids were used to create the site specifically linking protein–protein dimers, such as antibody-toxin conjugates and bispecific antibodies. The antibody-drug conjugate, trastuzumab-DM1, has shown biological activity and clinical efficacy in HERT2$^+$ breast cancer and other applications have also been discussed. Dr. Rabuka's review titled, *Antibody-Drug Conjugates: Can Coupling Cytotoxicity and Specificity Overcome Therapeutic Resistance?* discusses the exquisite selected antibody-drug conjugates (ADCs) for the target antigen and that kill cells at very low concentrations with little effect on normal tissues. This review presents the general properties of ADCs and their mode of action and how they can revert resistance to antibody therapeutics. The development of Mylotarg, gemtuzumab ozogamicin, was approved in 2000 and consists of an anti-CD33 mAb conjugated with a DNA-damaging agent, calicheamicin, for the treatment of $CD33^+$ leukemia. There are currently 20 new ADCs in clinical studies that should provide information about their therapeutic efficacy and their ability to reverse resistance.

I wish to acknowledge the assistance of Daphne Liang, Melissa Cao, Kathy Nguyen, and Suzie Vardanyan for their valuable assistance in the preparation and editing the various contributions in this volume.

Benjamin Bonavida, Ph.D.

Contents

Resistance to Anticancer Antibodies: From Mechanisms to Solutions 1
Lina Reslan and Charles Dumontet

Tumor Antigen-Specific Monoclonal Antibody-Based Immunotherapy, Cancer Initiating Cells and Disease Recurrence 25
Yangyang Wang, Francesco Sabbatino, Ling Yu, Elvira Favoino, Xinhui Wang, Matteo Ligorio, Soldano Ferrone, Joseph H. Schwab and Cristina R. Ferrone

Overcoming Resistance to Therapeutic Antibodies by Targeting Fc Receptors 49
Emily L. Williams, Sean H. Lim, Stephen A. Beers, Peter W. Johnson, Jonathan C. Strefford, Martin J. Glennie and Mark S. Cragg

Understanding the Mechanisms of Resistance to Rituximab: Paving the Road for the Development of Therapeutic Strategies to Overcome Rituximab-Resistance 73
Francisco J. Hernandez-Ilizaliturri and Myron S. Czuczman

Tumor Resistance to Antibody-Mediated Immunotherapy and Reversal of Resistance: Rituximab as Prototype 93
Benjamin Bonavida

Resistance to the Anti-EGFR Therapy, Beyond KRAS, in Patients with Metastatic Colorectal Cancer 125
Zacharenia Saridaki and John Souglakos

Overcoming Resistance of Melanoma to Immunotherapy with Monoclonal Antibodies Against Checkpoints Inhibitors 143
Peter Hersey, Stuart Gallagher and Branka Mijatov

Strategies to Overcome TRAIL Resistance in Cancer 157
Simone Fulda

Unnatural Amino Acid Antibody Conjugates as Next Generation Biologics 167
Vaughn Smider

Antibody-Drug Conjugates: Can Coupling Cytotoxicity and Specificity Overcome Therapeutic Resistance? 183
Penelope M. Drake and David Rabuka

Index 201

Contributors

Stephen A. Beers Antibody and Vaccine Group, Cancer Sciences Unit, University of Southampton, MP88, Tremona Road, Southampton SO16 6YD, UK

Benjamin Bonavida Department of Microbiology, Immunology and Molecular Genetics, David Geffen School of Medicine, Jonsson Comprehensive Cancer Center at UCLA, University of California, Los Angeles, CA 90095, USA

Mark S. Cragg Antibody and Vaccine Group, Cancer Sciences Unit, University of Southampton, MP88, Tremona Road, Southampton SO16 6YD, UK

Myron S. Czuczman Departments of Immunology and Medical Oncology, Roswell Park Cancer Institute, Elm and Carlton Streets, Buffalo, NY 14263, USA

Penelope M. Drake Redwood Bioscience, 5703 Hollis Street, Emeryville, CA 94608, USA

Charles Dumontet Université Lyon, F-69000 Lyon, France; Inserm U1052, Centre de Recherche en Cancérologie de Lyon, F-69000 Lyon, France; CNRS UMR5286, Centre de Recherche en Cancérologie de Lyon, F-69000 Lyon, France; Hospices Civils de Lyon, F-69003 Lyon, France; INSERM 590, Faculté Rockefeller, 8 avenue Rockefeller, 69008 Lyon, France

Elvira Favoino Department of Surgery, Massachusetts General Hospital, Boston, MA, USA

Cristina R. Ferrone Department of Surgery, Massachusetts General Hospital, Boston, MA, USA

Soldano Ferrone Department of Surgery, Massachusetts General Hospital, Boston, MA, USA

Simone Fulda Institute for Experimental Cancer Research in Pediatrics, Goethe-University, Komturstr. 3a, 60528 Frankfurt, Germany

Stuart Gallagher Kolling Institute of Medical Research, Royal North Shore Hospital, St Leonards, NSW 2065, Australia

Martin J. Glennie Antibody and Vaccine Group, Cancer Sciences Unit, University of Southampton, MP88, Tremona Road, Southampton SO16 6YD, UK

Peter Hersey Kolling Institute of Medical Research, Royal North Shore Hospital, St Leonards, NSW 2065, Australia

Francisco J. Hernandez-Ilizaliturri Departments of Immunology and Medical Oncology, Roswell Park Cancer Institute, Elm and Carlton Streets, Buffalo, NY 14263, USA

Peter W. Johnson CR UK Centre, Cancer Sciences Unit, University of Southampton, Southampton, UK

Matteo Ligorio Department of Surgery, Massachusetts General Hospital, Boston, MA, USA

Sean H. Lim Antibody and Vaccine Group, Cancer Sciences Unit, University of Southampton, MP88, Tremona Road, Southampton SO16 6YD, UK

Branka Mijatov Kolling Institute of Medical Research, Royal North Shore Hospital, St Leonards, NSW 2065, Australia

David Rabuka Redwood Bioscience, 5703 Hollis Street, Emeryville, CA 94608, USA

Lina Reslan Université Lyon, F-69000 Lyon, France; Inserm U1052, Centre de Recherche en Cancérologie de Lyon, F-69000 Lyon, France; CNRS UMR5286, Centre de Recherche en Cancérologie de Lyon, F-69000 Lyon, France; Hospices Civils de Lyon, F-69003 Lyon, France

Francesco Sabbatino Department of Surgery, Massachusetts General Hospital, Boston, MA, USA

Zacharenia Saridaki Department of Medical Oncology, University Hospital of Heraklion and Laboratory of Tumor Cell Biology, Medical School, University of Crete, Voutes and Stavrakia, 1352, 71110 Heraklion, Crete, Greece

Joseph H. Schwab Department of Orthopaedic Surgery, Massachusetts General Hospital, Boston, MA, USA

Vaughn Smider Department of Cell and Molecular Biology, The Scripps Research Institute, La Jolla, CA 92037, USA

Jonathan C. Strefford Cancer Genomics Group, Cancer Sciences Unit, University of Southampton, Southampton, UK

John Souglakos Department of Medical Oncology, University Hospital of Heraklion and Laboratory of Tumor Cell Biology, Medical School, University of Crete, Voutes and Stavrakia, 1352, 71110 Heraklion, Crete, Greece

Xinhui Wang Department of Surgery, Massachusetts General Hospital, Boston, MA, USA

Yangyang Wang Department of Surgery, Massachusetts General Hospital, Boston, MA, USA

Emily L. Williams Antibody and Vaccine Group, Cancer Sciences Unit, University of Southampton, MP88, Tremona Road, Southampton SO16 6YD, UK

Ling Yu Department of Surgery, Massachusetts General Hospital, Boston, MA, USA

Resistance to Anticancer Antibodies: From Mechanisms to Solutions

Lina Reslan and Charles Dumontet

Abstract Therapeutic monoclonal antibodies exert their antitumor effect through a variety of mechanisms, including apoptotic induction, extracellular mechanisms and the involvement of the innate and possibly the adaptative immune systems. Due to this complexity there are still few data regarding mechanisms of resistance to monoclonal antibody therapy. In this review, we discuss the available data for three of the best described antibodies, rituximab, trastuzumab and cetuximab. A variety of approaches and strategies has been suggested or are currently being tested to circumvent resistance to these antibodies.

Keywords Monoclonal antibodies · Rituximab · Trastuzumab · Cetuximab · Resistance

Abbreviations

ADCs	Antibody–drug conjugates
ADCC	Antibody-dependent cell-mediated cytotoxicity
ADCP	Antibody-dependent cellular phagocygtosis
CDC	Complement-dependent cytotoxicity
CLL	Chronic lymphocytic leukemia
CRP	Complement regulatory proteins

L. Reslan · C. Dumontet
Université Lyon, Lyon F-69000, France

L. Reslan · C. Dumontet
Inserm U1052, Centre de Recherche en Cancérologie de Lyon, F-69000 Lyon, France

L. Reslan · C. Dumontet
CNRS UMR5286, Centre de Recherche en Cancérologie de Lyon, F-69000 Lyon, France

L. Reslan · C. Dumontet
Hospices Civils de Lyon, Lyon F-69003, France

C. Dumontet (✉)
INSERM 590, Faculté Rockefeller, 8 avenue Rockefeller 69008 Lyon, France
e-mail: charles.dumontet@chu-lyon.fr

B. Bonavida (ed.), *Resistance to Immunotherapeutic Antibodies in Cancer*,
Resistance to Targeted Anti-Cancer Therapeutics 2, DOI: 10.1007/978-1-4614-7654-2_1,

DLBCL	Diffuse large B cell lymphoma
EGFR	Epidermal growth factor receptor
FcR	Fc receptor
FL	Follicular lymphoma
HER2	Human epidermal growth factor
HGF	Hepatocyte growth factor
GM-CSF	Granulocyte-macrophage colony-stimulating factor
IFN	Interferon
IL	Interleukin
IGF-1	Insulin-like growth factor 1
MAbs	Monoclonal antibodies
mTor	Mammalian target of rapamycin
MUC4	Mucin-4
NHL	Non-hodgkin lymphoma
NK	Natural killer
OS	Overall survival
PCD	Programmed cell death
PFS	Progression-free survival
RTK	Receptor tyrosine kinase
TKI	Tyrosine kinase inhibitor
VEGF	Vascular endothelial growth factor

Introduction

Anticancer immunotherapy in 2012 is still largely based on the production of monoclonal antibodies (MAbs) that bind with high specificity to secreted proteins or to the extracellular domain of membrane-bound proteins. The principle of the MAbs is to target molecules that are expressed at higher levels on neoplastic cells, with a lower expression on normal cells.

MAbs achieve their therapeutic effects through various mechanisms. The specific binding of the antibody to its target prevents the binding of ligand-receptor interaction, by blocking growth factor receptors, neutralizing the target antigen, disrupting or promoting receptor internalization, shedding of the extracellular portion of the receptor, or induction of apoptosis. In addition, evidence has shown that activation of the innate immune response against the targeted tumor cells, upon recognition of the bound antibody, can also account for their biological activity to induce complement-dependent cytotoxicity (CDC), antibody-dependent cell-mediated cytotoxicity (ADCC) and antibody-dependent cellular phagocytosis (ADCP). More recently, it has been shown that the full effect of *MAbs* may also involve an adaptative immune response.

Unfortunately, in most tumor types, tumors either possess an intrinsic resistance to targeted therapies or acquire resistance after having displayed an initial response. In both cases, patients eventually succumb to disease progression. Therefore, understanding resistance mechanisms will benefit patients in several ways. Patients more likely to respond to a specific targeted therapy would be selected on the basis of markers of response and resistance, thus allowing oncologists to make earlier decisions for treatment with more effective therapies. Patients with highly refractory disease could be oriented early on to novel experimental therapies. Furthermore, understanding novel mechanisms of tumor growth and resistance will contribute to novel therapeutic strategies or agents.

Information obtained from cellular models and relapsed patients have provided little knowledge on how cells adapt to the treatment, whether by reducing the expression or modifying the structure of the target protein or by activating alternative survival pathways. A better understanding of the functional interactions occurring within the target and the corresponding antibody is essential to efficiently target the individual tumor and to select appropriate patients for therapy, thereby maximizing drug efficacy and minimizing toxicity. Additionally, a deeper understanding of the role of the microenvironment will be decisive in improving the use of therapeutic MAbs.

Three MAbs, rituximab, trastuzumab and cetuximab, have been considered as pioneers in their abilities to change the landscape of different malignancies. In this chapter, we will provide the readers with recent mechanisms of resistance as well as novel potential therapies that will help in circumventing these mechanisms.

Rituximab

The introduction of rituximab in the management of B cell non-Hodgkin's lymphoma (NHL) as well as in Chronic Lymphocytic Leukemia (CLL) has improved the response rate, progression-free survival (PFS), and overall survival (OS) of patients [1]. Rituximab is routinely administered during all phases of conventional treatment, including first-line therapy, maintenance as well as salvage therapy. Although the clinical data testing its efficacy have shown variable response rates in different CD20+ malignancies [2], its effectiveness is sometimes unsatisfactory since a significant percentage of patients treated with rituximab-containing chemotherapy show relapse or progression [3]. The development of rituximab resistance is an emerging clinical problem. However, the mechanisms underlying the resistance to rituximab are mostly unresolved and the clinical significance of those mechanisms has remained obscure [4].

Rituximab-induced B cell lysis is thought to occur via a number of different mechanisms, including CDC, ADCC/ADCP and/or delivery of direct death signaling (apoptosis). Potential mechanisms of tumor resistance have been described in each of these major pathways of proposed rituximab action. While therapeutic MAbs share with small molecule anticancer agents possible resistance mechanisms such as altered pharmacokinetics or metabolism and reduced diffusion to the tumor site, monoclonals differ from the latter because of their much larger molecular weight which accentuates these resistance mechanisms as well as the importance of extracellular mechanisms (complement system and/or effector cells). Overall reported resistance mechanisms include alterations in rituximab pharmacokinetics, loss of CD20 expression, either through downregulation or through "shaving" of rituximab/CD20 complexes, and antigenic modulation that has recently been reconsidered as a mechanism of resistance.

The acquisition of phenotypic changes in cancer cells or host immune cells over time may affect rituximab responsiveness and underscores the complexity of the potential mechanisms of resistance to anti-CD20 MAbs. Among these, reduced CD20 antigen expression has been among the most extensively studied. The deregulation of CD20 protein expression has been reported to be associated with a decrease in rituximab sensitivity in B cell NHL [5, 6]. There are several potential mechanisms leading to reduced functional CD20 expression, including transcriptional or translational regulation, altered membrane environment, CD20 mutations and altered membrane half-life.

Unraveling the clinical relevance behind the phenotypic changes or the reduced level of CD20 expression in B cell lymphoma has been initiated by the Rituximab Extended Schedule or Retreatment (RESORT) trial which is an ongoing study of the frequency of phenotypic changes occurring in rituximab-resistant lymphoma. This study is aiming to define the optimal duration of treatment with rituximab as a single agent in patients with indolent CD20+ B cell lymphoma and low tumor burden [7]. Phenotypic changes can occur as a consequence of repeated exposure to rituximab, especially over prolonged periods of time in B cell lymphoma (such as in maintenance programs). A 70 % reduction in CD20 expression was observed in cell lines induced to be rituximab-resistant in vitro, even at very early stages in the process of acquiring resistance to rituximab.

There are currently few data regarding CD20 mutations in patients refractory to rituximab. Terui and colleagues identified CD20 gene mutations leading to C-terminus truncated forms of CD20 in a subset of patients with rituximab-relapsed/refractory lymphomas; thus, indicating that the C-terminal region of CD20 plays a critical role in presentation of the large loop in which the rituximab-binding site is located [8]. The same group demonstrated the possibility to predict the existence of lymphoma cells resistant to rituximab by using an antibody that recognizes N-terminal region of CD20 proteins including those having a mutation [9]. These authors suggested that the combination of antibodies that target two different epitopes could help identify the C-terminal CD20 mutations and thus help in deciding whether it is appropriate to switch to another treatment such as using a second-generation CD20 antibody that is effective against fewer CD20-expressing cells [10] or using an antibody targeting a different antigen such as CD22 [11].

Antigenic modulation of CD20 has been also demonstrated through two pathways, either internalization of CD20 into lysosomes in some types of B cell malignancies, leading to reduced macrophage recruitment, degradation of CD20/MAb complexes and shortening of MAb half life [12] or through "shaving" following rituximab exposure. The shaving mechanism occurred by removing rituximab/CD20 complexes from the B cell surface by monocytes through the Fc receptor (FcR) pathway resulting in antigen loss and rituximab resistance [13].

In preclinical models, resistant cell lines showed decreased expression of CD20 at both the pre- and post-translational levels [14, 15]. This decreased CD20 expression was associated with changes in lipid rafts and downstream signaling, suggesting that the impact of CD20 expression on rituximab resistance is more complex than simple antibody-antigen ratios [14]. It has also been reported that combining rituximab with statins, inhibitors of the cholesterol synthesis, significantly decreased rituximab-induced CDC and ADCC [16]. Furthermore, the lipid raft-associated ganglioside GM1 was found to correlate with rituximab sensitivity of primary B-NHL and CLL B cells [17]. Conversely, attempts have been made to enhance the expression of CD20. The relatively low level of CD20 expression detected in B cells from patients suffering from CLL has been correlated with the hypermethylation of the transcription factor *PU.1*-encoding gene [18]. This is in line with the study by Hiraga et al. [19] showing that the incubation of CD20– negative primary B-NHL cells with the demethylating agent 5-aza-20-deoxycytidine in vitro restored CD20 mRNA expression in relapsed patients with downregulated CD20.

Epigenetic silencing of the CD20 promoter or CD20-regulating transcription factors could be involved in resistance mechanisms to rituximab in B-NHL. Clinical intervention strategies focusing on the combination of rituximab with demethylating agents, such as histone deacetylase inhibitors (HDAC-I) will help gain understanding concerning their impact on CD20 expression levels and treatment response. The immune modulator bryostatin-1 was also found to induce the expression of CD20 protein via Extracellular Signal-Regulated Kinases 1 and 2 (ERK1/2) and Protein Kinase C (PKC)-dependent mechanisms and to sensitization of CLL B cells to rituximab [18].

The role of resistance to ADCC and CDC-mediated toxicity remains controversial since the role of these mechanisms of antitumor activity remains itself controversial. During ADCC, immune effector cells such as natural killer (NK) cells, macrophages and neutrophils, recognize the Fc portion of rituximab via their FcR. The activation of FcR leads to the release of perforin, granzymes and tumor necrosis factor (TNF), which can induce target cell death [20–22]. In ADCP, the tumor cell is phagocytosed by the effector cell. The Fc of rituximab is also recognized by the complement component C1q, which activates the classical complement pathway leading to cell lysis via formation of the membrane attack complex (MAC) [23–25]. Genetic polymorphisms in the gene for C1q have been linked to variations in rituximab efficacy in humans, again supporting a key role for CDC in rituximab efficacy. The polymorphism G267A in the *C1qA* gene was reported to affect rituximab-induced CDC and the clinical response to rituximab therapy in Follicular lymphoma (FL) [26]. On the other hand, the complement regulatory proteins (CRP) CD46, CD55, and CD59 have been shown to inhibit rituximab mediated cell kill by interfering with complement activation [27, 28]. Therefore, blocking of the CRPs CD46, CD55 or CD59 may increase the sensitivity to complement [29].

Several groups have investigated the infusion of fresh frozen plasma to replete complement levels as a means of overcoming rituximab resistance in CLL. This approach resulted in a "rapid and dramatic clinical response in all patients", lending support to the hypothesis that complement depletion plays a clinically significant role in rituximab resistance [30]. Another group reported similarly positive results by combining fresh frozen plasma with rituximab to overcome complement depletion and rituximab resistance in CLL patients [31]. These results are promising but remain to be confirmed in controlled trials.

Specific FcR profiles have been shown to correlate with reduced efficacy of rituximab-based immunotherapy. FcγRIIIa, a member of the leukocyte receptor family FcγRs, is known to be a major triggering receptor of ADCC in NK cells and may thus be one of the critical parameters determining antitumor activity [32]. FcγRIIIa on myeloid effectors appears critical in controlling antibody potency. Lymphoma patients bearing the higher affinity 158V allele in FcγRIIIa respond better to rituximab single agent therapy compared with those with the low affinity 158F allotype [33], leading many investigators to focus on augmenting the interaction of MAb with FcγRIIIa, for example via defucosylation [10].

Recently, a strong correlation between the internalization of rituximab and FcγRIIb expression on B cells was reported suggesting that FcγRIIb is a key participant in rituximab resistance mechanisms. Lim et al. [34] suggested that rituximab can crosslink CD20 and FcγRIIb predominantly on the same target B cell, resulting in phoshorylation of FcγRIIb, and internalization of CD20:rituximab:FcγRIIb complexes into lysosomes for degradation.

Response to anti-CD20 MAb therapy may be optimized using type II anti-CD20 MAbs such as obinutuzumab (GA101), which circumvent the limitations of internalization, regardless of FcγRIIb expression. It is similarly unclear, why type II anti-CD20 MAb tend neither to internalize nor to activate FcγRIIb, but this may relate to differences in orientation of type II MAb after binding or to the fact that type II antibodies do not lead to relocalization of CD20 in lipid rafts. A therapeutic approach could consist in the co-administration of an FcγRIIb inhibitor with rituximab. The evaluation of FcγRIIb expression by various types of effector cells and response to MAb immunotherapy in B cell neoplasms would be of particular interest.

A promising approach is to enhance ADCC by stimulating effector cells such as monocytes, granulocytes, and dendritic cell populations. This has been attempted with Interleukin-2 (IL-2), IL-12 or granulocyte-macrophage colony-stimulating factor (GM-CSF) [35]. GM-CSF plus rituximab results in high response rates, along with a tolerable safety profile in patients with relapsed or progressive FL [36]. However, the addition of GM-CSF to therapy with alemtuzumab and rituximab decreased the treatment efficacy and increased the rate of cytomegalovirus reactivation in high-risk CLL patients [37]. Alternatively, ADCC could indirectly be enhanced by changing the microenvironment of tumor cells, for example with CpG DNA sequences [38, 39]. These immunostimulatory sequences induce secretion of numerous cytokines (IL-12, IL-18, IFN-α, and IFN-h) by macrophages and dendritic cells [40].

In addition to dysregulations in CD20 protein expression, ADCC and CDC, alterations in the apoptotic pathway signaling have been described to induce resistance. Molecular mechanisms of acquired resistance to rituximab have been generated through repeated exposure to antibody using rituximab-resistant cell lines [41, 42]. These cell lines demonstrate resistance to apoptosis and lack sensitivity to multiple cytotoxic chemotherapeutic agents in addition to rituximab. These clones were found to exhibit upregulation of pro-proliferative and anti-apoptotic signaling pathways, such as hyperactivation of nuclear factor-κB (NF-κB), Phosphatidylinositol-3-Kinase (PI3 K)/protein kinase B (Akt) and ERK1/2. Moreover, up-regulation of the anti-apoptotic Bcl-2 protein family members Bcl-2, Bcl-xL and Mcl-1, as well as down-regulation of the essential pro-apoptotic Bak and Bax proteins have been observed [41, 43–45]. An in vivo model of resistance has also been reported by Dalle et al. [46]. This model was established by serial transplantion and rituximab exposure of a human FL cell line in immunodeficient mice. Analyses of these tumors revealed increased expression of the complement inhibitor CD59, the transcription factor Ying yang (YY1), and the anti-apoptotic protein Bcl-xL.

Many studies are ongoing based on combination therapies in order to modulate intracellular signal transduction, to inhibit proliferation and to induce apoptosis. Some of the most promising targets in intracellular signal transduction are within the PI3 K/Akt pathway. This can be partially blocked downstream of the serine/threonine kinase Akt using inhibitors of the mammalian target of Rapamycin (mTOR), such as temsirolimus and RAD00 [47]. Inhibitors of PI3 K or Akt are currently in clinical development for cancer therapy [48].

Pharmacologic mimetics of the BH3 domain, such as ABT-737 [49–51] or ABT-263 [52, 53] act by functional inhibition of antiapoptotic Bcl-2 and Bcl-xL. In particular, the latter agents bear high hopes for combination therapy of B-NHL and phase I studies have been reported in several entities. Agents including the pan-Bcl-2 inhibitor AT-101 or the Bcl-2 antisense oligodeoxynucleotide oblimersen which also targets Bcl-2 and sensitizes cells to induction of apoptosis [54, 55]. In addition to the intrinsic, 'mitochondrial' pathway of apoptotic caspase activation, the extrinsic, receptor-mediated pathway harbors therapeutic targets, such as Apo2L/TRAIL [56, 57], FasL [58] and their respective receptors, which can be stimulated by the corresponding recombinant ligands or agonistic antibodies. The combination of rituximab with such pro-apoptotic therapies appears very promising in the treatment of resistant B-NHL.

Besides these targetted therapies, broad acting pathway-unspecific inhibitors with anti-proliferative activities, such as the proteasome inhibitor bortezomib, have been combined with rituximab. Bortezomib and rituximab have shown additive activity in preclinical models of lymphoma, and have been shown to be active and generally well tolerated in a randomized phase II study in patients with follicular and marginal zone lymphomas. This regimen might represent a useful addition to the armamentarium, particularly for some subgroups of patients [59]. However, an unresolved question concerns the effect of these novel therapies on the microenvironment and the resulting consequences on tumor cell sensitivity to treatment. As the notion of a protective tumor "niche" appears to be more and more relevant in the clinic, the potential to pharmacologically target not only the tumor cells themselves but also their surroundings is becoming a priority.

Little knowledge of how to circumvent rituximab resistance is currently available as both the mechanisms of resistance and the mechanisms of action of rituximab remain incompletely elucidated. Variations in B cell lines, animal model systems, and techniques used to generate rituximab-resistant clones contribute to the complexity of synthesizing preclinical results. The lack of pharmacokinetic-driven clinical trials and the heterogeneity of patients with NHL and CLL further complicate the understanding of these mechanisms in vivo. Despite these limitations, a number of promising approaches have been explored to enhance the effectiveness of rituximab and to overcome rituximab resistance. Currently, there are several new-generation anti-CD20 MAbs undergoing clinical investigation (Table 1) [60]. The first difference to note of the next generation of MAbs is that they are humanized or fully human MAbs, unlike the chimeric rituximab. Some of these MAbs have been designed to enhance the effector functions including the enhancement of FcγR binding, cell death and CDC (obinutuzumab, ofatumumab, PRO13192, AME133 V; Table 1).

Well-designed clinical trials will help define and refine efficacy and provide further insights of which activ-ity of modified next generation anti-CD20 MAb will prevail to further improve anti-CD20 MAb therapy beyond rituximab [1, 3, 60–69].

Trastuzumab

Human-epidermal-growth-factor-receptor-2 (HER2) overexpressing breast cancers account for 20–25 % of invasive breast cancers and are associated with an aggressive biological behavior translating into poorer clinical outcomes [70]. Trastuzumab, targeting the extracellular domain IV (ECD) of the HER2 protein, has dramatically altered the natural history of HER2-positive breast cancer and ranks among the most significant advances in breast cancer therapeutics. The mechanisms of action of trastuzumab are still incompletely determined. Trastuzumab has been proposed to trigger HER2 internalization and degradation by promoting the activity of tyrosine kinase—ubiquitin ligase c-Cbl [71]. An important proposed mechanism of action of trastuzumab is ADCC, which is triggered through the detection of Fc portion of trastuzumab by the FcγR on immune effector cells, particularly NK cells, resulting in cell lysis of HER2-positive target cells bound to the antibody [72]. These observations are confirmed by in vivo data from a pilot study of 11 patients with HER2-positive early breast cancer, where a positive correlation was observed between responses to neoadjuvant trastuzumab and ADCC activity [73].

Musilino et al. [74] showed that FcγR polymorphisms plays a role in trastuzumab-mediated ADCC and may be a predictive tool for clinical outcome in

Table 1 Next-generation anti-CD20 MAbs in clinical development

	Antibody specificity	Activities compared to rituximab	Sponsor	Phase of development
Ofatumumab	Type I, fullly human IgG1	Increased CDC	Genmab, glaxo SmithKline	Approved in US 2009 for CLL and phase III trials in NHL and autoimmune diseases
Veltuzumab	Type I, humanized IgG1	Increased CDC	Immunomedics	Phase I/II of subcutaneous administration in NHL and CLL
Ocrelizumab	Type I, humanized IgG1	Increased binding to FcYRIIIa and ADCC, decreased CDC,	Genentech/Roche/ biogen	Phase II in NHL
Ocaratuzumab (AME-133v)	Type I, humanized IgG1	Increased binding to CD20, FcYRIIIa and ADCC	Applied molecular evolution/Eli Lilly	Phase I/II in NHL
PRO131921 (Version 114)	Type I, humanized IgG1	Increased FcYRIIIa binding and ADCC	Genentech	Phase I/II in NHL
Obinutuzumab (GA-101)	Type II, humanized IgG1	Enhanced FcYRIIIa binding, ADCC, PCD and decreased CDC	Glycart/Roche	Phase III in NHL and DLBCL

patients who are particularly FCγR158 V and/or FCγRIIa 131H homozygous. Conversely, Jung et al. [75] did not find a correlation between these polymorphisms and response to trastuzumab-based regimens.

In addition to ADCC, the best described effect of trastuzumab is the inhibition of the MAPK and PI3 K/Akt pathways which lead to an increase in cell cycle arrest, the suppression of cell growth and proliferation. It is widely accepted that by interfering with the dimerization of HER2, trastuzumab inhibits HER2 activation and suppresses Akt phosphorylation [76]. Other groups showed that trastuzumab, by binding to HER2, can block tyrosine kinase (Src) signaling leading to an increase in PTEN expression and activity, thereby, conferring considerable trastuzumab resistance in breast cancer cells [77]. Moreover, trastuzumab was demonstrated to induce cell cycle arrest by inducing p27 and suppressing CDK2 activity in BT474 and SKBR3 breast cancer cells.

Despite these multiple mechanisms, 70 % of patients with HER2-positive breast cancers demonstrate intrinsic or secondary resistance to trastuzumab, highlighting the importance of developing new therapies for this disease [78]. Molecular mechanisms that contribute to trastuzumab resistance include obstacles for trastuzumab binding upregulation of HER2 downstream signaling pathways and intracellular alterations. Steric hindrance caused by mucin-4 (MUC4), a highly O-glycosylated membrane protein, contributes to 'the masking' of the trastuzumab binding site on HER2 [79]. Similarly, preclinical studies have shown that a cleaved form of MUC1 protein, MUC1*, was associated with trastuzumab resistance in a breast cancer cell line [80]. Truncated forms of the HER2 receptor, lacking trastuzumab-binding epitopes, present another potential mechanism of resistance, and may thus have a potential role both as a prognostic and predictive biomarker. Patients overexpressing p95HER95 were found to have a higher incidence of lung metastases and experienced significantly shorter PFS and OS with trastuzumab treatment compared to patients expressing only the full-length receptor [81]. Similarly, a retrospective study showed a strong association between the presence of truncated p95HER2 and clinical resistance to trastuzumab treatment in metastatic breast cancer patients [82]. In those cases where resistance to trastuzumab is associated with reduced interaction with the target antigen, pharmacological inhibition could be of interest. Lapatinib is a reversible small-molecule tyrosine kinase inhibitor (TKI) of EGFR and HER2 which was found to possess antitumor activity in HER2-dependent cell lines [83]. This molecule could present a solution in the subset of p95HER2-overexpressing, trastuzumab-resistant breast tumors where it showed its potential activity [82, 84, 85].

Genetic aberrations in the PI3 K/Akt pathway significantly mediate trastuzumab resistance mainly through loss of PTEN and the activation of PI3 KCA mutations [86, 87]. Both of these have been associated with shorter time to progression and survival in a retrospective study of 256 trastuzumab treated HER-2 positive metastatic breast cancer patients [88]. As mTOR is a downstream component of the PTEN/PI3K pathway, inhibitors of mTOR are under investigation for HER2-positive cell lines. Everolimus, the most advanced mTOR inhibitor, is being developed in combination with existing HER2-directed therapies. The combination of the oral mTOR inhibitor everolimus (5 or 10 mg daily) and trastuzumab was associated with an overall response rate of 15 % and a PFS of 4.1 months in trastuzumab-pretreated patients [89]. Other mTOR inhibitors are in the developmental pipeline for the treatment of HER2 positive breast cancer such as deforolimus (AP23573) and temsirolimus (CCI-779) [90].

Increased signaling via the PI3 K/Akt pathway could also contribute to trastuzumab resistance because of the activation of multiple receptor pathways. The latter include HER2-related receptors or non-HER receptors such as the insulin-like growth factor 1 receptor (IGF1R), which appears to be involved in a cross-talk with HER2 in resistant cells [91]. The human anti-IGF1R MAb A12 (cixutumumab from ImClone) [92], MK 0646 (dalotuzumab from Merck) [93], and AMG 479 (ganitumumab from Amgen) [94] are novel IGF1R-targeted agents being tested in phase III clinical trials. Moreover, small molecule HER2 inhibitors/antagonists, currently in clinical development such as BMS-754807 [91], linsitinib (OSI-906) XL228 [95] and AXL1717 [96], have shown promising preliminary results.

Regarding intracellular signaling, various reports suggest that alterations in specific pathways can be associated with resistance to trastuzumab. MIG-6 mitogen-inducible gene 6 protein, has been shown to interact with and inhibit activation of EGFR and HER2, and to counteract the ability of ErbB ligands to promote trastuzumab resistance. A loss of RALT/MIG-6, a transcriptionally controlled feedback inhibitor of ErbB receptor tyrosine kinases, was found to favor resistance to trastuzumab [97]. T-DARPP, a protein associated with HER2, has been shown to regulate sensitivity to trastuzumab in preclinical breast cancer models [98].

Moreover, Liang et al. [99] found that recombinant human erythropoietin (rHuEPO), which has long been used to manage the anemia and fatigue caused by cancer treatment, antagonizes trastuzumab effects on breast cancer models both in vitro and in vivo. They found that the receptor for erythropoietin (EpoR) is co-expressed with HER2 in a significant percentage of human breast tumor specimens and breast cancer cell lines. The physical interaction and the co-expression of tyrosine kinase c-Met with HER2 in cell lines may also contribute to trastuzumab resistance through sustained Akt activation [100, 101]. c-MET is central to many processes of cancer cell migration, invasion, proliferation, and metastasis. It is activated by the ligand of the hepatocyte growth factor (HGF). Tivantinib, an oral and selective c-MET inhibitor, exhibited antitumor activity in preclinical models and was well tolerated in phase I clinical trial in patients with refractory advanced solid tumors [102]. Tivantinib is now being studied in a phase III trial (MARQUEE) that will enroll 988 patients with advanced, chemotherapy pre-treated non- non small cell lung carcinoma (NSCLC). MetMab is a monovalent antibody designed to inhibit HGF-mediated activation of the MET pathway. MetMab was recently studied in a controlled phase II study. Promising results are spurring phase III studies of this agent [103]. EGFR and HER3 expression was found substantially increased after long-term trastuzumab exposure in HER2-positive breast carcinoma-derived cell lines. Trastuzumab does not interfere with

HER2/HER3 heterodimerization and, therefore, does not block signaling from these heterodimers [104]. Pertuzumab, an anti-HER2 humanized MAb that binds to an epitope located in domain II of HER2, sterically blocks a binding pocket necessary for receptor dimerization and signaling. It therefore prevents HER2 dimerization, including HER2/HER3 heterodimerization. Pertuzumab is active against HER2-overexpressing cell lines and xenografts, and preclinical data suggest a potential synergism with trastuzumab [105]. Clinical trials testing pertuzumab in combination with trastuzumab in different settings, as well as pertuzumab with chemotherapy, are ongoing.

Since trastuzumab resistance may arise from cross-talk among other HER proteins resulting in lateral activation and incomplete inhibition of downstream signaling, one approach to overcome trastuzumab resistance is the simultaneous inhibition of multiple HER receptors [106]. Several novel HER2 small-molecule TKIs have demonstrated promising activity and are in various stages of clinical development. Neratinib (HKI-272), an orally administered, irreversible pan-HER (HER1, HER2 and HER4) receptor TKI, is one of the most advanced novel HER TKI in clinical development and offers more complete HER receptor blockade than lapatinib which inhibits only HER1 and HER2. Many clinical studies showed the efficacy of neratinib in HER2 positive metastatic breast cancer patients with prior trastuzumab treatment [107]. Other TKIs are now being investigated such as erlotinib and gefitinib [108]. Alternatively, bispecific antibodies could allow the simultaneous inhibition of two targets.

Another promising strategy for selectively targeting tumor cells involves coupling MAbs with potent cytotoxic agents, in the form of antibody–drug conjugates (ADCs). This approach is being investigated in a variety of settings and recently led to Food and Drug Administration approval for Brentuximab vedotin, an ADC targeting refractory CD30-positive lymphoma [109–111]. For HER2-positive breast cancer, trastuzumab–emtansine (also called T-DM1) is an ADC, which utilizes a stable thioether linkage to couple trastuzumab to a derivative of maytansine DM1, a microtubule-depolymerisation agent. Upon binding to the HER2 receptor, T-DM1 is internalized and DM1 is released intracellularly, enabling the selective delivery of the potent cytotoxic agent to HER-2 overexpressing cells with limited toxicity. In preclinical studies, trastuzumab–emtansine showed activity in trastuzumab-sensitive and trastuzumab-resistant models of HER2-positive breast cancer [112].

Several phase I studies have shown T-DM1 is safe, tolerable and has activity in trastuzumab- and lapatinib-pretreated breast cancer. Phase II studies are now being reported that confirm its safety and clinical efficacy in both the frontline and heavily pretreated settings [113] and a recently published phase III trial demonstrated the superiority of T-DM1 to lapatinib and capecitabine in patient having previously received trastuzumab and a taxane for advanced breast cancer [114].

Cetuximab

The epidermal growth factor receptor (EGFR) is a receptor tyrosine kinase belonging to the HER family of receptor tyrosine kinases (RTK). Upon natural ligand binding (TGF-alpha, amphiregulin and epiregulin), the receptor undergoes homodimerization or heterodimerization with other members of the ErbB family (HER2/neu, HER3 and HER4). These conformational changes activate the phosphorylation of tyrosine kinase leading to downstream activation of multiple signaling pathways including the Ras-Raf-MAP kinase pathway, the PI3 K pathway and the protein-serine/threonine kinase Akt pathway. Moreover, these events activate cellular proliferation and survival as well as increase the rate of tumor metastasis [115]. EGFR is overexpressed in a variety of solid tumors, suggesting an important role in the process of neoplastic transformation. Therefore, EGFR has been validated as a relevant therapeutic target in several human cancers, including metastatic colorectal cancer (mCRC) [116].

Cetuximab (an IgG1 MAb) and panitumumab (fully human IgG2 MAb) are the only MAbs against EGFR that are approved for treatment of mCRC. Cetuximab is a chimeric human-murine MAb that binds competitively and with high affinity to the EGFR [117]. Binding of cetuximab to the receptor results in its internalization and the termination of the signaling by preventing the phosphorylation of the ligand-mediated receptor tyrosine kinase. Moreover, its binding inhibits many cellular pathways such as the mitogen-activated protein kinase (MAPK), PI3 K and Akt [118]. It may also exert its antitumor effects through ADCC via its FcR.

Although EGFR is expressed in approximately 85 % of patients with mCRC, the clinical efficacy of treatment with anti-EGFR antibodies is limited to a subset of patients. Two polymorphisms FCGR2A-H131R and FCGR3A-V158F were independently associated with PFS and may be useful as molecular markers to predict clinical outcome in mCRC patients treated with cetuximab [119]. Mutations in several genes have recently emerged as the best predictive factors of low/absent response to EGFR-targeted therapy including cetuximab and panitumumab. Activating mutations at codons 12 and 13 in the *K-RAS* oncogene ($K\text{-}RAS^{G12V}$ and $K\text{-}RAS^{G13D}$) have emerged as the best predictive factors of low/absent response to these agents, either in the first-line or subsequent lines of treatment [120, 121]. No drugs are currently available for the specific and direct inhibition of K-RAS. However, the introduction of K-RAS testing as a diagnostic tool has been validated to select patients for EGFR-targeted treatment and is considered as one of the most important recent advances in the field of personalized CRC therapy. Although the presence of wild-type K-RAS seems to be a condition for response to EGFR-targeted therapy, up to 50–65 % of mCRC patients fail to benefit from this treatment, due to additional intrinsic resistance mechanisms. Recent data pointed out that *BRAF* and *PIK3CA* exon 20 mutations hamper response to EGFR-targeted treatment in mCRC [122, 123]. A number of agents designed to inhibit the kinase activity of BRAF are either already clinically approved or are progressing through the pipeline of phases I and II studies [124, 125].

Current data suggest the evaluation of not only KRAS mutations, but also BRAF and PIK3CA/PTEN alterations for selecting patients with mCRC who are unlikely to respond to anti-EGFR-targeted therapy. Furthermore, Montagut and coworkers have recently identified an acquired EGFR ectodomain mutation (S492R) that prevents cetuximab binding and confers resistance to this agent. Conversely, a patient harboring the S492R mutation responded to panitumumab treatment. This mutation may provide a molecular explanation for the clinical benefit of panitumumab in a subset of mCRC patients who do not respond to treatment with cetuximab. The specificity of the S492R mutation is expected to facilitate reliable testing to guide the clinical use of panitumumab after cetuximab failure and justifies prospective independent validation of the S492R EGFR mutation [126, 127]. Moreover, loss of PTEN expression has been reported to predict resistance to cetuximab in mCRC patients [128]. PTEN is degraded in cetuximab resistant cells, leading to constitutive activation of AKT [129].

Cetuximab resistance is partly due to the ability of cells to re-activate pro-angiogenic factors via alternative pathways. Several lines of investigation have identified inhibition of angiogenesis as part of the antitumor effect of cetuximab. Resistant cetuximab-tumor cells showed an increase in Cox-2, pMAPK, and vascular endothelial growth factor (VEGF) protein expression levels in a colon cancer cell line [130] as well as an increase in VEGFR-1 and -2 levels that result in increased migratory potential [131].

The combination of bevacizumab (a humanized anti-VEGF-A IgG1 MAb) and cetuximab in previously treated head and neck squamous cell carcinomas (HNSCC) demonstrated favorable response in these patients. Thus, the use of antibody targeting VEGF has the potential to increase the response of patients to cetuximab [132].

Preclinical data obtained with cetuximab-resistant clones in vitro following long-term exposure to cetuximab in two different cell lines (NSCLC (H226) and HNSCC (SCC-1) cell lines) showed strong activation of HER2, HER3 and cMET with dysregulation of EGFR internalization/degradation [133]. Acquired resistance in mCRC cells to cetuximab could thus develop via altered EGFR levels through promotion of EGFR ubiquitination and degradation and enhancement of Src kinase in collaboration with EGFR for supporting cell growth and survival [134].

MEHD7945A (Genentech; CA, USA) is a newly intravenous humanized EGFR/HER3 dual specific IgG1 MAb. This agent significantly inhibited the proliferation in tumor cells that express EGFR and HER3 and the growth of the EGFR resistant clones, suggesting that MEHD7945A may have an important role overcoming EGFR inhibitor acquired resistance [135, 136].

Benavente et al. [137] presented another model of resistance to cetuximab, gefitinib or erlotinib in head and neck tumor cells following chronic exposure to these agents where EGFR inhibitor-resistant lines showed increased proliferation rates and elevated levels of phosphorylated EGFR, MAPK, AKT and STAT3, with reduced apoptotic capacity. Further research on the mechanisms of secondary acquired resistance, such as alterations in other key elements of the EGFR-dependent signal cascade (MAPK or AKT1), or the presence of genetic alterations in RTK other than EGFR is also warranted to define additional signaling pathways to be targeted. The combination of cetuximab with other cell signaling pathway inhibitors such as mTor inhibitors will provide superior efficacy results. However, clinical trials will probably require the identification of the adequate subpopulation of patients by the analysis of molecular rearrangements present in their tumors.

Early small molecule RTK inhibitors of EGFR have proven disappointing to date in the treatment of patients with CRC. However, future generations of these classes of drugs are promising. These agents may replace or complete antibody-based therapy thanks to their oral administration and complementary mechanisms of action. Phase I clinical trials in solid tumors of an oral, small-molecule, irreversible HER family inhibitor afatinib (BIBW 2992, Boehringer Ingelheim; Ingelheim, Germany) that targets EGFR, HER-2, and HER-4 combined with cetuximab is now being tested. Combining foretinib (Glaxo Smithkline; London, United Kingdom), a multikinase inhibitor against MET and VEGF receptor-2 with erlotinib or lapatinib effectively decreased the phosphorylation of MET, EGFR, HER-2, HER-3, AKT, and ERK in these cells, suggesting a role for combining MET/HER inhibitors to overcome EGFR resistance.

Conclusion

An important clue to start unraveling molecular resistance is to find close links between preclinical observations and the clinic. These links will help to improve the clinical outcomes of patients treated with MAbs. As these latter are tested and compared in the clinic, they will hopefully provide more insights into their mechanisms of action. This is likely to include tumor profiling, analysis of the microenvironment, such as macrophage profiling, as well as an assessment of host immune effector function and genetic polymorphisms of FcγR.

Multiple mechanisms may act simultaneously to confer resistance to trastuzumab, due to the accumulation of intracellular alterations and the heterogeneity of breast cancer. Future efforts should therefore be directed towards the development of predictive biomarkers for optimal selection of HER2-directed therapies. Understanding the pathways involved in cetuximab resistance requires the identification of biomarkers that will accurately predict optimum responses to this agent and the identification of other key signaling pathways that can be targeted to enhance its activity. The analyses of some recent biomarkers have helped in predicting progression of disease with a high degree of accuracy and reproducibility; however, an important future challenge is the standardization of biomarkers assessment and the implementation and validation of promising molecular markers in large prospective clinical trial.

Conflicts of Interest
No potential conflicts of interest were disclosed.

References

1. Bello C, Sotomayor EM. Monoclonal antibodies for B-cell lymphomas: rituximab and beyond. Hematol Am Soc Hematol Educ Prog. 2007;2007:233–42.
2. Cvetkovic RS, Perry CM. Rituximab: a review of its use in non-Hodgkin's lymphoma and chronic lymphocytic leukaemia. Drugs. 2006;66:791–820.
3. Lim SH, Beers SA, French RR, Johnson PW, Glennie MJ, Cragg MS. Anti-CD20 monoclonal antibodies: historical and future perspectives. Haematologica. 2010;95:135–43.
4. Friedberg JW. Unique toxicities and resistance mechanisms associated with monoclonal antibody therapy. Hematol Am Soc Hematol Educ Prog. 2005;2005:329–34.
5. Haidar JH, Shamseddine A, Salem Z, Mrad YA, Nasr MR, Zaatari G, Bazarbachi A. Loss of CD20 expression in relapsed lymphomas after rituximab therapy. Eur J Haematol. 2003;70:330–2.
6. Kennedy GA, Tey SK, Cobcrft R, Marlton P, Cull G, Grimmett K, Thomson D, Gill D. Incidence and nature of CD20-negative relapses following rituximab therapy in aggressive B-cell non-Hodgkin's lymphoma: a retrospective review. Br J Haematol. 2002;119:412–6.
7. Kahl BS. Eastern Cooperative Oncology Group 4402: Rituximab Extended Schedule or Retreatment Trial (RESORT). Clin Lymphoma Myeloma. 2006;6:423–6.
8. Terui Y, Mishima Y, Sugimura N, Kojima K, Sakurai T, Mishima Y, Kuniyoshi R, Taniyama A, Yokoyama M, Sakajiri S, Takeuchi K, Watanabe C, Takahashi S, Ito Y, Hatake K. Identification of CD20 C-terminal deletion mutations associated with loss of CD20 expression in non-Hodgkin's lymphoma. Clin Cancer Res. 2009;15:2523–30.
9. Mishima Y, Terui Y, Takeuchi K, Matsumoto-Mishina Y, Matsusaka S, Utsubo-Kuniyoshi R, Hatake K. The identification of irreversible rituximab-resistant lymphoma caused by CD20 gene mutations. Blood Cancer J. 2011;1:e15.
10. Mossner E, Brunker P, Moser S, Puntener U, Schidt C, Herter S, Grau R, Gerdes C, Nopora A, van Puijenbroek E, Ferrara C, Sondermann P, Jager C, Strein P, Fertig G, Friess T, Schull C, Bauer S, Dal Porto J, Del Nagro C, Dabbagh K, Dyer MJ, Poppema S, Klein C, Umana P. Increasing the efficacy of CD20 antibody therapy through the engineering of a new type II anti-CD20 antibody with enhanced direct and immune effector cell-mediated B-cell cytotoxicity. Blood. 2009;115:4393–4402.
11. Dijoseph JF, Dougher MM, Armellino DC, Evans DY, Damle NK. Therapeutic potential of CD22-specific antibody-targeted chemotherapy using inotuzumab ozogamicin (CMC-544) for the treatment of acute lymphoblastic leukemia. Leukemia. 2007;21:2240–5.
12. Beers SA, French RR, Chan HT, Lim SH, Jarrett TC, Vidal RM, Wijayaweera SS, Dixon SV, Kim H, Cox KL, Kerr JP, Johnston DA, Johnson PW, Verbeek JS, Glennie MJ, Cragg MS. Antigenic modulation limits the efficacy of anti-CD20 antibodies: implications for antibody selection. Blood. 2010;115:5191–201.
13. Beum PV, Kennedy AD, Williams ME, Lindorfer MA, Taylor RP. The shaving reaction: rituximab/CD20 complexes are removed from mantle cell lymphoma and chronic lymphocytic leukemia cells by THP-1 monocytes. J Immunol. 2006;176:2600–9.
14. Czuczman MS, Olejniczak S, Gowda A, Kotowski A, Binder A, Kaur H, Knight J, Starostik P, Deans J, Hernandez-Illizaliturri FJ. Acquirement of rituximab resistance in lymphoma cell lines is associated with both global CD20 gene and protein down-regulation regulated at the pretranscriptional and posttranscriptional levels. Clin Cancer Res. 2008;14:1561–70.
15. Sarro SM, Unruh TL, Zuccolo J, Sanyal R, Luider JM, Auer-Grzesiak IA, Mansoor A, Deans JP. Quantification of CD20 mRNA and protein levels in chronic lymphocytic leukemia suggests a post-transcriptional defect. Leuk Res. 2010;34:1670–3.
16. Winiarska M, Bil J, Wilczek E, Wilczynski GM, Lekka M, Engelberts PJ, Mackus WJ, Gorska E, Bojarski L, Stoklosa T, Nowis D, Kurzaj Z, Makowski M, Glodkowska E, Issat T, Mrowka P, Lasek W, Dabrowska-Iwanicka A, Basak GW, Wasik M, Warzocha K, Sinski M, Gaciong Z, Jakobisiak M, Parren PW, Golab J. Statins impair antitumor effects of rituximab by inducing conformational changes of CD20. PLoS Med. 2008;5:e64.

17. Meyer zum Buschenfelde C, Feuerstacke Y, Gotze KS, Scholze K, Peschel C. GM1 expression of non-Hodgkin's lymphoma determines susceptibility to rituximab treatment. Cancer Res. 2008;68:5414–22.
18. Wojciechowski W, Li H, Marshall S, Dell'Agnola C, Espinoza-Delgado I. Enhanced expression of CD20 in human tumor B cells is controlled through ERK-dependent mechanisms. J Immunol. 2005;174:7859–68.
19. Hiraga J, Tomita A, Sugimoto T, Shimada K, Ito M, Nakamura S, Kiyoi H, Kinoshita T, Naoe T. Down-regulation of CD20 expression in B-cell lymphoma cells after treatment with rituximab-containing combination chemotherapies: its prevalence and clinical significance. Blood. 2009;113:4885–93.
20. Fischer L, Penack O, Gentilini C, Nogai A, Muessig A, Thiel E, Uharek L. The anti-lymphoma effect of antibody-mediated immunotherapy is based on an increased degranulation of peripheral blood natural killer (NK) cells. Exp Hematol. 2006;34:753–9.
21. Wang SY, Racila E, Taylor RP, Weiner GJ. NK-cell activation and antibody-dependent cellular cytotoxicity induced by rituximab-coated target cells is inhibited by the C3b component of complement. Blood. 2008;111:1456–63.
22. Hernandez-Ilizaliturri FJ, Jupudy V, Ostberg J, Oflazoglu E, Huberman A, Repasky E, Czuczman MS. Neutrophils contribute to the biological antitumor activity of rituximab in a non-Hodgkin's lymphoma severe combined immunodeficiency mouse model. Clin Cancer Res. 2003;9:5866–73.
23. Di Gaetano N, Cittera E, Nota R, Vecchi A, Grieco V, Scanziani E, Botto M, Introna M, Golay J. Complement activation determines the therapeutic activity of rituximab in vivo. J Immunol. 2003;171:1581–7.
24. Golay J, Cittera E, Di Gaetano N, Manganini M, Mosca M, Nebuloni M, van Rooijen N, Vago L, Introna M. The role of complement in the therapeutic activity of rituximab in a murine B lymphoma model homing in lymph nodes. Haematologica. 2006;91:176–83.
25. Zhou X, Hu W, Qin X. The role of complement in the mechanism of action of rituximab for B-cell lymphoma: implications for therapy. Oncologist. 2008;13:954–66.
26. Racila E, Link BK, Weng WK, Witzig TE, Ansell S, Maurer MJ, Huang J, Dahle C, Halwani A, Levy R. A polymorphism in the complement component C1qA correlates with prolonged response following rituximab therapy of follicular lymphoma. Clin Cancer Res. 2008;14:6697–703.
27. Golay J, Zaffaroni L, Vaccari T, Lazzari M, Borleri GM, Bernasconi S, Tedesco F, Rambaldi A, Introna M. Biologic response of B lymphoma cells to anti-CD20 monoclonal antibody rituximab in vitro: CD55 and CD59 regulate complement-mediated cell lysis. Blood. 2000;95:3900–8.
28. Golay J, Lazzari M, Facchinetti V, Bernasconi S, Borleri G, Barbui T, Rambaldi A, Introna M. CD20 levels determine the in vitro susceptibility to rituximab and complement of B-cell chronic lymphocytic leukemia: further regulation by CD55 and CD59. Blood. 2001;98:3383–9.
29. Bellosillo B, Villamor N, Lopez-Guillermo A, Marce S, Esteve J, Campo E, Colomer D, Montserrat E. Complement-mediated cell death induced by rituximab in B-cell lymphoproliferative disorders is mediated in vitro by a caspase-independent mechanism involving the generation of reactive oxygen species. Blood. 2001;98:2771–7.
30. Klepfish A, Gilles L, Ioannis K, Rachmilewitz EA, Schattner A. Enhancing the action of rituximab in chronic lymphocytic leukemia by adding fresh frozen plasma: complement/ rituximab interactions & clinical results in refractory CLL. Ann NY Acad Sci. 2009;1173:865–73.
31. Xu W, Miao KR, Zhu DX, Fang C, Zhu HY, Dong HJ, Wang DM, Wu YJ, Qiao C, Li JY. Enhancing the action of rituximab by adding fresh frozen plasma for the treatment of fludarabine refractory chronic lymphocytic leukemia. Int J Cancer. 2011;128:2192–201.
32. Uchida J, Hamaguchi Y, Oliver JA, Ravetch JV, Poe JC, Haas KM, Tedder TF. The innate mononuclear phagocyte network depletes B lymphocytes through Fc receptor-dependent mechanisms during anti-CD20 antibody immunotherapy. J Exp Med. 2004;199:1659–69.

33. Weng WK, Levy R. Two immunoglobulin G fragment C receptor polymorphisms independently predict response to rituximab in patients with follicular lymphoma. J Clin Oncol. 2003;21:3940–7.
34. Lim SH, Vaughan AT, Ashton-Key M, Williams EL, Dixon SV, Chan HT, Beers SA, French RR, Cox KL, Davies AJ, Potter KN, Mockridge CI, Oscier DG, Johnson PW, Cragg MS, Glennie MJ. Fc gamma receptor IIb on target B cells promotes rituximab internalization and reduces clinical efficacy. Blood. 2011;118:2530–40.
35. Gluck WL, Hurst D, Yuen A, Levine AM, Dayton MA, Gockerman JP, Lucas J, Denis-Mize K, Tong B, Navid D, Difrancesco A, Milan S, Wilson SE, Wolin M. Phase I studies of interleukin (IL)-2 and rituximab in B-cell non-hodgkin's lymphoma: IL-2 mediated natural killer cell expansion correlations with clinical response. Clin Cancer Res. 2004;10:2253–64.
36. Cartron G, Zhao-Yang L, Baudard M, Kanouni T, Rouille V, Quittet P, Klein B, Rossi JF. Granulocyte-macrophage colony-stimulating factor potentiates rituximab in patients with relapsed follicular lymphoma: results of a phase II study. J Clin Oncol. 2008;26:2725–31.
37. Zent CS, Wu W, Bowen DA, Hanson CA, Pettinger AM, Shanafelt TD, Kay NE, Leis JF, Call TG. Addition of granulocyte macrophage colony stimulating factor does not improve response to early treatment of high-risk chronic lymphocytic leukemia with alemtuzumab and rituximab. Leuk Lymphoma. 2013;54:476–82.
38. Askew D, Chu RS, Krieg AM, Harding CV. CpG DNA induces maturation of dendritic cells with distinct effects on nascent and recycling MHC-II antigen-processing mechanisms. J Immunol. 2000;165:6889–95.
39. Zent CS, Smith BJ, Ballas ZK, Wooldridge JE, Link BK, Call TG, Shanafelt TD, Bowen DA, Kay NE, Witzig TE, Weiner GJ. Phase I clinical trial of CpG oligonucleotide 7909 (PF-03512676) in patients with previously treated chronic lymphocytic leukemia. Leuk Lymphoma. 2011;53:211–7.
40. Hacker G, Redecke V, Hacker H. Activation of the immune system by bacterial CpG-DNA. Immunology. 2002;105:245–51.
41. Jazirehi AR, Vega MI, Bonavida B. Development of rituximab-resistant lymphoma clones with altered cell signaling and cross-resistance to chemotherapy. Cancer Res. 2007;67:1270–81.
42. Vega MI, Jazirehi AR, Huerta-Yepez S, Bonavida B. Rituximab-induced inhibition of YY1 and Bcl-xL expression in Ramos non-Hodgkin's lymphoma cell line via inhibition of NF-kappa B activity: role of YY1 and Bcl-xL in Fas resistance and chemoresistance, respectively. J Immunol. 2005;175:2174–83.
43. Suzuki E, Umezawa K, Bonavida B. Rituximab inhibits the constitutively activated PI3 K-Akt pathway in B-NHL cell lines: involvement in chemosensitization to drug-induced apoptosis. Oncogene. 2007;26:6184–93.
44. Tomita A, Hiraga J, Kiyoi H, Ninomiya M, Sugimoto T, Ito M, Kinoshita T, Naoe T. Epigenetic regulation of CD20 protein expression in a novel B-cell lymphoma cell line, RRBL1, established from a patient treated repeatedly with rituximab-containing chemotherapy. Int J Hematol. 2007;86:49–57.
45. Olejniczak SH, Hernandez-Ilizaliturri FJ, Clements JL, Czuczman MS. Acquired resistance to rituximab is associated with chemotherapy resistance resulting from decreased Bax and Bak expression. Clin Cancer Res. 2008;14:1550–60.
46. Dalle S, Dupire S, Brunet-Manguat S, Reslan L, Plesa A, Dumontet C. In vivo model of follicular lymphoma resistant to rituximab. Clin Cancer Res. 2009;15:851–7.
47. Wanner K, Hipp S, Oelsner M, Ringshausen I, Bogner C, Peschel C, Decker T. Mammalian target of rapamycin inhibition induces cell cycle arrest in diffuse large B cell lymphoma (DLBCL) cells and sensitises DLBCL cells to rituximab. Br J Haematol. 2006;134:475–84.
48. Garcia-Echeverria C, Sellers WR. Drug discovery approaches targeting the PI3 K/Akt pathway in cancer. Oncogene. 2008;27:5511–26.
49. Oltersdorf T, Elmore SW, Shoemaker AR, Armstrong RC, Augeri DJ, Belli BA, Bruncko M, Deckwerth TL, Dinges J, Hajduk PJ, Joseph MK, Kitada S, Korsmeyer SJ, Kunzer AR, Letai A, Li C, Mitten MJ, Nettesheim DG, Ng S, Nimmer PM, O'Connor JM, Oleksijew A, Petros

AM, Reed JC, Shen W, Tahir SK, Thompson CB, Tomaselli KJ, Wang B, Wendt MD, Zhang H, Fesik SW, Rosenberg SH. An inhibitor of Bcl-2 family proteins induces regression of solid tumors. Nature. 2005;435:677–81.
50. Konopleva M, Contractor R, Tsao T, Samudio I, Ruvolo PP, Kitada S, Deng X, Zhai D, Shi YX, Sneed T, Verhaegen M, Soengas M, Ruvolo VR, McQueen T, Schober WD, Watt JC, Jiffar T, Ling X, Marini FC, Harris D, Dietrich M, Estrov Z, McCubrey J, May WS, Reed JC, Andreeff M. Mechanisms of apoptosis sensitivity and resistance to the BH3 mimetic ABT-737 in acute myeloid leukemia. Cancer Cell. 2006;10:375–88.
51. van Delft MF, Wei AH, Mason KD, Vandenberg CJ, Chen L, Czabotar PE, Willis SN, Scott CL, Day CL, Cory S, Adams JM, Roberts AW, Huang DC. The BH3 mimetic ABT-737 targets selective Bcl-2 proteins and efficiently induces apoptosis via Bak/Bax if Mcl-1 is neutralized. Cancer Cell. 2006;10:389–99.
52. Tse C, Shoemaker AR, Adickes J, Anderson MG, Chen J, Jin S, Johnson EF, Marsh KC, Mitten MJ, Nimmer P, Roberts L, Tahir SK, Xiao Y, Yang X, Zhang H, Fesik S, Rosenberg SH, Elmore SW. ABT-263: a potent and orally bioavailable Bcl-2 family inhibitor. Cancer Res. 2008;68:3421–8.
53. Ackler S, Xiao Y, Mitten MJ, Foster K, Oleksijew A, Refici M, Schlessinger S, Wang B, Chemburkar SR, Bauch J, Tse C, Frost DJ, Fesik SW, Rosenberg SH, Elmore SW, Shoemaker AR. ABT-263 and rapamycin act cooperatively to kill lymphoma cells in vitro and in vivo. Mol Cancer Ther. 2008;7:3265–74.
54. Pro B, Leber B, Smith M, Fayad L, Romaguera J, Hagemeister F, Rodriguez A, McLaughlin P, Samaniego F, Zwiebel J, Lopez A, Kwak L, Younes A. Phase II multicenter study of oblimersen sodium, a Bcl-2 antisense oligonucleotide, in combination with rituximab in patients with recurrent B-cell non-Hodgkin lymphoma. Br J Haematol. 2008;143:355–60.
55. Ramanarayanan J, Hernandez-Ilizaliturri FJ, Chanan-Khan A, Czuczman MS. Pro-apoptotic therapy with the oligonucleotide Genasense (oblimersen sodium) targeting Bcl-2 protein expression enhances the biological anti-tumor activity of rituximab. Br J Haematol. 2004;127:519–30.
56. Maddipatla S, Hernandez-Ilizaliturri FJ, Knight J, Czuczman MS. Augmented antitumor activity against B-cell lymphoma by a combination of monoclonal antibodies targeting TRAIL-R1 and CD20. Clin Cancer Res. 2007;13:4556–64.
57. Daniel D, Yang B, Lawrence DA, Totpal K, Balter I, Lee WP, Gogineni A, Cole MJ, Yee SF, Ross S, Ashkenazi A. Cooperation of the proapoptotic receptor agonist rhApo2L/TRAIL with the CD20 antibody rituximab against non-Hodgkin lymphoma xenografts. Blood. 2007;110:4037–46.
58. Stel AJ, Ten Cate B, Jacobs S, Kok JW, Spierings DC, Dondorff M, Helfrich W, Kluin-Nelemans HC, de Leij LF, Withoff S, Kroesen BJ. Fas receptor clustering and involvement of the death receptor pathway in rituximab-mediated apoptosis with concomitant sensitization of lymphoma B cells to fas-induced apoptosis. J Immunol. 2007;178:2287–95.
59. Coiffier B, Osmanov EA, Hong X, Scheliga A, Mayer J, Offner F, Rule S, Teixeira A, Walewski J, de Vos S, Crump M, Shpilberg O, Esseltine DL, Zhu E, Enny C, Theocharous P, van de Velde H, Elsayed YA, Zinzani PL. LYM-3001 study investigators. Bortezomib plus rituximab versus rituximab alone in patients with relapsed, rituximab-naive or rituximab-sensitive, follicular lymphoma: a randomised phase 3 trial. Lancet Oncol. 2011;12:773–84.
60. Czuczman MS, Gregory SA. The future of CD20 monoclonal antibody therapy in B-cell malignancies. Leuk Lymphoma. 2010;51:983–94.
61. Alduaij W, Illidge TM. The future of anti-CD20 monoclonal antibodies: are we making progress? Blood. 2010;117:2993–3001.
62. Hagenbeek A, Gadeberg O, Johnson P, Pedersen LM, Walewski J, Hellmann A, Link BK, Robak T, Wojtukiewicz M, Pfreundschuh M, Kneba M, Engert A, Sonneveld P, Flensburg M, Petersen J, Losic N, Radford J. First clinical use of ofatumumab, a novel fully human anti-CD20 monoclonal antibody in relapsed or refractory follicular lymphoma: results of a phase 1/2 trial. Blood. 2008;111:5486–95.

63. Salles G, Morschhauser F, Lamy T, Milpied N, Thieblemont C, Tilly H, Bieska G, Asikanius E, Carlile D, Birkett J, Pisa P, Cartron G. Phase 1 study results of the type II glycoengineered humanized anti-CD20 monoclonal antibody obinutuzumab (GA101) in B-cell lymphoma patients. Blood. 2012;119:5126–32.
64. Sehn LH, Assouline SE, Stewart DA, Mangel J, Gascoyne RD, Fine G, Frances-Lasserre S, Carlile DJ, Crump M. A phase 1 study of obinutuzumab induction followed by 2 years of maintenance in patients with relapsed CD20-positive B-cell malignancies. Blood. 2012;119:5118–25.
65. Morschhauser F, Marlton P, Vitolo U, Lindén O, Seymour JF, Crump M, Coiffier B, Foà R, Wassner E, Burger HU, Brennan B, Mendila M. Results of a phase I/II study of ocrelizumab, a fully humanized anti-CD20 mAb, in patients with relapsed/refractory follicular lymphoma. Ann Oncol. 2010;21:1870–6.
66. Vugmeyster Y, Beyer J, Howell K, Combs D, Fielder P, Yang J, Qureshi F, Sandlund B, Kawaguchi L, Dummer W, Lowman H, McKeever K. Depletion of B cells by a humanized anti-CD20 antibody PRO70769 in *Macaca fascicularis*. J Immunother. 2005;28:212–9.
67. Goldenberg DM, Rossi EA, Stein R, Cardillo TM, Czuczman MS, Hernandez-Ilizaliturri FJ, Hansen HJ, Chang CH. Properties and structure-function relationships of veltuzumab (hA20), a humanized anti-CD20 monoclonal antibody. Blood. 2009;113:1062–70.
68. Morschhauser F, Leonard JP, Fayad L, Coiffier B, Petillon MO, Coleman M, Schuster SJ, Dyer MJ, Horne H, Teoh N, Wegener WA, Goldenberg DM. Humanized anti-CD20 antibody, veltuzumab, in refractory/recurrent non-Hodgkin's lymphoma: phase I/II results. J Clin Oncol. 2009;27:3346–53.
69. Bowles JA, Wang SY, Link BK, Allan B, Beuerlein G, Campbell MA, Marquis D, Ondek B, Wooldridge JE, Smith BJ, Breitmeyer JB, Weiner GJ. Anti-CD20 monoclonal antibody with enhanced affinity for CD16 activates NK cells at lower concentrations and more effectively than rituximab. Blood. 2006;108:2648–54.
70. Slamon DJ, Clark GM, Wong SG, Levin WJ, Ullrich A, McGuire WL. Human breast cancer: correlation of relapse and survival with amplification of the HER-2/neu oncogene. Science. 1987;235:177–82.
71. Klapper LN, Waterman H, Sela M, Yarden Y. Tumor-inhibitory antibodies to HER-2/ErbB-2 may act by recruiting c-Cbl and enhancing ubiquitination of HER-2. Cancer Res. 2000;60:3384–8.
72. Spector NL, Blackwell KL. Understanding the mechanisms behind trastuzumab therapy for human epidermal growth factor receptor 2-positive breast cancer. J Clin Oncol. 2009;27:5838–47.
73. Gennari R, Menard S, Fagnoni F, Ponchio L, Scelsi M, Tagliabue E, Castiglioni F, Villani L, Magalotti C, Gibelli N, Oliviero B, Ballardini B, Da Prada G, Zambelli A, Costa A. Pilot study of the mechanism of action of preoperative trastuzumab in patients with primary operable breast tumors overexpressing HER2. Clin Cancer Res. 2004;10:5650–5.
74. Musolino A, Naldi N, Bortesi B, Pezzuolo D, Capelletti M, Missale G, Laccabue D, Zerbini A, Camisa R, Bisagni G, Neri TM, Ardizzoni A. Immunoglobulin G fragment C receptor polymorphisms and clinical efficacy of trastuzumab-based therapy in patients with HER-2/neu-positive metastatic breast cancer. J Clin Oncol. 2008;26:1789–96.
75. Jung M, Koo JS, Moon YW, Park BW, Kim SI, Park S, Lee SH, Hong S, Rha SY, Chung HC, Kim JH, Sohn J. Overexpression of class III beta tubulin and amplified HER2 gene predict good response to paclitaxel and trastuzumab therapy. PLoS ONE. 2012;7:e45127.
76. Junttila TT, Akita RW, Parsons K, Fields C, Lewis Phillips GD, Friedman LS, Sampath D, Sliwkowski MX. Ligand-independent HER2/HER3/PI3 K complex is disrupted by trastuzumab and is effectively inhibited by the PI3 K inhibitor GDC-0941. Cancer Cell. 2009;15:429–40.
77. Zhang S, Huang WC, Li P, Guo H, Poh SB, Brady SW, Xiong Y, Tseng LM, Li SH, Ding Z, Sahin AA, Esteva FJ, Hortobagyi GN, Yu D. Combating trastuzumab resistance by targeting SRC, a common node downstream of multiple resistance pathways. Nat Med. 2011;17:461–9.

78. Arribas J, Baselga J, Pedersen K, Parra-Palau JL. p95HER2 and breast cancer. Cancer Res. 2011;71:1515–9.
79. Nagy P, Friedländer E, Tanner M, Kapanen AI, Carraway KL, Isola J, Jovin TM. Decreased accessibility and lack of activation of ErbB2 in JIMT-1, a herceptin-resistant, MUC4-expressing breast cancer cell line. Cancer Res. 2005;65:473–82.
80. Fessler SP, Wotkowicz MT, Mahanta SK, Bamdad C. MUC1* is a determinant of trastuzumab (Herceptin) resistance in breast cancer cells. Breast Cancer Res Treat. 2009;118:113–24.
81. Sperinde J, Jin X, Banerjee J, Penuel E, Saha A, Diedrich G, Huang W, Leitzel K, Weidler J, Ali SM, Fuchs EM, Singer CF, Köstler WJ, Bates M, Parry G, Winslow J, Lipton A. Quantitation of p95HER2 in paraffin sections by using a p95-specific antibody and correlation with outcome in a cohort of trastuzumab-treated breast cancer patients. Clin Cancer Res. 2010;16:4226–35.
82. Scaltriti M, Rojo F, Ocaña A, Anido J, Guzman M, Cortes J, Di Cosimo S, Matias-Guiu X, Ramon y Cajal S, Arribas J, Baselga J. Expression of p95HER2, a truncated form of the HER2 receptor, and response to anti-HER2 therapies in breast cancer. J Natl Cancer Inst. 2007;99:628–38.
83. Xia W, Mullin RJ, Keith BR, Liu LH, Ma H, Rusnak DW, Owens G, Alligood KJ, Spector NL. Anti-tumor activity of GW572016: a dual tyrosine kinase inhibitor blocks EGF activation of EGFR/erbB2 and downstream Erk1/2 and AKT pathways. Oncogene. 2002;21:6255–63.
84. Scaltriti M, Chandarlapaty S, Prudkin L, Aura C, Jimenez J, Angelini PD, Sánchez G, Guzman M, Parra JL, Ellis C, Gagnon R, Koehler M, Gomez H, Geyer C, Cameron D, Arribas J, Rosen N, Baselga J. Clinical benefit of lapatinib-based therapy in patients with human epidermal growth factor receptor 2-positive breast tumors coexpressing the truncated p95HER2 receptor. Clin Cancer Res. 2010;16:2688–95.
85. Burstein HJ, Storniolo AM, Franco S, Forster J, Stein S, Rubin S, Salazar VM, Blackwell KL. A phase II study of lapatinib monotherapy in chemotherapy-refractory HER2-positive and HER2-negative advanced or metastatic breast cancer. Ann Oncol. 2008;19:1068–74.
86. Berns K, Horlings HM, Hennessy BT, Madiredjo M, Hijmans EM, Beelen K, Linn SC, Gonzalez-Angulo AM, Stemke-Hale K, Hauptmann M, Beijersbergen RL, Mills GB, van de Vijver MJ, Bernards R. A functional genetic approach identifies the PI3 K pathway as a major determinant of trastuzumab resistance in breast cancer. Cancer Cell. 2007;12:395–402.
87. Kataoka Y, et al. Association between gain-of-function mutations in PIK3CA and resistance to HER2-targeted agents in HER2-amplified breast cancer cell lines. Ann Oncol. 2010;21:255–62.
88. Razis E, Bobos M, Kotoula V, Eleftheraki AG, Kalofonos HP, Pavlakis K, Papakostas P, Aravantinos G, Rigakos G, Efstratiou I, Petraki K, Bafaloukos D, Kostopoulos I, Pectasides D, Kalogeras KT, Skarlos D, Fountzilas G. Evaluation of the association of PIK3CA mutations and PTEN loss with efficacy of trastuzumab therapy in metastatic breast cancer. Breast Cancer Res Treat. 2011;128:447–56.
89. Morrow PK, Wulf GM, Ensor J, Booser DJ, Moore JA, Flores PR, Xiong Y, Zhang S, Krop IE, Winer EP, Kindelberger DW, Coviello J, Sahin AA, Nuñez R, Hortobagyi GN, Yu D, Esteva FJ. Phase I/II study of trastuzumab in combination with everolimus (RAD001) in patients with HER2-overexpressing metastatic breast cancer who progressed on trastuzumab-based therapy. J Clin Oncol. 2011;29:3126–32.
90. Wong AL, Lee SC. Mechanisms of resistance to trastuzumab and novel therapeutic strategies in HER2-positive breast cancer. Int J Breast Cancer. 2012;2012:415170.
91. Carboni JM, Wittman M, Yang Z, Lee F, Greer A, Hurlburt W, Hillerman S, Cao C, Cantor GH, Dell-John J, Chen C, Discenza L, Menard K, Li A, Trainor G, Vyas D, Kramer R, Attar RM, Gottardis MM. BMS-754807, a small molecule inhibitor of insulin-like growth factor-1R/IR. Mol Cancer Ther. 2009;8:3341–9.

92. Yee D. Insulin-like growth factor receptor inhibitors: baby or the bathwater? J Natl Cancer Inst. 2012;104:975–81.
93. Atzori F, Tabernero J, Cervantes A, Prudkin L, Andreu J, Rodríguez-Braun E, Domingo A, Guijarro J, Gamez C, Rodon J, Di Cosimo S, Brown H, Clark J, Hardwick JS, Beckman RA, Hanley WD, Hsu K, Calvo E, Roselló S, Langdon RB, Baselga J. A phase I pharmacokinetic and pharmacodynamic study of dalotuzumab (MK-0646), an anti-insulin-like growth factor-1 receptor monoclonal antibody, in patients with advanced solid tumors. Clin Cancer Res. 2011;17:6304–12.
94. Tolcher AW, Sarantopoulos J, Patnaik A, Papadopoulos K, Lin CC, Rodon J, Murphy B, Roth B, McCaffery I, Gorski KS, Kaiser B, Zhu M, Deng H, Friberg G,Puzanov I. Phase I, pharmacokinetic, and pharmacodynamic study of AMG 479, a fully human monoclonal antibody to insulin-like growth factor receptor 1. J Clin Oncol. 2009;27:5800–7.
95. Scagliotti GV, Novello S. The role of the insulin-like growth factor signaling pathway in non-small cell lung cancer and other solid tumors. Cancer Treat Rev. 2012;38:292–302.
96. Ekman S, Frödin JE, Harmenberg J, Bergman A, Hedlund A, Dahg P, Alvfors C, Ståhl B, Bergström S, Bergqvist M. Clinical Phase I study with an Insulin-like Growth Factor-1 receptor inhibitor: experiences in patients with squamous non-small cell lung carcinoma. Acta Oncol. 2011;50:441–7.
97. Anastasi S, Sala G, Huiping C, Caprini E, Russo G, Iacovelli S, Lucini F, Ingvarsson S, Segatto O. Loss of RALT/MIG-6 expression in ERBB2-amplified breast carcinomas enhances ErbB-2 oncogenic potency and favors resistance to Herceptin. Oncogene. 2005;24:4540–8.
98. Belkhiri A, Dar AA, Peng DF, Razvi MH, Rinehart C, Arteaga CL, El-Rifai W. Expression of t-DARPP mediates trastuzumab resistance in breast cancer cells. Clin Cancer Res. 2008;14:4564–71.
99. Liang K, Esteva FJ, Albarracin C, Stemke-Hale K, Lu Y, Bianchini G, Yang CY, Li Y, Li X, Chen CT, Mills GB, Hortobagyi GN, Mendelsohn J, Hung MC, Fan Z. Recombinant human erythropoietin antagonizes trastuzumab treatment of breast cancer cells via Jak2-mediated Src activation and PTEN inactivation. Cancer Cell. 2010;18:423–35.
100. Shattuck DL, Miller JK, Carraway KL 3rd, Sweeney C. Met receptor contributes to trastuzumab resistance of Her2-overexpressing breast cancer cells. Cancer Res. 2008;68:1471–7.
101. Agarwal S, Zerillo C, Kolmakova J, Christensen JG, Harris LN, Rimm DL, Digiovanna MP, Stern DF. Association of constitutively activated hepatocyte growth factor receptor (Met) with resistance to a dual EGFR/Her2 inhibitor in non-small-cell lung cancer cells. Br J Cancer. 2009;100:941–9.
102. Rosen LS, Senzer N, Mekhail T, Ganapathi R, Chai F, Savage RE, Waghorne C, Abbadessa G, Schwartz B, Dreicer R. A phase I dose-escalation study of Tivantinib (ARQ 197) in adult patients with metastatic solid tumors. Clin Cancer Res. 2011;17:7754–64.
103. Spigel DR, et al. Final efficacy results from OAM4558 g, a randomized phase II study evaluating MetMAb or placebo in combination with erlotinib in advanced NSCLC. J Clin Oncol. 2011;29 (suppl) Abstract 7505.
104. Narayan M, Wilken JA, Harris LN, Baron AT, Kimbler KD, Maihle NJ. Trastuzumab-induced HER reprogramming in "resistant" breast carcinoma cells. Cancer Res. 2009;69:2191–4.
105. Sendur MA, Aksoy S, Altundag K. Pertuzumab in HER2-positive breast cancer. Curr Med Res Opin. 2012;28:1709–16.
106. Jones KL, Buzdar AU. Evolving novel anti-HER2 strategies. Lancet Oncol. 2009;10:1179–87.
107. Burstein HJ, Elias AD, Rugo HS, Cobleigh MA, Wolff AC, Eisenberg PD, Lehman M, Adams BJ, Bello CL, DePrimo SE, Baum CM, Miller KD. Phase II study of sunitinib malate, an oral multitargeted tyrosine kinase inhibitor, in patients with metastatic breast cancer previously treated with an anthracycline and a taxane. J Clin Oncol. 2008;26:1810–6.

108. Yu HA, Riely GJ. Who should receive EGFR tyrosine-kinase inhibitors? Lancet Oncol. 2012;13:1074–6.
109. Mullen TD, Hannun YA, Obeid LM. Ceramide synthases at the centre of sphingolipid metabolism and biology. Biochem J. 2012;441:789–802.
110. Katz J, Janik JE, Younes A. Brentuximab vedotin (SGN-35). Clin Cancer Res. 2011;17:6428–36.
111. Younes A, Bartlett NL, Leonard JP, Kennedy DA, Lynch CM, Sievers EL, Forero-Torres A. Brentuximab vedotin (SGN-35) for relapsed CD30-positive lymphomas. N Engl J Med. 2010;363:1812–21.
112. Lewis Phillips GD, Li G, Dugger DL, Crocker LM, Parsons KL, Mai E, Blättler WA, Lambert JM, Chari RV, Lutz RJ, Wong WL, Jacobson FS, Koeppen H, Schwall RH, Kenkare-Mitra SR, Spencer SD, Sliwkowski MX. Targeting HER2-positive breast cancer with trastuzumab-DM1, an antibody-cytotoxic drug conjugate. Cancer Res. 2008; 68:9280–90.
113. Burris HA 3rd, Rugo HS, Vukelja SJ, Vogel CL, Borson RA, Limentani S, Tan-Chiu E, Krop IE, Michaelson RA, Girish S, Amler L, Zheng M, Chu YW, Klencke B, O'Shaughnessy JA. Phase II study of the antibody drug conjugate trastuzumab-DM1 for the treatment of human epidermal growth factor receptor 2 (HER2)-positive breast cancer after prior HER2-directed therapy. J Clin Oncol. 2011;29:398–405.
114. Hurvitz SA, Kakkar R. The potential for trastuzumab emtansine in human epidermal growth factor receptor 2 positive metastatic breast cancer: latest evidence and ongoing studies. Ther Adv Med Oncol. 2012;4:235–45.
115. Mendelsohn J, Baselga J. Status of epidermal growth factor receptor antagonists in the biology and treatment of cancer. J Clin Oncol. 2003;21:2787–99.
116. Mendelsohn J, Baselga J. Epidermal growth factor receptor targeting in cancer. Semin Oncol. 2006;33:369–85.
117. Kim ES, Khuri FR, Herbst RS. Epidermal growth factor receptor biology (IMC-C225). Curr Opin Oncol. 2011;13:506–13.
118. Yarden Y, Sliwkowski MX. Untangling the ErbB signalling network. Nat Rev Mol Cell Biol. 2001;2:127–37.
119. Zhang W, Gordon M, Schultheis AM, Yang DY, Nagashima F, Azuma M, Chang HM, Borucka E, Lurje G, Sherrod AE, Iqbal S, Groshen S, Lenz HJ. FCGR2A and FCGR3A polymorphisms associated with clinical outcome of epidermal growth factor receptor expressing metastatic colorectal cancer patients treated with single-agent cetuximab. J Clin Oncol. 2007;25:3712–8.
120. Karapetis CS, Khambata-Ford S, Jonker DJ, O'Callaghan CJ, Tu D, Tebbutt NC, Simes RJ, Chalchal H, Shapiro JD, Robitaille S, Price TJ, Shepherd L, Au HJ, Langer C, Moore MJ, Zalcberg JR. K-ras mutations and benefit from cetuximab in advanced colorectal cancer. N Engl J Med. 2008;359:1757–65.
121. Normanno N, Tejpar S, Morgillo F, De Luca A, Van Cutsem E, Ciardiello F. Implications for KRAS status and EGFR-targeted therapies in metastatic CRC. Nat Rev Clin Oncol. 2009;6:519–27.
122. Sartore-Bianchi A, Bencardino K, Cassingena A, Venturini F, Funaioli C, Cipani T, Amatu A, Pietrogiovanna L, Schiavo R, Di Nicolantonio F, Artale S, Bardelli A, Siena S. Therapeutic implications of resistance to molecular therapies in metastatic colorectal cancer. Cancer Treat Rev. 2010;36(Suppl 3):S1–5.
123. De Roock W, Claes B, Bernasconi D, De Schutter J, Biesmans B, Fountzilas G, Kalogeras KT, Kotoula V, Papamichael D, Laurent-Puig P, Penault-Llorca F, Rougier P, Vincenzi B, Santini D, Tonini G, Cappuzzo F, Frattini M, Molinari F, Saletti P, De Dosso S, Martini M, Bardelli A, Siena S, Sartore-Bianchi A, Tabernero J, Macarulla T, Di Fiore F, Gangloff AO, Ciardiello F, Pfeiffer P, Qvortrup C, Hansen TP, Van Cutsem E, Piessevaux H, Lambrechts D, Delorenzi M, Tejpar S. Effects of KRAS, BRAF, NRAS, and PIK3CA mutations on the efficacy of cetuximab plus chemotherapy in chemotherapy-refractory metastatic colorectal cancer: a retrospective consortium analysis. Lancet Oncol. 2010;11:753–62.

124. Hoeflich KP, Herter S, Tien J, Wong L, Berry L, Chan J, O'Brien C, Modrusan Z, Seshagiri S, Lackner M, Stern H, Choo E, Murray L, Friedman LS, Belvin M. Antitumor efficacy of the novel RAF inhibitor GDC-0879 is predicted by BRAFV600E mutational status and sustained extracellular signal-regulated kinase/mitogen-activated protein kinase pathway suppression. Cancer Res. 2009;69:3042–51.
125. Kopetz S, et al. PLX4032 in metastatic colorectal cancer patients with mutant BRAF tumors. J Clin Oncol. 2010;28(suppl):3534.
126. Montagut C, Dalmases A, Bellosillo B, Crespo M, Pairet S, Iglesias M, Salido M, Gallen M, Marsters S, Tsai SP, Minoche A, Seshagiri S, Serrano S, Himmelbauer H, Bellmunt J, Rovira A, Settleman J, Bosch F, Albanell J. Identification of a mutation in the extracellular domain of the epidermal growth factor receptor conferring cetuximab resistance in colorectal cancer. Nat Med. 2012;18:1445.
127. Saif MW, Kaley K, Chu E, Copur MS. Safety and efficacy of panitumumab therapy after progression with cetuximab: experience at two institutions. Clin Colorectal Cancer. 2010;9:315–8.
128. Perrone F, Lampis A, Orsenigo M, Di Bartolomeo M, Gevorgyan A, Losa M, Frattini M, Riva C, Andreola S, Bajetta E, Bertario L, Leo E, Pierotti MA, Pilotti S. PI3KCA/PTEN deregulation contributes to impaired responses to cetuximab in metastatic colorectal cancer patients. Ann Oncol. 2009;20:84–90.
129. Kim SM, Kim JS, Kim JH, Yun CO, Kim EM, Kim HK, Solca F, Choi SY, Cho BC. Acquired resistance to cetuximab is mediated by increased PTEN instability and leads cross-resistance to gefitinib in HCC827 NSCLC cells. Cancer Lett. 2010;296:150–9.
130. Ciardiello F, Bianco R, Caputo R, Caputo R, Damiano V, Troiani T, Melisi D, De Vita F, De Placido S, Bianco AR, Tortora G. Antitumor activity of ZD6474, a vascular endothelial growth factor receptor tyrosine kinase inhibitor, in human cancer cells with acquired resistance to antiepidermal growth factor receptor therapy. Clin Cancer Res. 2004;10:784–93.
131. Bianco R, Rosa R, Damiano V, Daniele G, Gelardi T, Garofalo S, Tarallo V, De Falco S, Melisi D, Benelli R, Albini A, Ryan A, Ciardiello F, Tortora G. Vascular endothelial growth factor receptor-1 contributes to resistance to anti-epidermal growth factor receptor drugs in human cancer cells. Clin Cancer Res. 2008;14:5069–80.
132. Kies M, Gibson M, Kim S. Cetuximab (C) and bevacizumab (B) in patients with recurrent or metastatic head and neck squamous cell carcinoma (SCCHN). An interim analysis. J Clin Oncol. 2008;26(15S):6072.
133. Wheeler DL, Huang S, Kruser TJ, Nechrebecki MM, Armstrong EA, Benavente S, Gondi V, Hsu KT, Harari PM. Mechanisms of acquired resistance to cetuximab: role of HER (ErbB) family members. Oncogene. 2008;27:3944–56.
134. Lu Y, Li X, Liang K, Luwor R, Siddik ZH, Mills GB, Mendelsohn J, Fan Z. Epidermal growth factor receptor (EGFR) ubiquitination as a mechanism of acquired resistance escaping treatment by the anti-EGFR monoclonal antibody cetuximab. Cancer Res. 2007;67:8240–7.
135. Kamath AV, Lu D, Gupta P, Jin D, Xiang H, Wong A, Leddy C, Crocker L, Schaefer G, Sliwkowski MX, Damico-Beyer LA. Preclinical pharmacokinetics of MEHD7945A, a novel EGFR/HER3 dual-action antibody, and prediction of its human pharmacokinetics and efficacious clinical dose. Cancer Chemother Pharmacol. 2012;69:1063–9.
136. Huang S, Li C, Sliwkowski M. MEHD7945A, an EGFR/ErbB3 dual specific antibody, overcomes acquired resistance to EGFR inhibitors in head and neck and lung tumors. In: 102nd American association for cancer research, Orlando (Abstract 637).
137. Benavente S, Huang S, Armstrong EA, Chi A, Hsu KT, Wheeler DL, Harari PM. Establishment and characterization of a model of acquired resistance to epidermal growth factor receptor targeting agents in human cancer cells. Clin Cancer Res. 2009;15:1585–92.

Tumor Antigen-Specific Monoclonal Antibody-Based Immunotherapy, Cancer Initiating Cells and Disease Recurrence

Yangyang Wang, Francesco Sabbatino, Ling Yu, Elvira Favoino, Xinhui Wang, Matteo Ligorio, Soldano Ferrone, Joseph H. Schwab and Cristina R. Ferrone

Abstract Immunotherapy with tumor antigen (TA)-specific monoclonal antibody (mAb) has been shown to be effective in the treatment of several types of cancer. However, its efficacy is limited by the lack of response in some of the treated patients and by disease recurrence. In this chapter, following a short description of the characteristics of cancer initiating cells (CICs) and the markers used for their identification in various types of cancer, we will provide *in vitro* evidence to suggest that disease recurrence is caused by the lack of eradication of CICs by the TA-specific mAb-based immunotherapy. In addition, we will describe potential strategies to overcome this resistance mechanism which is a major obstacle to the successful application of TA-specific mAb-based immunotherapy.

Keywords Cancer initiating cells · Monoclonal antibody · Tumor antigen · Head and neck cancer · Breast cancer · Pancreatic cancer · Osteosarcoma · Disease recurrence · Combinatorial therapy

---

Yangyang Wang and Francesco Sabbatino equally contributed to this manuscript.

Y. Wang · F. Sabbatino · L. Yu · E. Favoino · X. Wang · M. Ligorio · S. Ferrone (✉)
C. R. Ferrone
Department of Surgery, Massachusetts General Hospital, Boston, MA, USA
e-mail: sferrone@partners.org

Y. Wang
e-mail: ywang54@partners.org

F. Sabbatino
e-mail: fsabbatino@partners.org

J. H. Schwab
Department of Orthopaedic Surgery, Massachusetts General Hospital, Boston, MA, USA

B. Bonavida (ed.), *Resistance to Immunotherapeutic Antibodies in Cancer*,
Resistance to Targeted Anti-Cancer Therapeutics 2, DOI: 10.1007/978-1-4614-7654-2_2,

Abbreviations

ADCC	Antibody-dependent cell-mediated cytotoxicity
ALDH	Aldeyde dehydrogenase
BAAA	BODIPY^{TM}-aminoacetaldehyde
CDC	Complement-dependent cytotoxicity
CICs	Cancer initiating cells
CSPG4	Chondroitin sulfate proteoglycan 4
CTL	Cytotoxic T cells
DEAB	Diethylaminobenzaldehyde
Grp94	Glucose-regulated protein of 94 kDa
HSP	Heat shock protein
mAb	Monoclonal antibody
MCSP	Melanoma-associated chondroitin sulfate proteoglycan
MDSC	Myeloid-derived suppressor cells
MFI	Mean fluorescence intensity
NG2	Neuron-glial antigen 2
PDAC	Pancreas ductal adenocarcinoma
SCID	Severe combined immunodeficiency
SHH	Sonic Hedgehog Homologue
T regs	T regulatory cells
TA	Tumor antigen
TNBC	Triple negative breast cancer

Introduction

The hybridoma methodology has greatly facilitated the identification of a large number of human tumor antigens (TAs) by providing highly specific probes. Several of the identified TAs meet the criteria in terms of high expression on tumor cells, restricted distribution in normal tissues and functional properties to be used as targets of monoclonal antibody (mAb)-based immunotherapy for the treatment of malignant diseases [1]. A large body of clinical evidence in conjunction with the results of studies in animal model systems have convincingly shown that targeting TA with mAbs may represent an effective strategy for the treatment of many types of cancer [1]. The therapeutic efficacy of TA-specific mAbs is in general enhanced by combination with chemo- and/or radio-therapy [1]. Nevertheless, immunotherapy with TA-specific mAbs is not effective in all the treated patients and in most patients its efficacy is limited in time because of disease recurrence and/or metastases [1]. These clinical findings have stimulated interest in defining the molecular mechanism(s) underlying the innate and acquired resistance of tumor cells to TA-specific mAb-based immunotherapy with the expectation that this

Table 1 Mechanism of cancer resistance to antibody treatment

Mechanism of resistance	Mediated mechanism	Alteration	Cancer	References
Amplification of downstream signaling and alternative signaling pathways	Independent growth stimulatory effects	(1) KRAS mutation (codon 12 or 13) (2) BRAF mutation (V600E) (3) PIK3CA mutation (4) PTEN loss (5) Overexpression of other HER family receptors (6) Increased IGF-IR activity	Breast, colon, cancer	[40–45]
Expression of immune inhibitory molecules	Inhibition of NK cells-mediated lysis by mAbs Inhibition of ADCC	Increased HLA-G or HLA-E expression	Colon, ovarian, cancer	[46, 47]
Expression of membrane-bound complement regulatory proteins	Inhibition of CDC	Increased CD46, CD55, and CD59 expressions	Breast, lung, colon cancer and hematological malignancies	[48–51]
Impairment of proper antigen presentation	Evasion to destruction by MHC-restricted CTLs response mediated by mAbs	Down-regulation of MHC I expression	Breast cancer, colon cancer	[52–54]
Increased inhibitory signals by intratumoral Tregs or MDSCs	Suppression of the anti-cancer immune response mediated by mAbs	Apoptosis of immune effectors cells by increased production of perforin and granzyme, by expression of indolamine 2,3 dioxygenase and by production of soluble mediators such as TGF-β and IL-10	Breast cancer, hematological malignancies	[55–57]
Reduction of binding affinity of TA	Reduction of TA recognition	(1) FcγRII and FcγIII polymorphism (2) CD20 mutation (ANPS and YCYSI, at positions 170 to 173 and 182 to 185)	Breast cancer, colon cancer, hematological malignancies	[58–60]
Reduction or loss of TA expression	Reduction or loss of tumor cell recognition	(1) Genetic instability of tumor cells (2) MAPK pathway activation (3) increased histone deacetylase activity	Colon cancer and hematological malignancies	[61–65]
Impaired access to TA or production of antagonist TA	Reduction of TA recognition	(1) Expression of extracellular domain-truncated HER2 (p95 HER2) (2) Overexpression of MUC4	Breast cancer	[66, 67]

information will contribute to the rational design of targeted therapeutic strategies to counteract these resistances.

Multiple mechanisms have been shown to underlie the resistance of tumor cells to TA-specific mAb-based immunotherapy. As recently reviewed by other groups (see Table 1) and discussed in many chapters of this book, they include loss of the targeted TA, mutations in the targeted TA, upregulation of complement component inhibitors, etc. In addition, recent evidence demonstrated that the therapeutic activity of TA-specific mAbs may be mediated by induction or enhancement of TA-specific cytotoxic T cells (CTL). If this is the case, defects in antigen presentation by tumor cells to cognate CTL or suppression of their functional properties may represent mechanisms of resistance of tumor cells to mAb-based immunotherapy.

In the present paper, utilizing our recent *in vitro* data, we will discuss the possibility that disease recurrence in patients treated with TA-specific mAb-based immunotherapy in combination with radio- and/or chemo-therapy may be caused by the resistance of cancer initiating cells (CICs) to this type of therapy. Specifically, we will describe (1) the characteristics of CICs in the tumors we have investigated; (2) the effects of TA-specific mAbs with chemo- and/or radio-therapy on CICs; and (3) strategies to overcome this resistance.

Resistance of Cancer Initiating Cells from TA-Specific mAb-based Immunotherapy

1. Characteristics of CICs in Various Types of Tumors

According to the cancer stem cell theory, CICs are a subpopulation of tumor cells that, like normal stem cells, are "multipotent" since they can give rise to all cell types found in a particular cancer sample, are asymmetrically self-renewing, can divide indefinitely, and are able to generate tumor spheres and are tumorigenic in low numbers in immunodeficient mice [2]. Relevant to the data that we are going to present, CICs are chemo-and radio-resistant and are believed to play a major role in both the metastatic spread and disease recurrence, the major causes of patients morbidity and mortality [3]. Therefore, CICs cells have to be eradicated in order to "cure" a malignant disease.

Several markers have been reported to identify CICs in various types of tumors. They include $CD44^{high}CD24^{low}$ in breast cancer [4], CD133 in pancreas ductal adenocarcinoma (PDAC) [5] and in osteosarcoma [6], and the activity of the aldeyde dehydrogenases (ALDHs) in head and neck, breast, lung, pancreas, colon, prostate, and ovary cancers and osteosarcoma [2, 7–13].

According to the information in the literature and our own data, the ALDH activity appears to be a reliable marker. Since this marker has been used in studies we are going to present, we will first give some background about the ALDH activity in normal and cancer cells. ALDHs are a family of enzymes involved in the maintenance of cellular homeostasis by metabolizing both endogenous and exogenous reactive compounds [14]. They oxidize aldehydes to the corresponding carboxylic acids using either Nicotinamide adenine dinucleotide (NAD) or nicotinamide adenine dinucleotide phosphate (NADP) as a coenzyme [15]. These enzymes are known to modulate several cell functions, including proliferation, differentiation and survival as well as the cellular response to oxidative stress. How ALDHs modulate these processes still remain to be determined. Nineteen ALDH genes have been found in the human genome [16]. They are clustered in 11 families and 4 subfamilies with distinct chromosomal locations. ALDHs, namely, ALDH1A2, ALDH1A3, ALDH1A7, ALDH2*2, ALDH3A1, ALDH4A1, ALDH5A1, ALDH6 and ALDH9A1 display high enzymatic activity in normal and cancer stem cells. Therefore, these enzymes may be considered a marker for these cells and may well play a functional role in terms of self protection, differentiation, and/or expansion of stem cell populations.

The detection of ALDH in a cell relies on the measurement of its enzymatic activity. This has been facilitated by the availability of a specific substrate which can be detected by fluorescence analysis (ALDEFLUOR). It is noteworthy that this substrate does not discriminate among different isoforms of ALDHs. Therefore, as ALDH isoforms have a wide substrate spectrum, it has been possible to determine that ALDH positivity, evidenced in various types of stem cells, including cancer stem cells, is not due to the expression of the same isoforms. It is believed that this heterogeneity indicates that the isoform responsible for Adelfluor activity in the case of normal cells depends on the type of the cell and on the tissue of origin in the case of cancer cells [17]. That is why most studies on ALDHs and stem cells do not specify the ALDH isoform, but speak rather generically of ALDH. However, ALDHA1 has been identified as a marker for the isolation and identification of normal or cancer stem cells [2], and along with ALDH3A1, which it has been shown to play a role in differentiation and cell proliferation [15]. Indeed, a reduction in cell proliferation has been observed when the enzyme is directly inhibited by the administration of synthetic specific inhibitors, antisense oligonucleotides, or siRNA.

Several lines of evidence indicate that cells which display high activity of ALDH ($ALDH^{bright}$) are normal or cancer stem cells. The enzymatic activity of ALDHs in human hematopoietic progenitor cells has been shown to be higher than in more mature hematopoietic cells [18]. In addition, it has been associated with an enhanced repopulating function and cellular resistance to cytotoxic drugs such as alkylating agents. As multipotent cells, $ALDH^{bright}$ cells isolated from bone marrow have been demonstrated to include hematopoietic, endothelial, mesenchymal, and neural progenitor cells, which are crucial in repair protocols for various pathological conditions. Like human hematopoietic progenitor cells, several other types of normal stem cells have been shown to display high levels of cytosolic ALDH expression. They include neural cells, myogenic cells, mammary cells, prostate cells, and intestinal crypt cells. These cells have been shown to be multipotent, self-renewing, and able to generate spheres and epithelial stem-like cells in culture.

Increased ALDH activity in cancer stem cells was first reported in acute myeloid leukemia. Subsequently, similar observations have been reported for several types of solid cancers, including breast, colon, prostate, lung, pancreas and ovary. Our data as well as data from the literature demonstrate that ALDH^{bright} cells in head and neck, triple negative breast and pancreatic cancers have the characteristic of CICs, such as *in vitro* self-renewal, chemo- and radio-resistance, ability to divide indefinitely, aberrant regulation of several stem cell signaling pathways (such as Hedgehog and MAPK, Notch, PI3K/AKT, TGF-β and Wnt), expression of stem cell markers, tumor cell sphere formation, and high tumorigenicity at low cell numbers in SCID mice [19–21].

ALDH^{bright} cells are analyzed using the ALDEFLUOR™ reagent kit. The activated ALDEFLUOR™ Reagent, BODIPY™-aminoacetaldehyde (BAAA), is a fluorescent non-toxic substrate for ALDH, which freely diffuses into intact and viable cells. In the presence of ALDH, BAAA is converted into BODIPY™-aminoacate (BAA), which is retained inside the cells. The amount of fluorescent reaction product is proportional to the ALDH activity in the cells and is measured using a flow cytometer. The active efflux of the reaction product is inhibited by an efflux inhibitor in the ALDEFLUOR™ Assay Buffer. A specific inhibitor of ALDH, diethylaminobenzaldehyde (DEAB), is used to control for background fluorescence as the gating reference standard of the ALDH^{neg} population. Thus, ALDH^{bright} cells are those ALDH^{+} cells with twice the mean fluorescence intensity (MFI) of the ALDH^{+} cell population (Fig. 1). The frequency of ALDH^{bright} cells varies among cell lines of different tumor types as well as among cell lines from the same type of tumor. Table 2 presents the results we have obtained with different human cancer cell lines analyzed for the content of ALDH^{bright} cells. It is noteworthy that this frequency is influenced by the culture conditions such as cell confluency, cell starvation and hypoxia [22]. Viable ALDH^{bright} cells can be

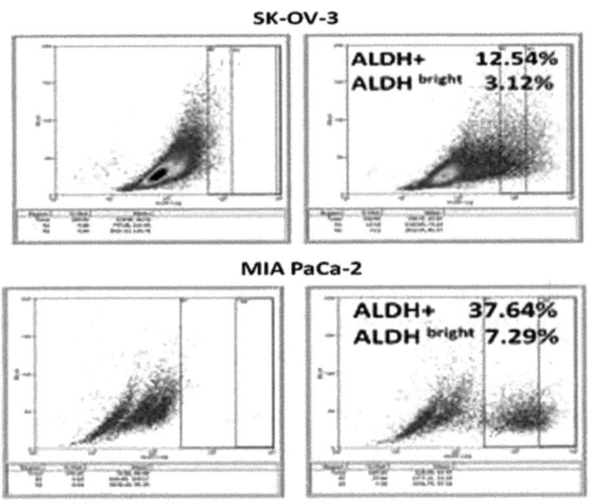

Fig. 1 ALDH activity expression as a marker of CICs in the human ovarian cancer cell line SK-OV-3 and in the human PDAC cell line MIA PaCa-2. SK-OV-3 and MIA PaCa-2 cells (2.5×10^5) were cultured in complete medium at 37 °C, 5 % CO_2. Then, the cells were harvested and stained with ALDEFLUOR with or without the DEAB inhibitor to identify ALDH^{bright} cells. ALDH^{bright} cells were identified as those ALDH^{+} cells with twice the mean fluorescence intensity (MFI) of the ALDH^{+} cell population

Table 2 Expression of $ALDH^+$ and $ALDH^{bright}$ cells in different types of cancer

Cell line	$ALDH^+$ cells (%)	$ALDH^{bright}$ cells (%)
Head and neck cancer		
PCI-4A	23.2	6.3
PCI-13	11.3	1.9
PCI-30	0.3	0.1
PCI-37A	1.2	0.1
SCC-4	5.4	1.1
SCC-90	1.6	0.2
SCC-104	0.5	0.1
UD-SCC-4	0.5	0.1
UD-SCC-6	0.3	0.1
FaDu	1.8	0.1
Breast cancer		
MDA-MB-231	18.2	0.7
SUM-149	22.1	1.5
UACC-812	4.7	0.3
Pancreatic cancer		
MIA PaCa-2	43.2	4.6
S2-LM7-AA	19.3	1.6
PDAC1	21.3	2.5
PDAC2	14.4	2.3
PDAC3	38.2	8.0
PDAC5	5.7	0.8

further isolated using a cell sorter and can be tested for their ability to form tumor spheres *in vitro* and for their tumorigenicity in low number in immunodeficient mice. As shown in Fig. 2, $ALDH^{bright}$ cells sorted from the head and neck cancer PCI-13 cell line, the PDAC MIA PaCa-2 cell line, and the TNBC MDA-MB-231-Luc cell line orthotopically injected at a low number (500 cells/mouse) in immunodeficient mice induce tumors in most if not in all of the injected mice. On the other hand, the $ALDH^{neg}$ cells failed to induce tumors.

2. Characteristics of the TA Utilized to Target Differentiated Tumor Cells and CICs in Our Laboratory

We have focused our work aiming at developing immunotherapy of solid tumors with TA-specific mAbs on three types of TA which are characterized by a high expression on the tumor cell membrane, a restricted distribution in normal tissue and the ability to modulate multiple signaling pathways. We will describe the characteristics of these TAs which are most relevant for the experiments discussed below.

A. *Chondroitin Sulfate Proteoglycan 4*

In the late 70s, utilizing mAb elicited in mice immunized with cultured human melanoma cells, we identified a TA with high expression on the membrane of melanoma cells and with a restricted distribution in normal tissues. This TA, which is highly conserved through phylogenetic evolution, consists of an N linked

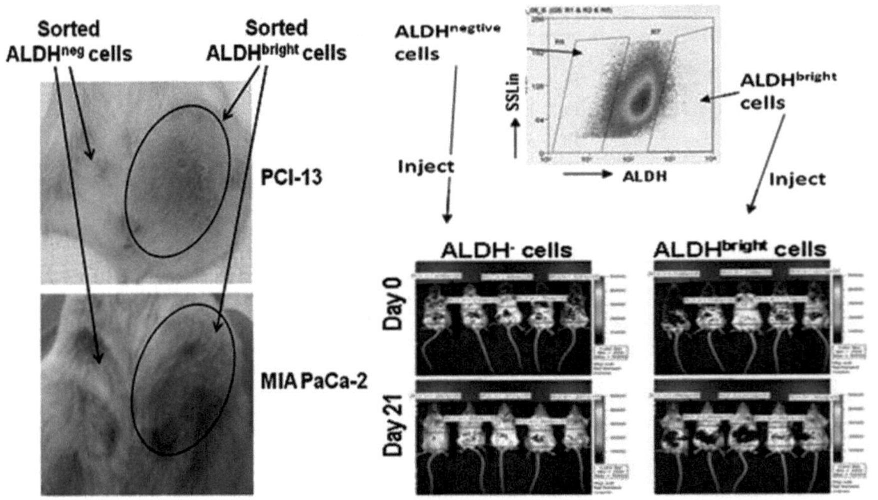

Fig. 2 Tumorigenicity of ALDH^{bright} cells sorted from human carcinoma cell lines. Immunodeficient NOD/SCID mice were challenged in the right and left flanks with 500 sorted ALDH^{bright} or ALDH^{neg} PCI-13 or MIA PaCa-2 cells isolated from human carcinoma cell lines and established xenografts and photographs of representative mice are shown. Xenografts were established in 3/3 mice challenged with ALDH^{bright} PCI-13 and 2/3 mice challenged with ALDH^{bright} MIA PaCa-2 cells (*left* panel). Sorted ALDH^{bright} and ALDH^{neg} MDA-MB-231-luc-D3H1 (Xenogen Corp) cells (500/mouse) were mixed with irradiated unsorted MDA-MB-231 cells (10,000/mouse) and Matrigel and injected (total final vol. 100 μl) intraperitoneally (i.p.) into 2 groups of NOD/SCID mice. Tumor growth was monitored in each mouse weekly by Bioluminescence imaging (*right* panel)

280 kDa glycoprotein and a 450 kDa chondroitin sulfate proteoglycan, the two components have the same polypeptide moiety [23]. Because of its large size, we named this TA high molecular weight- melanoma associated antigen. This TA, also known as cell surface chondroitin sulfate proteoglycan 4 (CSPG4), melanoma-associated chondroitin sulfate proteoglycan (MCSP) or neuron-glial antigen 2 (NG2), is expressed not only on melanoma but also on head and neck cancer, TNBC, mesothelioma, chordoma, chondrosarcoma and osteosarcoma [24]. In the tumors which have been analyzed, CSPG4 has been found to be expressed not only on differentiated cancer cells but also on CICs, defined as ALDH^{bright} cells, in head and neck cancer, triple negative breast cancer and osteosarcoma. A representative example of a double staining of ALDH^{bright} cells with a CSPG4-specific mAb in the TNBC MDA-MB-231 cell line is shown in Fig. 3. The expression of CSPG4 on CICs is also corroborated by functional data. Specifically, CSPG4 specific-mAb can inhibit the proliferation and the migration of TNBC and osteosarcoma cell lines *in vitro* (Figs. 4 and 5) and their ability to metastasize when injected in immunodeficient mice [25]. Furthermore, CSPG4-specific mAb could suppress disease recurrence and prolong survival in mice which have been grafted with the TNBC cell line MDA-MB-231 and then subjected to surgical removal of the primary tumor (Fig. 6). As already discussed, CICs play a major role in disease

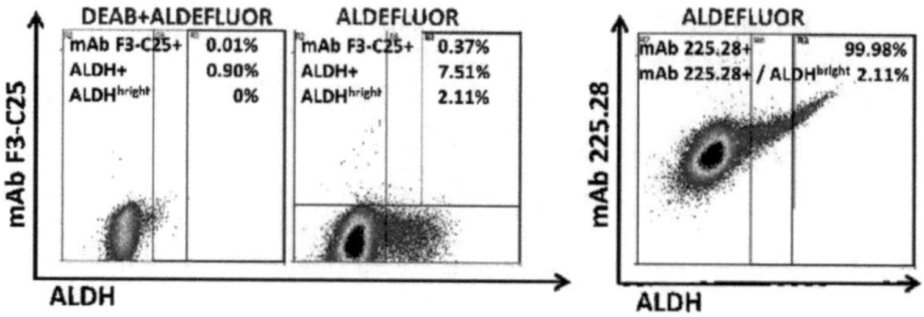

Fig. 3 CSPG4 expression on human TNBC CICs. The TNBC cells MDA-MB-231 were incubated with ALDEFLUOR (Stem Cell Technologies) to detect ALDH activity and stained with the CSPG4-specific mAb 225.28. DEAB, a specific inhibitor of ALDH, was used to establish the baseline fluorescence of these cells. The isotype matched mAb F3-C25 was used as a control for the CSPG4-specific mAb 225.28. The $ALDH^{bright}$ cells were identified as those $ALDH^{+}$ cells with twice the mean fluorescence intensity (MFI) of the $ALDH^{+}$ cell population. The % of cells stained by ALDEFLUOR and/or by mAbs is shown

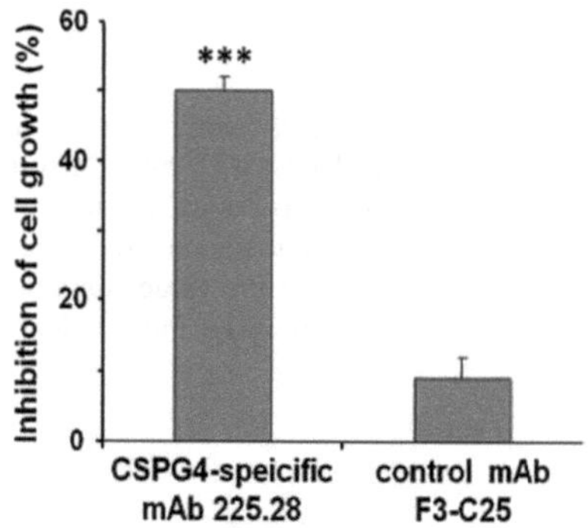

Fig. 4 Inhibition of human osteosarcoma U2OS carcinoma cell growth. Human osteosarcoma U2OS cells were serum starved 3 days and incubated either with 0.25 mg/ml CSPG4-specific mAb 225.28 or control mAb F3-C25 in a 3-D (matrigel) setting for 10 days. PBS, which was used as the solvent for both mAbs, was used as a reference for 100 % cell growth. Cells in each well were harvested from the matrigel using the Cell Recovery Solution (BD Pharmingen) and counted by two individuals using Trypan Blue. The results are expressed as % inhibition of cell growth, utilizing the values obtained for cells grown in PBS, as a reference. The values shown are the mean of three independent experiments. *** indicates $p < 0.001$

recurrence and metastatic spread. The effects of immunotherapy with the CSPG4-specific mAb are mediated by the inhibition of the activation of multiple signaling components of pathways involved in proliferation, survival and antiapoptotic signals as well as in migration of cancer cells including CICs (Fig. 7). The potential clinical relevance of these data is indicated by the beneficial effect of the clinical course of the disease of CSPG4-specific antibodies induced by CSPG4 mimics in patients with melanoma.

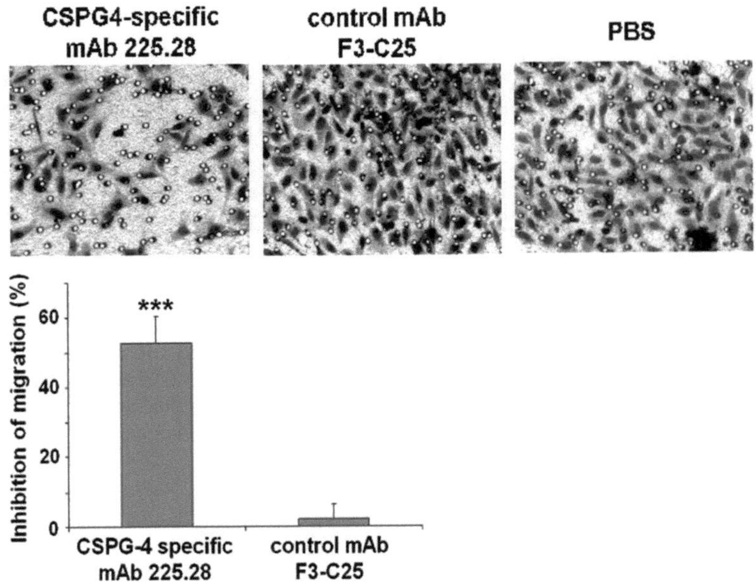

Fig. 5 Inhibition of human osteosarcoma U2OS carcinoma cell migration. U2OS cells were serum starved 3 days and seeded and incubated with either 0.5 mg/ml CSPG4-specific mAb 225.28, control mAb F3-C25 or PBS in a migration assay. Pictures of each well were taken with a Zeiss Inverted Fluorescence Microscope (AxioVision Software) (×200). The results are expressed as % inhibition of migration, utilizing the values obtained in PBS without mAb as a reference. The values shown are the mean of three independent experiments. *** indicates $p < 0.001$

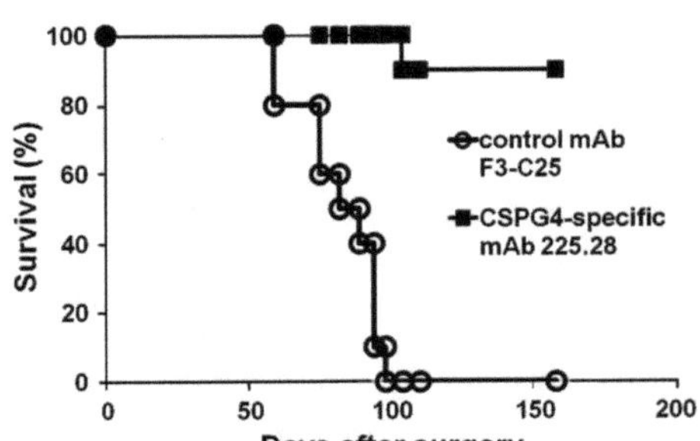

Fig. 6 Prolongation of mice survival by the CSPG4-specific mAb after surgical removal of the primary tumor derived by TNBC MDA-MB-231 cells. TNBC MDA-MB-231 cells (2×10^6 cells/mouse) were injected orthotopically into 20 SCID mice. After 63 days, mice were divided into two groups ($n = 10$/group) using a stratified randomization strategy, such that the mean tumor volume was not statistically significantly different between two groups. On day 63, all primary tumors were surgically removed. Starting from day 66, mice were treated intravenously (i.v.) with CSPG4-specific mAb 225.28 (200 μg/mouse/twice per week) or control mAb F3-C25 (200 μg/mouse/twice per week). The survival of mice was analyzed using the Kaplan–Meier survival curve

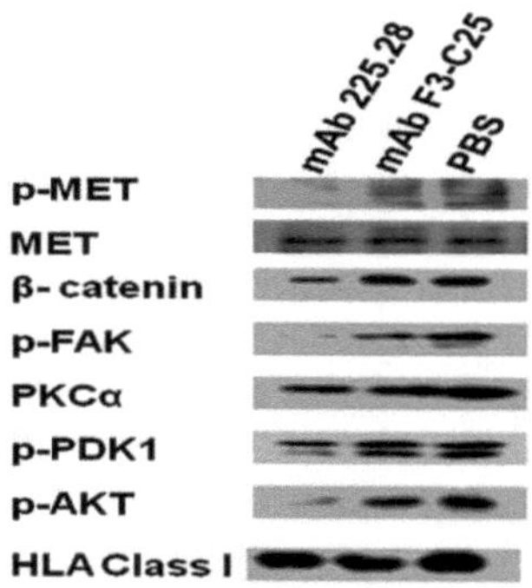

Fig. 7 Effect of the CSPG4-specific mAb 225.28 on multiple signaling pathways *in vitro* in the human osteosarcoma MG-63 cell line. The human ostersarcoma cell line MG-63 was incubated with either the CSPG4-specific mAb 225.28, the isotype control mAb F3-C25 or PBS for 72 h at 37 °C. Cell lysates were tested in western blot with anti-phosphorylated (p)-MET, MET, β-catenin, p-FAK, PKCα, p-PDK1, p-AKT antibodies. HLA class I heavy chain (HLA class I) was used as the loading control

B. *Glucose-regulated Protein of 94 kDa*

The heat shock protein (HSP) glucose-regulated protein of 94 kDa (Grp94) is a member of the HSP90 family [26, 27]. Similar to other members of this family, the molecular chaperone Grp94 is required for the stability and activity of client proteins involved in the activation of signaling pathways associated with tumor cell survival and proliferation [27–29]. These functional properties of Grp94 provide a molecular mechanism for the anti-proliferative effect and the induction of apoptosis of malignant cells by Grp94 inhibitors. The potential clinical relevance of these findings is suggested by the clinical responses observed in patients treated with inhibitors of HSP90 [30–32], which display a high degree of homology with Grp94. However, the clinical use of HSP90 inhibitors is hampered by the significant side effects they cause because of their lack of selectivity and the ubiquitous intracellular expression of HSP90. To overcome these limitations, we have isolated a Grp94-specific single chain Fv fragment from a phage display antibody library. This single chain has the unique specificity to recognize an extracellular epitope of Grp94 which is selectively expressed on the membrane of many types of malignant cells, but has a restricted distribution in normal cells. In the tumors we have analyzed, Grp94 has been found to be expressed not only on differentiated cancer cells but also on CICs, defined as $ALDH^{bright}$ cells. A representative example of a double staining of $ALDH^{bright}$ cells with a Grp94-specific mAb in the PDAC MIA-PaCa-2 cell line is shown in Fig. 8. The Grp94-specific mAb inhibits the proliferation and the migration of malignant cells and induces their apoptosis. These effects are mediated by inhibition of the activation of several components of signaling pathways involved in proliferation, survival and antiapoptosis as well as in migration of cancer cells including CICs (data not shown).

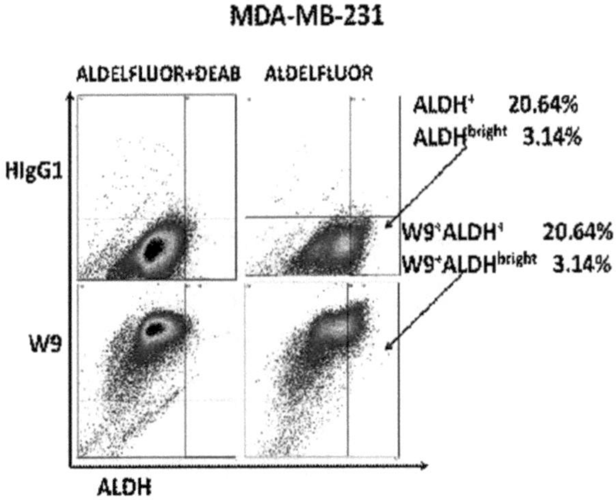

Fig. 8 Grp94 expression on human TNBC CICs. The TNBC cells MDA-MB-231 were incubated with ALDEFLUOR (Stem Cell Technologies) to detect ALDH activity and stained with the Grp94-specific mAb W9. DEAB, a specific inhibitor of ALDH, was used to establish the baseline fluorescence of these cells. The isotype matched mAb HIgG1 was used as a control for the mAb W9. $ALDH^{bright}$ cells were identified as those $ALDH^{+}$ cells with twice the mean fluorescence intensity (MFI) of the $ALDH^{+}$ cell population. The % of cells stained by ALDEFLUOR and/or by mAbs is shown

C. B7-H3

B7-H3 known also as CD276 is a member of the B7 family; it shares 20–27 % amino acid sequence homology with other members of the B7 family [33]. To detect B7-H3, we use the mAb 376.96, an IgG2a generated from a BALB/c mouse hyperimmunized with cultured human melanoma cells. The specificity of mAb 376.96 for B7-H3 has been recently shown by the following lines of evidence. First, mass spectrometry analysis of the peptides generated by trypsin digestion of the 94 kDa glycoprotein immunoprecipitated by mAb 376.96 from cultured human melanoma Colo38 cells has demonstrated a high degree of homology with that of B7-H3. Second, the mAb 376.96 specifically reacts with purified B7-H3 in binding assays. Third, the mAb 376.96 stains CHO cells transfected with human B7-H3 (2Ig) or B7-H3 (4Ig) cDNA; the epitope recognized by the mAb 376.96 is expressed on both 2 and 4Ig human B7-H3. Immunohistochemical staining with the B7-H3-specific mAb 376.96 has shown that the corresponding epitope has a broad distribution on several types of cancer including head and neck, breast, pancreatic, ovarian, prostate cancer and osteosarcoma. In contrast, this epitope has a more restricted distribution than the B7-H3 molecules in normal tissues since several tissues which express the B7-H3 molecule are not stained by the B7-H3-specific mAb 376.96. In the tumors we have analyzed, the B7-H3-specific mAb 376.96 has been found to be expressed not only on differentiated cancer cells but also on CICs, defined as $ALDH^{bright}$ cells. A representative example of a double

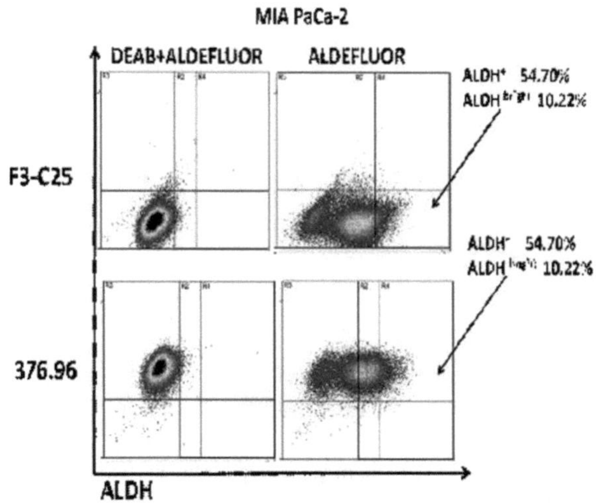

Fig. 9 B7-H3-specific mAb 376.96 expression on human PDAC MIA PaCa-2 CICs. MIA PaCa-2 cells were incubated with ALDEFLUOR (Stem Cell Technologies) to detect ALDH activity and stained with the B7-H3-specific mAb 376.96. DEAB, a specific inhibitor of ALDH, was used to establish the baseline fluorescence of these cells. The isotype matched mAb F3-C25 was used as a control for the mAb 376.96. $ALDH^{bright}$ cells were identified as those $ALDH^+$ cells with twice the mean fluorescence intensity (MFI) of the $ALDH^+$ cell population. The % of cells stained by ALDEFLUOR and/or by mAbs is shown

staining of $ALDH^{bright}$ cells with the B7-H3-specific mAb 376.96 in the PDAC Mia-PaCa-2 cell line is shown in Fig. 9. The mAb 376.96 displays an antiproliferative effect *in vitro* with various types of cell lines including TNBC, PDAC and ovarian cancers. These results are paralleled by the inhibition of PDAC cell growth grafted in immunodeficient mice (Fig. 10). Studies in progress suggest that this effect is mediated by the inhibition of the activation of several components of signaling pathways involved in proliferation, survival and antiapoptosis as well as in migration of cancer cells including CICs (Fig. 11).

Effects of TA-specific MAbs in Combination with Chemo-radio-therapy on CICs

The results shown above in the previous sections indicate that TA-specific mAbs have anti-tumor effects by inhibiting cell growth, cell migration, and inducing apoptosis *in vitro*. These effects are paralleled by an inhibition but not complete suppression of metastatic spread and disease recurrence in immunodeficient mice grafted with human cancer cell lines. These findings are likely to reflect the inability of TA-specific mAbs to eliminate CICs. This possibility is supported by our *in vitro* data which have shown that incubation of cell lines with the

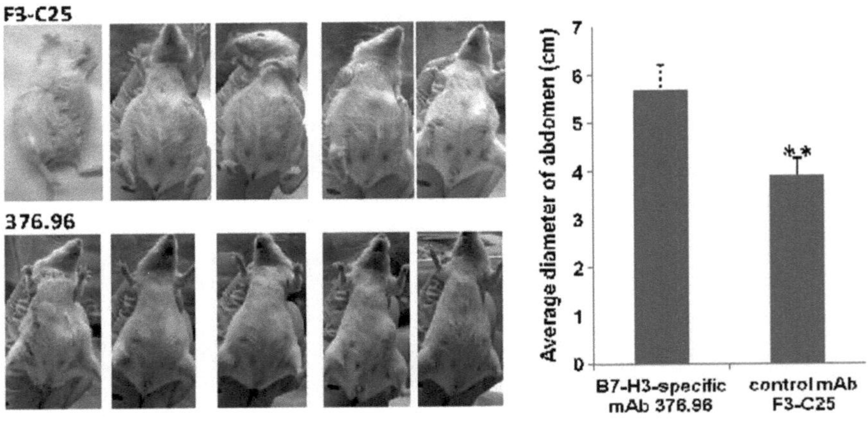

Fig. 10 Inhibition by the B7-H3-specific mAb 376.96 on the growth of tumors derived from the human PDAC MIA PaCa-2 cells grafted in SCID mice. Ten SCID mice were orthotopically challenged by the human PDAC cell line MIA PaCa-2 (2×10^6/mouse). After 28 days, the mice were randomly divided into 2 groups ($n = 5$/group). One group was treated i.v. with the B7-H3-specific mAb 376.96 (200 μg/mouse) and the other group was treated i.v. with the control mAb F3-C25 (200 μg/mouse) twice per week. After a total of 8 treatments, one mouse from the control group was dead and all other mice in the control group have ascites. In contrast, no mouse in the mAb 376.96-treated group had ascites. The pictures of mice on day 56 are shown in the left panel and the average diameters of the abdomen from both groups are shown in the right panel. **: p value < 0.01

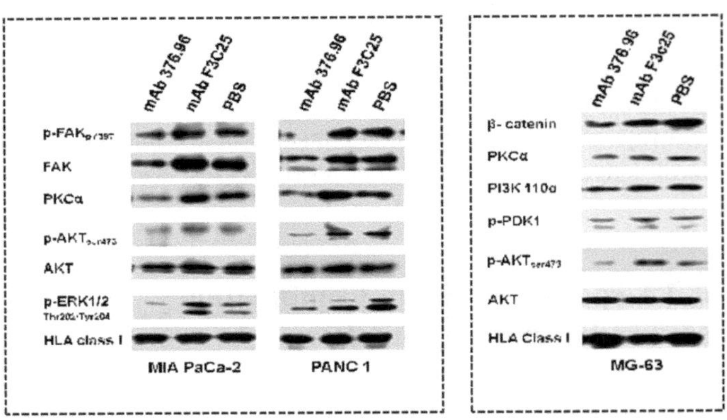

Fig. 11 Effect of the B7-H3-specific mAb 376.96 on multiple signaling pathways *in vitro* in the human osteosarcoma MG-63 cell line The human PDAC cells MIA PaCa-2, PANC 1 and the human ostersarcoma cell line MG-63 were incubated for 48 h (MIA PaCa-2 and PANC 1) or 72 h (MG-63) at 37 °C with either the B7-H3-specific mAb 376.96 or the control mAb F3-C25. Cells incubated in medium without mAbs were used as control. Cell lysates were tested by western blot with phosphorylated (p)-FAK, FAK, PKCα, p-ERK1/2, ERK1/2, p-AKT, AKT, β-catenin, PI3 K 110α and p-PDK1 mAbs. HLA class I was used as a loading control

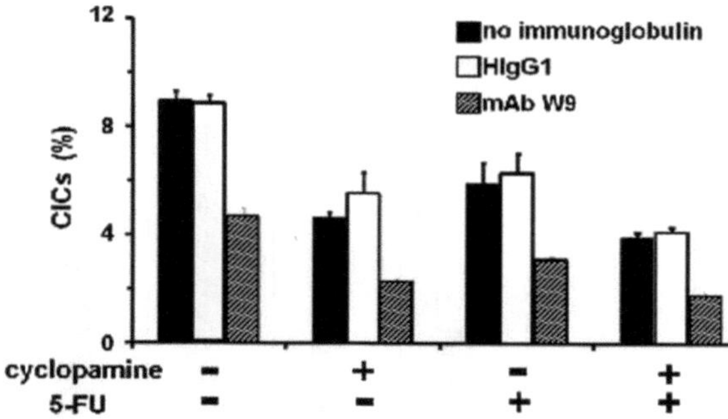

Fig. 12 Inhibition of pancreatic CICs *in vitro* proliferation by the Grp94-specific mAb W9. The PDAC MIA PaCa-2 cells were incubated with the mAb W9 (20 μg/ml), cyclopamine (20 μM), and 5-FU (10 μM) for 48 h at 37 °C. Cells were then harvested and stained with ALDEFLUOR with or without DEAB. HIgG1 was used as an isotype control. The triple combination of mAb W9, cyclopamine and 5-FU was significantly ($p < 0.05$) more effective than the triple combination of HIgG1, cyclopamine and 5-FU, double combinations and individual agents. The double combination of mAb W9 and cyclopamine was significantly ($p < 0.05$) more effective than the other combinations of two agents and individual agents. Cyclopamine was significantly ($p < 0.05$) more effective than the other individual agents

CSPG4/Grp94/B7-H3-specific mAbs can reduce the percentage of $\text{ALDH}^{\text{bright}}$ cells but not completely eliminate them. Representative examples of the effect of TA-specific mAbs on CICs are shown in Figs. 12 and 13. The detrimental effect of TA-specific mAbs on the percentage of CICs can be enhanced by combining the mAbs with chemotherapeutic agents, novel targeted agents and/or radiotherapy. Representative examples are shown in Figs. 12 and 13. The antiproliferative activity of the Grp94-specific mAb on differentiated PDAC cells as well as on pancreatic CICs is significantly enhanced when PDAC cells are incubated with the Grp94-specific mAb in combination with 5FU or with radiation (Fig. 14).

Enhancement by Signaling of the CICs Pathway Inhibitor of the Detrimental Effects of TA-specific MAb on CICs

The antitumor effects of TA-specific mAbs on both differentiated cancer cells and CICs have been shown to be enhanced by combining TA-specific mAbs with chemotherapeutic agents, targeted agents or radiotherapy. However, these types of combinatorial strategies do not completely eliminate CICs from a tumor cell population. These *in vitro* results provide an explanation for the limited duration of clinical objective responses of tumor-bearing hosts treated with TA-specific mAbs in combination with chemotherapeutic agents, targeted agents or radiotherapy. The fraction of CICs which is not eradicated by this combinatorial therapy may cause disease recurrence. These findings emphasize the need to develop novel and

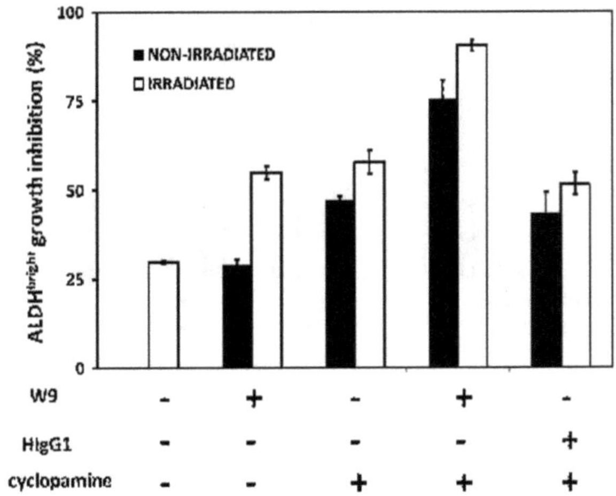

Fig. 13 Inhibition of pancreatic CICs *in vitro* proliferation by the Grp94-specific mAb W9. The PDAC MIA PaCa-2 cells were incubated with the mAb W9 (20 μg/ml), cyclopamine (20 μM), and radiotherapy (20 Gy). Following a 72 h incubation at 37 °C, the cells were harvested and stained with ALDEFLUOR with or without DEAB. HIgG1 was used as isotype control. The triple combination of mAb W9, cyclopamine and 20 Gy was significantly ($p < 0.05$) more effective than the triple combination of HIgG1, cyclopamine and 20 Gy, double combinations and individual treatment. The double combination of mAb W9 and cyclopamine was significantly ($p < 0.05$) more effective than the other combinations of two agents and individual agents. Cyclopamine was significantly ($p < 0.05$) more effective than the other individual treatments

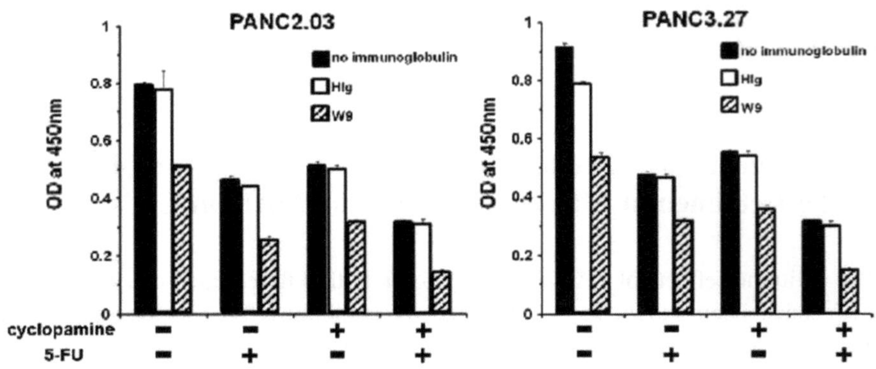

Fig. 14 Inhibition of cell growth in PDAC cells by the mAb W9, cyclopamine and 5-FU Cells (4×10^5/ml) were starved for 3 h, then incubated with the mAb W9 (20 μg/ml), cyclopamine (20 μM), and 5-FU (10 μM) in RPMI 1,640 medium containing 1.5 % FCS. Cells were then tested by the MTT assay. HIgG1 was used as a negative control. Results were shown as OD value and error bars were presented as standard deviation. The mAb W9, cyclopamine, and 5-FU combination was significantly ($p < 0.01$) more effective than the HIgG1, cyclopamine, and 5-FU combination, dual-agent combinations, and individual agents

effective therapeutic strategies which completely eradicate differentiated cancer cells and CICs. In addressing this need, we have been guided by the realization that signaling pathways involved in proliferation and survival are aberrantly activated in CICs. Inhibition of these signaling pathways has been shown to suppress CICs growth *in vitro* and in immunodeficient mice. However, also in this case, the eradication of CICs is not complete. Therefore, we have tested whether the detrimental effect on CICs by TA-specific mAbs could be enhanced by combination with chemotherapy or radiotherapy and by inhibitors of the CIC signaling pathways. Several pathways have been shown to be activated in CICs. They include the Sonic Hedgehog Homologue (SHH), MAPK, Notch, PI3 K/AKT, TGF-β and Wnt pathways [34, 35]. Since in the types of tumors that we investigated the SHH pathway has been found to be aberrantly activated in CICs, we have tested whether combining TA-specific mAbs and/or chemoradio-therapy with cyclopamine, an inhibitor of the SHH pathway, could eradicate CICs. Our *in vitro* results demonstrate that this is indeed the case at least in the tumor we have investigated. A representative example is shown in Figs. 12 and 13. Treatment of the PANC2.03, PANC3.27 and Mia-PaCa2 PDAC cell lines with the Grp94-specific mAb in combination with 5FU or radiotherapy and cyclopamine eliminate more than 90 % of the CICs in a tumor cell population. This effect is mediated by the inhibition of activation of multiple components of signaling pathways involved in proliferation, survival, antiapoptotic signals and CICs proliferation (Fig. 15).

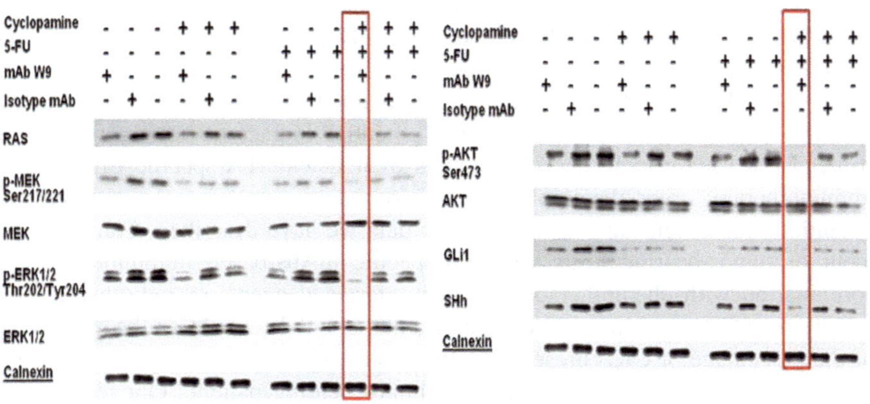

Fig. 15 Inhibition of signaling pathways in MIA PaCa-2 PDAC cells by the mAb W9, cyclopamine and 5-FU. The MIA PaCa-2 cells were incubated with the Grp94-specific mAb W9 (20 μg/ml), cyclopamine (20 μM) and 5-FU (10 μM) for 48 h at 37 °C. Cell lysates were then prepared and tested by western blot with the corresponding antibodies (Cell Signaling Technology). Calnexin was used as the loading control. Cells incubated with the mAb W9 alone, with the mAb W9 and cyclopamine, with cyclopamine alone, with the mAb W9 and 5-FU and with 5-FU alone were used as controls

Conclusions

Convincing experimental and clinical evidence indicate that TA-specific mAbs represent valuable reagents for the treatment of various types of cancer. However, a major limitation of this type of immunotherapy is its limited efficacy in time because of the occurrence of metastatic spread and/or disease recurrence, the two major causes of patients morbidity and mortality. According to the cancer stem cell theory, both complications may be mediated by CICs, a cellular subpopulation that displays stem cell properties and drives and maintains the growth of many types of cancer. In the experiments described in this chapter, we have tested this possibility by assessing the sensitivity of CICs to the detrimental effects of TA-specific mAbs. The *in vitro* data we have obtained utilizing three TA systems in several types of solid tumors indicate that CICs have a limited sensitivity to the detrimental effects of TA-specific mAbs even when they are combined with chemotherapeutic agents, targeted agents or radiotherapy. These combinations can eliminate only part of the CICs present in a tumor cell population. Whether the differential sensitivity of CICs to TA-specific mAbs in combination with chemotherapy, targeted therapy or radiotherapy reflects differences in their differentiation stage and/or epigenetic changes remains to be determined. Whatever the mechanism, if these *in vitro* findings reflect what happens in tumor-bearing hosts treated with TA based immunotherapy, then our data provide a mechanism for the disease recurrence which frequently occurs in patients treated with TA-specific mAb-based immunotherapy. Our *in vitro* data also suggest that the ability of TA-specific mAbs in combination with chemotherapeutic agents, targeted agents or radiotherapy to eradicate CICs can be markedly enhanced by inhibitors of signal transduction pathways that are aberrantly activated in CICs. These results have to be interpreted with caution since they were obtained with established cell lines and *in vitro* experiments. Nevertheless, the potential impact of this combinatorial strategy on disease recurrence in patients treated with TA-specific mAbs-based immunotherapy urges the implementation of *in vivo* experiments to assess the potential clinical relevance of the *in vitro* data we have described. Can the treatment of tumor-bearing hosts with TA-specific mAbs-based immunotherapy in combination with chemotherapeutic agents, targeted agents or radiotherapy and inhibitors of CIC signaling pathways cure a malignant disease? Can the monitoring of the percentage of CICs present in a tumor-bearing host be used to optimize the combinatorial therapy administered to a tumor bearing patient? Our results may also provide a mechanism for the failure observed in clinical trials which have tested the clinical efficacy of CIC signaling pathway inhibitors. An example is represented by the lack of clinical efficacy which has been reported for cyclopamine in patients with PDAC. Our *in vitro* results suggest that this failure can reflect the limited efficacy of cyclopamine [36] in eliminating differentiated cancer cells and CICs when it is used as a single agent. However, our data argue that this compound enhances the ability of TA-specific mAbs in combination with chemotherapeutic agents, targeted agents or radiotherapy in eliminating CICs.

This finding is not unique of cyclopamine since a recent clinical trial has demonstrated that agents which inhibit CIC signaling pathways such as cabozantinib, a c-Met inhibitor, and Trastuzumab, a HER2-specific mAb, have clinical efficacy in advanced castration-resistant prostatic cancer when they are used in combination, although the two agents failed when used as single agents [37–39].

In summary, our *in vitro* data strongly suggest that lack of complete elimination of CICs by TA-specific mAbs in combination with chemotherapeutic agents, targeted agents or radiotherapy plays a major role in disease recurrence which represents a significant obstacle to the successful clinical efficacy of TA-specific mAbs. The *in vivo* relevance of these *in vitro* data has to be tested in animal model systems since the resulting information may represent a useful background for a rational design of an effective clinical strategy.

Acknowledgments This work was supported by PHS grants RO1CA138188 and RO1CA110249 awarded by the National Cancer Institute and Susan Komen Post Doctoral Fellowship KG111486 awarded by the Susan G. Komen for the Cure Foundation.

Conflicts of Interest

No potential conflicts of interest were disclosed.

References

1. Ferris RL, Jaffee EM, Ferrone S. Tumor antigen-targeted, monoclonal antibody-based immunotherapy: clinical response, cellular immunity, and immuno escape. J Clin Oncol: Official J Am Soc Clin Oncol. 2010;28:4390–9.
2. Ginestier C, Hur MH, Charafe-Jauffret E, Monville F, Dutcher J, Brown M, Jacquemier J, Viens P, Kleer CG, Liu S, Schott A, Hayes D, Birnbaum D, Wicha MS, Dontu G. ALDH1 is a marker of normal and malignant human mammary stem cells and a predictor of poor clinical outcome. Cell Stem Cell. 2007;1:555–67.
3. Wicha MS, Liu S, Dontu G. Cancer stem cells: an old idea–a paradigm shift. Cancer research. 2006;66:1883–90, discussion 95–6.
4. Wicha MS. Cancer stem cell heterogeneity in hereditary breast cancer. Breast Cancer Res: BCR. 2008;10:105.
5. Matsuda Y, Kure S, Ishiwata T. Nestin and other putative cancer stem cell markers in pancreatic cancer. Med Mol Morphol. 2012;45:59–65.
6. Li J, Zhong XY, Li ZY, Cai JF, Zou L, Li JM, et al. CD133 expression in osteosarcoma and derivation of CD133(+) cells. Mol Med Rep. 2013;7:577–84.
7. Visus C, Ito D, Amoscato A, Maciejewska-Franczak M, Abdelsalem A, Dhir R, Shin DM, Donnenberg VS, Whiteside TL, DeLeo AB. Identification of human aldehyde dehydrogenase 1 family member A1 as a novel CD8+ T-cell-defined tumor antigen in squamous cell carcinoma of the head and neck. Cancer Res. 2007;67:10538–45.
8. Huang CP, Tsai MF, Chang TH, Tang WC, Chen SY, Lai HH, Lin TY, Yang JC, Yang PC, Shih JY, Lin SB. ALDH-positive lung cancer stem cells confer resistance to epidermal growth factor receptor tyrosine kinase inhibitors. Cancer Lett. 2013;328:144–51.
9. Kim MP, Fleming JB, Wang H, Abbruzzese JL, Choi W, Kopetz S, McConkey DJ, Evans DB, Gallick GE. ALDH activity selectively defines an enhanced tumor-initiating cell population relative to CD133 expression in human pancreatic adenocarcinoma. PLoS One. 2011;6:e20636.

10. Deng S, Yang X, Lassus H, Liang S, Kaur S, Ye Q, Li C, Wang LP, Roby KF, Orsulic S, Connolly DC, Zhang Y, Montone K, Bützow R, Coukos G, Zhang L. Distinct expression levels and patterns of stem cell marker, aldehyde dehydrogenase isoform 1 (ALDH1), in human epithelial cancers. PLoS ONE. 2010;5:e10277.
11. Sanders MA, Majumdar AP. Colon cancer stem cells: implications in carcinogenesis. Front Biosci: J Virtual Library. 2011;16:1651–62.
12. Li T, Su Y, Mei Y, Leng Q, Leng B, Liu Z, Stass SA, Jiang F. ALDH1A1 is a marker for malignant prostate stem cells and predictor of prostate cancer patients' outcome. Lab Invest; J Tech Methods pathol. 2010;90:234–44.
13. Honoki K, Fujii H, Kubo A, Kido A, Mori T, Tanaka Y, Tsujiuchi T. Possible involvement of stem-like populations with elevated ALDH1 in sarcomas for chemotherapeutic drug resistance. Oncol Rep. 2010;24:501–5.
14. Vasiliou V, Pappa A, Estey T. Role of human aldehyde dehydrogenases in endobiotic and xenobiotic metabolism. Drug Metab Rev. 2004;36:279–99.
15. Muzio G, Maggiora M, Paiuzzi E, Oraldi M, Canuto RA. Aldehyde dehydrogenases and cell proliferation. Free Radical Biol Med. 2012;52:735–46.
16. Jackson B, Brocker C, Thompson DC, Black W, Vasiliou K, Nebert DW, Vasiliou V. Update on the aldehyde dehydrogenase gene (ALDH) superfamily. Human Genom. 2011;5:283–303.
17. Marcato P, Dean CA, Giacomantonio CA, Lee PW. Aldehyde dehydrogenase: its role as a cancer stem cell marker comes down to the specific isoform. Cell Cycle. 2011;10:1378–84.
18. Storms RW, Trujillo AP, Springer JB, Shah L, Colvin OM, Ludeman SM, Smith C. Isolation of primitive human hematopoietic progenitors on the basis of aldehyde dehydrogenase activity. Proc Natl Acad Sci USA. 1999;96:9118–23.
19. Clarke MF, Dick JE, Dirks PB, Eaves CJ, Jamieson CH, Jones DL, Visvader J, Weissman IL, Wahl GM. Cancer stem cells–perspectives on current status and future directions: AACR Workshop on cancer stem cells. Cancer Res. 2006;66:9339–44.
20. Lauth M. RAS and Hedgehog–partners in crime. Front Biosci. 2011;17:2259–70.
21. Visvader JE. Cells of origin in cancer. Nature. 2011;469:314–22.
22. Tavaluc RT, Hart LS, Dicker DT, El-Deiry WS. Effects of low confluency, serum starvation and hypoxia on the side population of cancer cell lines. Cell Cycle. 2007;6:2554–62.
23. Campoli MR, Chang CC, Kageshita T, Wang X, McCarthy JB, Ferrone S. Human high molecular weight-melanoma-associated antigen (HMW-MAA): a melanoma cell surface chondroitin sulfate proteoglycan (MSCP) with biological and clinical significance. Crit Rev Immunol. 2004;24:267–96.
24. Campoli M, Ferrone S, Wang X. Functional and clinical relevance of chondroitin sulfate proteoglycan 4. Adv Cancer Res. 2010;109:73–121.
25. Wang X, Osada T, Wang Y, Yu L, Sakakura K, Katayama A, McCarthy JB, Brufsky A, Chivukula M, Khoury T, Hsu DS, Barry WT, Lyerly HK, Clay TM, Ferrone S. CSPG4 protein as a new target for the antibody-based immunotherapy of triple-negative breast cancer. J Natl Cancer Inst. 2010;102:1496–512.
26. McLaughlin M, Vandenbroeck K. The endoplasmic reticulum protein folding factory and its chaperones: new targets for drug discovery? Br J Pharmacol. 2011;162:328–45.
27. Marzec M, Eletto D, Argon Y. GRP94: An HSP90-like protein specialized for protein folding and quality control in the endoplasmic reticulum. Biochim Biophys Acta. 2011;1823:774–87.
28. Argon Y, Simen BB. GRP94, an ER chaperone with protein and peptide binding properties. Semin Cell Dev Biol. 1999;10:495–505.
29. Yang Y, Li Z. Roles of heat shock protein gp96 in the ER quality control: redundant or unique function? Mol Cells. 2005;20:173–82.
30. de Bono JS, Kristeleit R, Tolcher A, Fong P, Pacey S, Karavasilis V, Mita M, Shaw H, Workman P, Kaye S, Rowinsky EK, Aherne W, Atadja P, Scott JW, Patnaik A. Phase I pharmacokinetic and pharmacodynamic study of LAQ824, a hydroxamate histone deacetylase inhibitor with a heat shock protein-90 inhibitory profile, in patients with advanced solid tumors. Clin Cancer Res: Official J Am Assoc Cancer Res. 2008;14:6663–73.

31. Tse AN, Klimstra DS, Gonen M, Shah M, Sheikh T, Sikorski R, Carvajal R, Mui J, Tipian C, O'Reilly E, Chung K, Maki R, Lefkowitz R, Brown K, Manova-Todorova K, Wu N, Egorin MJ, Kelsen D, Schwartz GK. A phase 1 dose-escalation study of irinotecan in combination with 17-allylamino-17-demethoxygeldanamycin in patients with solid tumors. Clin Cancer Res: Official J Am Assoc Cancer Res. 2008;14:6704–11.
32. Solit DB, Osman I, Polsky D, Panageas KS, Daud A, Goydos JS, Teitcher J, Wolchok JD, Germino FJ, Krown SE, Coit D, Rosen N, Chapman PB. Phase II trial of 17-allylamino-17-demethoxygeldanamycin in patients with metastatic melanoma. Clin Cancer Res: Official J Am Assoc Cancer Res. 2008;14:8302–7.
33. Chapoval AI, Ni J, Lau JS, Wilcox RA, Flies DB, Liu D, Dong H, Sica GL, Zhu G, Tamada K, Chen L. B7–H3: a costimulatory molecule for T cell activation and IFN-gamma production. Nat Immunol. 2001;2:269–74.
34. Merchant AA, Matsui W. Targeting Hedgehog–a cancer stem cell pathway. Clin Cancer Res: Official J Am Assoc Cancer Res. 2010;16:3130–40.
35. Dreesen O, Brivanlou AH. Signaling pathways in cancer and embryonic stem cells. Stem Cell Rev. 2007;3:7–17.
36. Keeler RF, Baker DC. Oral, osmotic minipump, and intramuscular administration to sheep of the Veratrum alkaloid cyclopamine. Proceedings of the society for experimental biology and medicine society for experimental biology and medicine. 1989;192:153–156.
37. Ziada A, et al. The use of trastuzumab in the treatment of hormone refractory prostate cancer; phase II trial. Prostate. 2004;60:332–7.
38. Ryan CJ, et al. Targeted MET inhibition in castration-resistant prostate cancer: a randomized phase II study and biomarker analysis with rilotumumab plus mitoxantrone and prednisone. Clin Cancer Res: Official J Am Assoc Cancer Res. 2013;19:215–24.
39. Smith DC, Smith MR, Sweeney C, Elfiky AA, Logothetis C, Corn PG, Vogelzang NJ, Small EJ, Harzstark AL, Gordon MS, Vaishampayan UN, Haas NB, Spira AI, Lara PN Jr, Lin CC, Srinivas S, Sella A, Schöffski P, Scheffold C, Weitzman AL, Hussain M. Cabozantinib in patients with advanced prostate cancer: results of a phase II randomized discontinuation trial. J Clin Oncol: Official J Am Soc Clin Oncolo. 2013;31:412–9.
40. Bardelli A, Siena S. Molecular mechanisms of resistance to cetuximab and panitumumab in colorectal cancer. J Clin Oncol: Official J Am Soc Clin Oncol. 2010;28:1254–61.
41. Berns K, Horlings HM, Hennessy BT, Madiredjo M, Hijmans EM, Beelen K, Linn SC, Gonzalez-Angulo AM, Stemke-Hale K, Hauptmann M, Beijersbergen RL, Mills GB, van de Vijver MJ, Bernards R. A functional genetic approach identifies the PI3 K pathway as a major determinant of trastuzumab resistance in breast cancer. Cancer Cell. 2007;12:395–402.
42. Nagata Y, Lan KH, Zhou X, Tan M, Esteva FJ, Sahin AA, Klos KS, Li P, Monia BP, Nguyen NT, Hortobagyi GN, Hung MC, Yu D. PTEN activation contributes to tumor inhibition by trastuzumab, and loss of PTEN predicts trastuzumab resistance in patients. Cancer Cell. 2004;6:117–27.
43. Lu Y, Zi X, Zhao Y, Mascarenhas D, Pollak M. Insulin-like growth factor-I receptor signaling and resistance to trastuzumab (Herceptin). J Natl Cancer Inst. 2001;93:1852–7.
44. Desbois-Mouthon C, Baron A. Blivet-Van Eggelpoel MJ, Fartoux L, Venot C, Bladt F, Housset C, Rosmorduc O. Insulin-like growth factor-1 receptor inhibition induces a resistance mechanism via the epidermal growth factor receptor/HER3/AKT signaling pathway: rational basis for cotargeting insulin-like growth factor-1 receptor and epidermal growth factor receptor in hepatocellular carcinoma. Clin Cancer Res: Official J Am Assoc Cancer Res. 2009;15:5445–56.
45. Koutras AK, Fountzilas G, Kalogeras KT, Starakis I, Iconomou G, Kalofonos HP. The upgraded role of HER3 and HER4 receptors in breast cancer. Critical Rev Oncol/hematology. 2010;74:73–8.
46. Lin A, Yan WH, Xu HH, Gan MF, Cai JF, Zhu M, Zhou MY. HLA-G expression in human ovarian carcinoma counteracts NK cell function. Ann Oncol. 2007;18:1804–9.

47. Levy EM, Sycz G, Arriaga JM, Barrio MM, von Euw EM, Morales SB, González M, Mordoh J, Bianchini M. Cetuximab-mediated cellular cytotoxicity is inhibited by HLA-E membrane expression in colon cancer cells. Innate Immun. 2009;15:91–100.
48. Fishelson Z, Donin N, Zell S, Schultz S, Kirschfink M. Obstacles to cancer immunotherapy: expression of membrane complement regulatory proteins (mCRPs) in tumors. Mol Immunol. 2003;40:109–23.
49. Jurianz K, Maslak S, Garcia-Schuler H, Fishelson Z, Kirschfink M. Neutralization of complement regulatory proteins augments lysis of breast carcinoma cells targeted with rhumAb anti-HER2. Immunopharmacology. 1999;42:209–18.
50. You T, Hu W, Ge X, Shen J, Qin X. Application of a novel inhibitor of human CD59 for the enhancement of complement-dependent cytolysis on cancer cells. Cell Mol Immunol. 2011;8:157–63.
51. Dzietczenia J, Wrobel T, Mazur G, Poreba R, Jazwiec B, Kuliczkowski K. Expression of complement regulatory proteins: CD46, CD55, and CD59 and response to rituximab in patients with CD20+ non-Hodgkin's lymphoma. Med Oncol. 2010;27:743–6.
52. Chang CC, Campoli M, Ferrone S. Classical and nonclassical HLA class I antigen and NK Cell-activating ligand changes in malignant cells: current challenges and future directions. Adv Cancer Res. 2005;93:189–234.
53. Taylor C, Hershman D, Shah N, Suciu-Foca N, Petrylak DP, Taub R, Vahdat L, Cheng B, Pegram M, Knutson KL, Clynes R. Augmented HER-2 specific immunity during treatment with trastuzumab and chemotherapy. Clin Cancer Res: Official J Am Assoc Cancer Res. 2007;13:5133–43.
54. Algarra I, Garcia-Lora A, Cabrera T, Ruiz-Cabello F, Garrido F. The selection of tumor variants with altered expression of classical and nonclassical MHC class I molecules: implications for tumor immune escape. Cancer Immunol, Immunotherapy: CII. 2004;53:904–10.
55. Zou W. Regulatory T cells, tumour immunity and immunotherapy. Nat Rev Immunol. 2006;6:295–307.
56. Nagaraj S, Gupta K, Pisarev V, Kinarsky L, Sherman S, Kang L, Herber DL, Schneck J, Gabrilovich DI. Altered recognition of antigen is a mechanism of CD8 + T cell tolerance in cancer. Nat Med. 2007;13:828–35.
57. Xue SA, Stauss HJ. Enhancing immune responses for cancer therapy. Cell Mol Immunol. 2007;4:173–84.
58. Musolino A, Naldi N, Bortesi B, Pezzuolo D, Capelletti M, Missale G, Laccabue D, Zerbini A, Camisa R, Bisagni G, Neri TM, Ardizzoni A. Immunoglobulin G fragment C receptor polymorphisms and clinical efficacy of trastuzumab-based therapy in patients with HER-2/neu-positive metastatic breast cancer. J Clin Oncol: Official J Am Soc Clin Oncol. 2008;26:1789–96.
59. Zhang W, Gordon M, Schultheis AM, Yang DY, Nagashima F, Azuma M, Chang HM, Borucka E, Lurje G, Sherrod AE, Iqbal S, Groshen S, Lenz HJ. FCGR2A and FCGR3A polymorphisms associated with clinical outcome of epidermal growth factor receptor expressing metastatic colorectal cancer patients treated with single-agent cetuximab. J Clin Oncol: Official J Am Soc Clin Oncol. 2007;25:3712–8.
60. Binder M, Otto F, Mertelsmann R, Veelken H, Trepel M. The epitope recognized by rituximab. Blood. 2006;108:1975–8.
61. Pejawar-Gaddy S, Finn OJ. Cancer vaccines: accomplishments and challenges. Crit Rev Oncology/hematology. 2008;67:93–102.
62. Lopez-Albaitero A, Lee SC, Morgan S, Grandis JR, Gooding WE, Ferrone S, Ferris RL. Role of polymorphic Fc gamma receptor IIIa and EGFR expression level in cetuximab mediated, NK cell dependent in vitro cytotoxicity of head and neck squamous cell carcinoma cells. Cancer Immunol, immunotherapy: CII. 2009;58:1853–64.
63. Kurai J, Chikumi H, Hashimoto K, Yamaguchi K, Yamasaki A, Sako T, Touge H, Makino H, Takata M, Miyata M, Nakamoto M, Burioka N, Shimizu E. Antibody-dependent cellular

cytotoxicity mediated by cetuximab against lung cancer cell lines. Clin Cancer Res: Official J Ame Assoc Cancer Res. 2007;13:1552–61.
64. Burtness B, Goldwasser MA, Flood W, Mattar B, Forastiere AA. Eastern cooperative oncology G. Phase III randomized trial of cisplatin plus placebo compared with cisplatin plus cetuximab in metastatic/recurrent head and neck cancer: an eastern cooperative oncology group study. J Clin Oncol: Official J Am Soc Clin Oncol. 2005;23:8646–54.
65. Zhao WL, Wang L, Liu YH, Yan JS, Leboeuf C, Liu YY, Wu WL, Janin A, Chen Z, Chen SJ. Combined effects of histone deacetylase inhibitor and rituximab on non-Hodgkin's B-lymphoma cells apoptosis. Exp Hematol. 2007;35:1801–11.
66. Mukohara T. Mechanisms of resistance to anti-human epidermal growth factor receptor 2 agents in breast cancer. Cancer Sci. 2011;102:1–8.
67. Neller MA, Lopez JA, Schmidt CW. Antigens for cancer immunotherapy. Semin Immunol. 2008;20:286–95.

Overcoming Resistance to Therapeutic Antibodies by Targeting Fc Receptors

Emily L. Williams, Sean H. Lim, Stephen A. Beers, Peter W. Johnson, Jonathan C. Strefford, Martin J. Glennie and Mark S. Cragg

Abstract Monoclonal antibodies (mAb) are now at the forefront of cancer therapy. Their mechanisms of action remain the focus of intense investigation as it offers the prospect of increased potency through antibody engineering or adjuvant therapy. Although roles for complement and the induction of direct cell death remain controversial, the importance of Fc gamma receptors (FcγR) to the efficacy of therapeutic antibodies is irrefutable. However, the biology of these receptors is complex and it is now clear that in certain instances inappropriate expression or upregulation of FcγR can be detrimental. This complexity is compounded by recent exciting data showing that FcγR on both the effector and the target cell help govern therapeutic potency. In this review the ability of FcγR to elicit and modulate antibody therapy will be discussed alongside potential strategies to overcome the associated resistance.

Keywords Antibodies · Fc receptors · FcγRIIb · Modulation · Immunotherapy · CD20 · Tumour resistance

Abbreviations

ADCC	Antibody-dependent cellular cytotoxicity
ADCP	Antibody-dependent cellular phagocytosis
CDC	Complement-dependent cytotoxicity
CLL	Chronic lymphocytic leukaemia

E. L. Williams · S. H. Lim · S. A. Beers · M. J. Glennie · M. S. Cragg (✉)
Antibody and Vaccine Group, Cancer Sciences Unit, University of Southampton, MP88, Tremona Road, Southampton SO16 6YD, UK
e-mail: msc@soton.ac.uk

P. W. Johnson
CR UK Centre, Cancer Sciences Unit, University of Southampton, Southampton, UK

J. C. Strefford
Cancer Genomics Group, Cancer Sciences Unit, University of Southampton, Southampton, UK

B. Bonavida (ed.), *Resistance to Immunotherapeutic Antibodies in Cancer*, Resistance to Targeted Anti-Cancer Therapeutics 2, DOI: 10.1007/978-1-4614-7654-2_3,

CNV	Copy number variation
DLBCL	Diffuse large B cell lymphoma
FcγR	Fc gamma receptor
IC	Immune complexes
ITAM	Immunoreceptor tyrosine-based activation motif
ITIM	Immunoreceptor tyrosine-based inhibitory motif
mAb	Monoclonal antibodies
MCL	Mantle cell lymphoma
NHL	Non Hodgkins Lymphoma
TAM	Tumour-associated macrophages
TGF-β	Transforming growth factor-β
TLR	Toll-like receptor

Introduction

Over the last decade, monoclonal antibodies (mAbs) have become a highly effective class of therapeutics [1, 2]. More than 30 are now approved for use in humans, targeting a range of different diseases, including cancer. It is, therefore, clear that mAb immunotherapy is a viable approach for human treatment [1–3]. The drive now is to better understand their key mechanisms of action and identify the reasons why certain patients do not respond or become resistant to therapy.

Much of the success of anti-cancer mAbs derives from their high level of specificity, long biological half-life and ability to recruit numerous effector mechanisms [3]. Initially, it was supposed that all anti-tumour mAb would function in a similar way by engaging two of the main host immune effector systems. The complement system can result in cellular lysis through the insertion of the membrane attack complex (complement-dependent cytotoxicity; CDC) and innate effector cells such as Natural Killer (NK) cells and macrophages can kill the target by releasing cytotoxic granules, triggering Fas-dependent cell death or by physical engulfment and digestion (antibody-dependent cellular cytotoxicity; ADCC or antibody-dependent cellular phagocytosis; ADCP). However, not all mAb are capable of triggering effective target cell deletion through engaging these systems and eliciting therapeutic responses in man [3–5].

In fact, a very limited range of mAb specificities have been translated into clinical practice. Of these, mAb to CD20, in particular rituximab, have been the most successful, perhaps representing the most important advances in the treatment of lymphoproliferative disorders in the last 30 years [6–8]. The success of the anti-CD20 mAb rituximab in Non Hodgkins Lymphoma (NHL) has heralded in a plethora of second and third generation mAb [9]. Initially, development and technical refinement focused on reducing the immunogenicity of the mAb, moving from part-murine chimeric mAb such as rituximab to fully human or humanized reagents such as ofatumumab. Subsequent to these advances, the next generation of developments has focused on maximizing the various potential effector mechanisms available to mAbs.

Pre-clinical and clinical work have investigated the main effector pathways, including complement-dependent cytotoxicity (CDC) and direct programmed cell death (PCD), but the importance of both these pathways in patients remains controversial [10]. Recent evidence indicates that engaging complement may even be detrimental [11] by augmenting 'shaving' [12–14] and blocking the Fc gamma receptor (FcγR) IIIA on NK cells, hence impairing ADCC [15]. Similarly, in our most recent studies, we showed that mouse B cells expressing the *Bcl-2* transgene were just as susceptible to deletion by rituximab in vivo as B cells lacking the transgene [16]. Clearly, in this fully syngeneic model, induction of the intrinsic apoptosis pathway is not important for B cell depletion. However, although the evidence regarding the involvement of CDC and PCD remains inconclusive and contentious, it is clear that Fc:FcR interactions are critical for the success of mAb immunotherapy [16–20]. Almost all of the mAb approved or being developed for anti-cancer therapy are of the IgG class, which function through their interaction with the various members of the FcγR family (Fig. 1).

The FcγR Family

The FcγR family of receptors is composed of multiple members in both man and mouse. They are expressed on a wide range of effector cells such as macrophages, neutrophils and NK cells, and can be broadly divided into two types: activatory receptors (human: FcγRI, FcγRIIA, FcγRIIC and FcγRIIIA; mouse: FcγRI, FcγRIIIA and FcγRIV) which signal via an immunoreceptor tyrosine-based activation motif (ITAM), and an inhibitory receptor [human: FcγRIIB and mouse: FcγRII (both hereafter referred to as FcγRIIB for simplicity)] which signals via an immunoreceptor tyrosine-based inhibitory motif (ITIM). Although homology exists between the mouse and human receptors, alternative forms of human FcγR (hFcγR) exist that are not observed in the mouse such as the GPI-linked FcγRIIIB expressed on neutrophils. As this receptor lacks an intracellular domain, its designation as an activatory or inhibitory receptor is unclear. FcγRs can also be discriminated based upon their affinity for IgG, with only FcγRI capable of binding soluble monomeric IgG and the others referred to as low/moderate affinity receptors, with preferential binding to IgG in the context of immune complexes (IC) [21]. As such, it is anticipated that FcγRI is typically occupied by circulating IgG, whereas the low-moderate affinity human receptors are only triggered in the presence of ICs or mAb-opsonised targets. For further details see excellent reviews elsewhere [22, 23]. To add a further level of complexity, differing isoforms of a certain FcγR also exist. A clear example of this, is the inhibitory FcγRIIB which

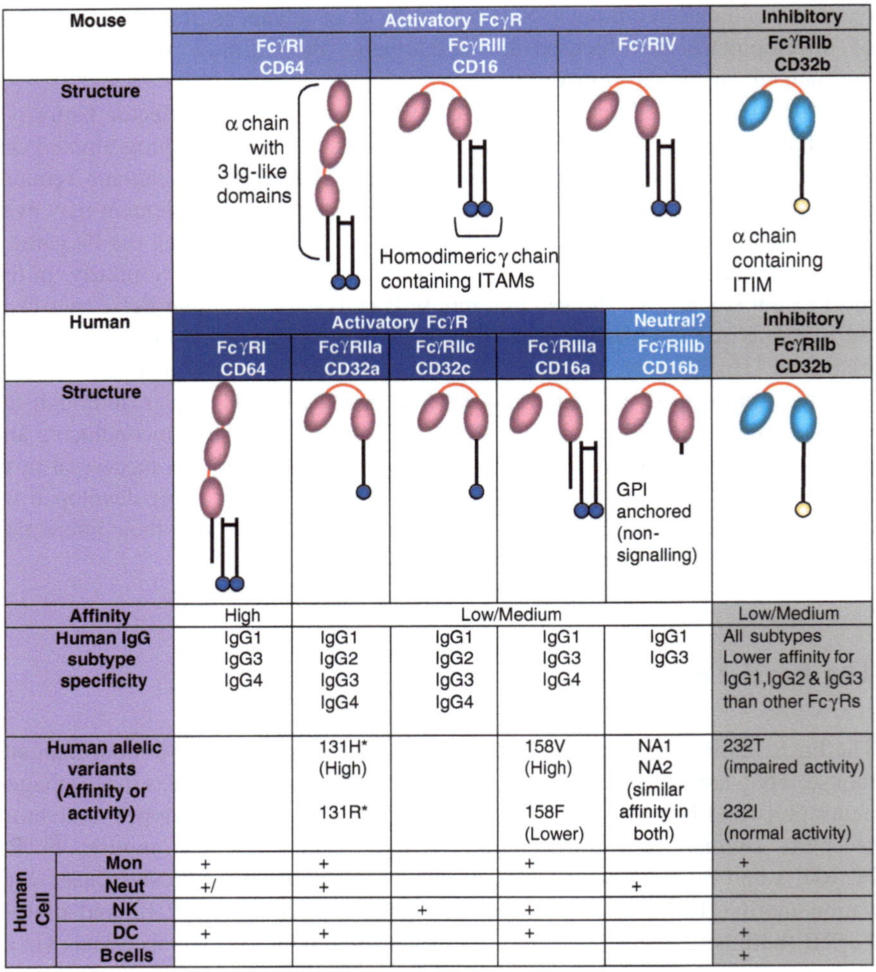

Fig. 1 The FcγR family. The figure describes the structure of human and mouse FcγR, their affinity to IgG, preferential subtype specificity, common and significant allelic variants and expression on haematopoietic cells. *Mon* monocytes; *Neut* neutrophils. Based upon data from [22, 23]

displays b1 and b2 isoforms through differential mRNA splicing [24, 25]. The two isoforms show very specific patterns of expression with FcγRIIB-b1 predominantly expressed by B cells and FcγRIIB-b2 mainly expressed by monocytes and macrophages [26–28]. It is thought that these two isoforms have different functional properties with only FcγRIIB-b2 able to undergo rapid receptor endocytosis upon ligation [29] resulting in differential consequences of receptor engagement.

Result of FcγR Engagement

Once appropriate FcγR engagement has occurred it can lead to inflammatory mediator release and/or killing/phagocytosis of opsonised target cells as discussed above [3]. However, the outcome of mAb: FcγR binding varies dependent on a number of factors, including cell type, mAb isotype, and the balance of activatory and inhibitory FcγR signalling induced as discussed in further detail below [21, 30–33]. The observation that distinct FcγR have widely varying affinities for different IgG subclasses (reviewed in [23]) helps explain the contrasting efficacy of mAb isotypes in vivo. As such, in the mouse, mIgG2a binds strongly to the activatory FcγRs and comparatively weakly to FcγRIIB, whereas mIgG1 does not engage the activatory FcγRI or IV but binds with equal affinity to the inhibitory FcγRII and activatory FcγRIII. This differential binding led to the concept of the activatory:inhibitory (A:I) ratio or index and the notion that therapy with direct targeting mAb could be augmented with its elevation. Similarly, in humans IgG1 binds relatively strongly to hFcγRI, IIA and IIIA but to a lesser extent to the inhibitory hFcγRIIB, thereby, possessing a high A:I ratio.

Role of Fc:FcγR in Immunoatherapy

In mouse models the therapeutic activity of a range of direct-targeting anti-cancer mAbs has been clearly shown to correlate with their isotypes and ability to bind preferentially to activatory FcγR [19, 34–37]. Furthermore, removing all activating FcγR by genetic deletion of the common signalling gamma chain eliminates almost all the therapeutic activity of most anti-cancer mAbs, including rituximab [17], findings which have been recapitulated by several groups and in fully syngeneic model systems [16, 36, 38, 39]. Conversely, deleting the inhibitory FcγRIIB generally promotes mAb therapeutic activity [17, 40], presumably by reducing inhibitory signalling in the effector cells and augmenting the A:I ratio in these cells.

Indirectly, these data also indicate that NK cells, which do not express FcγRIIB, are not involved in this improvement to mAb efficacy [41] This is an important point as in humans, in vitro experiments with blood borne effector cells point to the NK cell as a prominent effector in ADCC [42, 43], but whether this also applies in tissues is unclear, particularly given the relative abundance of myeloid cells in lymphoid tissues. Similarly, whether FcγRIIIb-expressing neutrophils, the predominant leucocyte in peripheral blood, play a role in providing therapy in vivo remains to be clarified [44]. In the mouse there is good agreement that monocytes/macrophages are the key FcγR-expressing effector cells responsible for the efficacy of anti-CD20 mAb [16, 36, 38, 39]. Depleting these cells using liposome-encapsulated clodronate [45] results in decreased mAb efficacy [36, 38, 39] and their repopulation correlates with subsequent target-cell deletion [16], but the removal of neutrophils or natural killer cells has no impact.

Although the key effector cell population has not yet been determined for humans, it is clear that FcγR-expressing effectors are critical in regulating mAb therapy. Evidence for this relies upon the observation that certain FcγR gene single nucleotide polymorphisms (SNPs) affect the receptor's affinity for mAb and are associated with response to mAb immunotherapy [30, 31, 46]. For example, a SNP encoding for valine rather than phenylalanine at position 158 in FcγRIIIA results in higher affinity for IgG1, and patients with the former allele are more likely to have durable responses following treatment with rituximab monotherapy. Similar observations have been made concerning high (histidine-131) or low (arginine-131) affinity variants of FcγRIIA [31]. It is not clear why this latter polymorphism should influence a rituximab-mediated response since it is an IgG1 mAb and should not be influenced by this allelic difference which principally effects binding to IgG2 [47]. However, allelic polymorphisms need not just affect affinity but may also be linked to other phenotypic differences; for example the valine-158 variant of FcγRIIIA is also associated with higher receptor expression [48]. Furthermore, there is evidence that certain SNPs such as the 158 V of FcγRIIIA and the 131H variant of FcγRIIA are linked in terms of their inheritance with the functional allele of FcγRIIC [49, 50]. Therefore, in some instances the prognostic significance of a certain SNP may relate to their association with other alleles. Functional SNP also exist in the inhibitory FcγRIIB. For example, the $I > T$ SNP at position 232 results in a reduced ability of this receptor to partition into lipid rafts which decreases its ability to inhibit activatory FcγR or B cell receptor signalling [51]. Although the 232TT genotype has been shown to predispose to autoimmune diseases such as Systemic Lupus Erythematosus [52], its effect on antibody immunotherapy has yet to be proven [53], potentially due to its relative rarity.

A further level of complexity relating to FcγR biology and expression that has recently been highlighted is that relating to copy number variation (CNV). Initially, qPCR approaches identified variation at the FcγRIIIB locus in populations from different ethnic backgrounds and linked changes in CNV with autoimmune disease [54–56]. Subsequently, multiplex ligation-dependent probe amplification (MLPA) and paralogue ratio tests (PRT) confirmed CNV at the FcγRIIIB locus and also showed variation of the *FcγRIIIA* and *FcγRIIC* genes [57]. Importantly, CNV has been shown to affect the expression and function of these receptors [54, 57]. As predicted, fewer copies of the gene for a relevant receptor result in a decrease in functional response (for example NK cells from a donor carrying a single copy of FcγRIIIA elicit less ADCC compared to NK cells taken from donors with 2 or 3 copies [57]). However, the relationship between CNV and mAb immunotherapy has not yet been assessed.

Regulation of FcγR Expression

As detailed above, the expression of FcγR on the cell surface and ensuing cellular response is tightly controlled by a multitude of factors, including the nature of the cell, prior activation status, cytokine milieu and microenvironment. It has long been known that inflammatory mediators, such as LPS or IFN-γ upregulate the expression of activatory FcγR on both human [58] and mouse [32, 59] monocytes and also on human mast cells [60] in vitro. In addition, studies have shown that IFN-α and -β in mice, but not in humans, increase FcγR expression [58, 61]. Conversely, IFN-γ reduces FcγRIIB expression, as does Complement 5a (C5a), which was also shown to increase activatory FcγRIII expression in mouse cells in vitro [62]. This suggests that within a pro-inflammatory environment FcγR-expressing cells are likely to be directed towards an activatory phenotype. It also suggests that cytokine or Toll-like receptor (TLR) manipulation might result in a more optimal FcγR profile with the ability to overcome treatment resistance and augment immunotherapy. Recently, a TLR7 agonist in combination with radiation was shown to prime durable anti-tumour immune responses in mouse models of lymphoma [63] and it is attractive to suggest that similar synergy may be achieved with mAbs.

In contrast, anti-inflammatory cytokines, such as IL-4, IL-10 and transforming growth factor-β (TGF-β) produced by T_H2 cells, suppress activatory FcγR expression on innate immune effector cells and increase FcγRIIb expression. Tridandapani et al. [64] demonstrated that treatment of human myeloid cells with TGF-β resulted in a down-regulation of the activatory FcγR and associated decrease in FcγR-dependent effector function, i.e. phagocytosis. Alongside this, it has been established that monocytes and polymorphonuclear leukocytes (PMN) treated with IL-4 up-regulate FcγRIIb but suppress expression of FcγRIIa [65], as well as other activatory FcγRs [32, 66]. These studies also confirmed that IFN-γ treatment abrogated FcγRII expression, but enhanced activatory FcγR expression. It was also demonstrated that similar to the effects of IL-4, IL-10 treatment also upregulated FcγRIIb expression on myeloid cells [26]. Intriguingly, it is exactly these cytokines that are proposed to drive the conversion of macrophages towards an immunosuppressive, wound healing M2 phenotype (see below). Therefore, an attractive proposal is that mAb immunotherapy might be augmented through the blockade of immunosuppressive cytokines such as these. However, it should be noted that this may prove to be far from straightforward. IL-4 for example has differential effects on FcγRII expression depending upon the cell type. Indeed, Rudge et al. [67] demonstrated that whilst IL-4 upregulated FcγRII on myeloid cells, it down regulated the receptor on activated B cells. Therefore, the outcomes of such manipulating strategies will need to consider how they affect the tumour target cell, effector cell population as well as the immune system as a whole in order to correctly identify strategies which will enhance mAb efficacy in patients.

Ectopic Expression of FcγR in Cancer

In addition to regulation by cytokines and various other immunomodulatory molecules in vitro and in mouse models, abnormal expression of FcγR has been observed in patients in several lymphoid and non-lymphoid cancers [68]. Furthermore, FcγR expression has also been shown to be increased on peripheral blood mononuclear cells (PBMCs) in patients with cancer. In some instances, the increase in FcγR expression on PBMCs correlated both with an increase in tumour mass and decrease in survival in patients with metastatic disease [69, 70]. It was therefore thought that the FcγR expressing cells in the tumour mass were tumour infiltrating lymphocytes or inflammatory cells [71]. However, a study by Ran et al. [72] confirmed that both infiltrating cells and the tumour cells themselves expressed FcγR.

The reason behind abnormal expression of FcγR on tumour cells has not been determined in many cases. One exception is for FcγRIIB in malignant lymphoma, where in one study FcγRIIB-b2 was shown to be upregulated due to a t(1;22) chromosomal translocation in Follicular lymphoma (FL) [73]. This is potentially important as it has also been recently demonstrated that it is specifically the abnormal expression of the inhibitory FcγR by tumour cells that can confer enhanced tumourigenicity in certain cancers [74–76]. Similarly, 3T3 cells transfected with the b1 isoform of FcγRIIB (FcγRIIB-b1) were shown to be more tumourgenic than FcγRIIB-b1-negative cells. These authors also observed that if the tumour was comprised of FcγRIIB-negative and -positive cells, then the FcγRIIB-positive cells would outgrow the negative ones in the tumour cell population in vivo [75]. This suggests that FcγRIIB expression provides a selective advantage for tumour cell growth. However, contrary to this, it has also been shown that tumours of long latency, i.e. those which took longer to establish in mice, had increased expression of FcγRIIB [74, 77], implying that FcγRIIB expression may be gained by tumour cells during the pathogenic process.

Immunohistochemical analysis of a panel of primary tumours and metastases from those tumours has demonstrated that ectopic FcγRIIB expression is observed in a variety of cancers. In melanoma for, example, FcγRIIB has been shown to be overexpressed on metastatic tumour cells in 34 % of cases, with a lower percentage of ovary, brain and colon tumours (14, 5 and 4 %, respectively) also demonstrating abnormal FcγRIIB expression in comparison with normal tissue [78]. Alongside this, B cell tumours have also been shown to overexpress FcγRIIB in comparison with normal B cells, as determined by immunohistochemistry and recently by our laboratory using flow cytometry [9]. Similar to the example of metastatic melanoma, in some cases an increase in FcγRIIB expression on B cell tumours has been linked to tumour transformation and disease progression [79]. Interestingly, Cassard et al. [77] also observed that FcγRIIB expression correlated with tumour progression, in particular noting an increased percentage of FcγRIIB expressing tumour cells at various sites of metastasis, confirming that tumours of longer latency express FcγRIIB (above), and suggesting that expression is gained during disease progression. They discovered that the highest percentage of FcγRIIB expressing tumour cells could be found within the liver, followed by lymph nodes, lung and skin [78]. In addition, examination of tumour biopsies from both primary and metastatic sites from a single patient during disease, consistently demonstrated an absence of FcγRIIB in the primary tumour, but expression of FcγRIIB in the liver and lymph nodes. Taken together, these studies propose that not only does FcγRIIB expression confer a selective advantage for tumour cell growth, but that this is likely to contribute to disease progression and prognosis.

How and why FcγRIIB becomes upregulated, particularly in non-lymphoid tumours has not yet been established, but it has been suggested that environmental factors may play a part, either in response to IgG (within IC) or as a result of interactions with the tumour microenvironment [80, 81]. The latter is supported by evidence showing that FcγRIIB expression was lost during in vitro culture, but restored after treatment with IFN-γ [70]. In terms of tumour escape, it has been suggested that FcγRIIB might interfere with the anti-tumour response and as a result, protect the tumour from deletion via the immune system [82, 83]. Specifically, it has been postulated that FcγRIIB might function by sequestering the Fc portion of mAb and as such limit FcγR-dependent effector functions [68, 78], thereby allowing the tumour cells to evade the immune system and acquire metastatic potential. Although an attractive possibility, with clear implications for mAb immunotherapy, definitive supporting data are currently lacking.

Modulation as a Mechanism of Resistance

We recently observed a new facet of FcγRIIB biology that relates to this overexpression of FcγRIIB that directly impinges on the efficacy of certain therapeutic mAb. Rituximab and other type I anti-CD20 mAbs [84] such as the recently approved ofatumumab, can be internalized and cleared from the cell surface in a largely FcγRIIB-dependent manner [9]. Such internalization results in both reduced Fc on the target cell surface and accelerated mAb consumption in vivo, at least in pre-clinical models [16]. These findings reveal a mechanism through which overexpression of FcγRIIB on the tumour , not effector, can regulate mAb efficacy (Fig. 2). Intriguingly, when we investigated the nature of the FcγRIIb overexpression in the CLL and MCL samples detailed above, we noted that whilst both b1 and b2 isoforms of FcγRIIb were detected, the CLL cells seemed to express more IIb2 than IIb1 contrary to the relationship in MCL and normal B cells ([9] and data not shown). As all of the samples with equivalent expression of FcγRIIb were equally capable of internalizing rituximab, it suggested that although the b1 isoform is reported as being non-endocytic, both FcγRIIb isoforms are functionally similar at promoting anti-CD20 mAb internalization. Using cell-lines over-expressing either the b1 or b2 isoform of FcγRIIb we have recently formally proven this and demonstrated that they have equivalent ability to promote the internalization of rituximab (Vaughan et al. manuscript under revision Blood 2013).

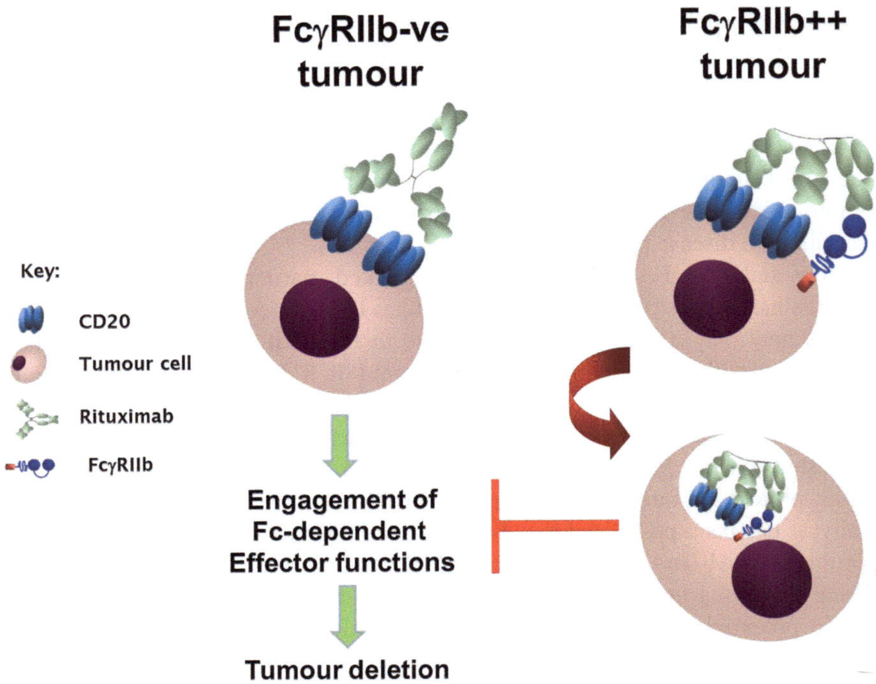

Fig. 2 Schematic of the ability of FcγRIIb to impair mAb efficacy. Following treatment of FcγRIIb-ve tumours with rituximab or other Type I anti-CD20 mAb, Fc dependent effector functions are engaged (potentially including CDC, ADCC and ADCP) resulting in deletion of the tumour cells. However, treatment of FcγRIIb +ve tumours, results in a cis-engagement of rituximab and FcγRIIb, resulting in its internalisation along with CD20, into early endosomes and subsequent destruction by lysosomes [9]. This removal of mAb from the cell surface precludes engagement of Fc-dependent effector functions and potentially reduces mAb half-life, resulting in diminished therapeutic efficacy [16]

Our preliminary findings further indicate a strong inverse correlation between the readiness of a tumour to internalise mAb and its therapeutic response to rituximab monotherapy. FL and diffuse large B cell lymphoma (DLBCL) tend to respond better to rituximab and generally internalize rituximab slowly, whereas chronic lymphocytic leukaemia (CLL) and mantle cell lymphoma (MCL) generally respond less well and internalize rituximab rapidly [16]. Furthermore, there is a strong positive correlation within lymphoid tumours between expression of FcγRIIB and internalisation of rituximab [9]. Our data also showed that the expression level of FcγRIIB on MCL correlated with poorer responses following chemoimmunotherapy, albeit in a very small cohort. These data suggest that FcγRIIB may provide a biomarker of rituximab response, indicating that controlling its expression may serve to help improve treatment. Furthermore, some FL display atypically high expression of FcγRIIB and internalize extremely rapidly. Our most recent data assessing a trial of 133 FL patients indicates this adversely affects the median time of failure-free survival following rituximab monotherapy (22.1 vs. 7 months in the negative/low versus medium/high FcγRIIb expression cohort, $p = 0.0227$) [85].

Intriguingly, Type II anti-CD20 mAb such as GA101 (obinutuzumab) and tositumumab, are not as affected by this process. The molecular basis behind this difference is currently unknown but given that the main discriminatory property of Type I and II mAbs is the interaction with lipid rafts, we currently favour a model whereby raft redistribution of Type I mAbs provides a favourable orientation of Fc regions for cis-based interactions with FcγRIIB on the same cell. This also brings about the question of whether other therapeutic mAbs will be susceptible to similar modulation through FcγRIIB. Our ongoing studies reveal that CD20 is certainly not unique in this aspect and that anti-CD19 and -CD38 mAbs are also affected (Vaughan et al. manuscript under revision Blood 2013). For anti-CD20 mAbs and perhaps for other target specificities, it may well be that a Type II mAb that does not interact with FcγRIIB (and therefore does not rapidly internalize) is required to overcome this resistance mechanism.

Role of Tumour Microenvironment

Despite the potential of enhancing mAb efficacy through the careful design and selection of target antigen, antibody specificity, type, isotype and further through Fc engineering there is clearly great potential in strategies beyond those concentrated on optimising the mAb alone. We would suggest that none of these strategies are likely to overcome any inherent deficiencies in the resident effector population within the patient. These deficiencies might include effector exhaustion, depletion, or inhibition as a result of other therapeutic interventions or the tumour microenvironment itself. In this latter regard, it has become increasingly clear over the last decade that tumours can suppress the innate and adaptive arms of the immune system through various means including regulation of myeloid cells [86, 87]. Central to this suppressive capacity is their regulation of macrophages. Macrophages can be broadly classified as inflammatory (M1) or anti-inflammatory (M2) according to their state of activation and a number of key characteristics [87]. Tumours are able to direct tumour-associated macrophages (TAM) to become polarized towards an anti-inflammatory, pro-angiogenic, M2 phenotype promoting tumour growth [88]. High TAM numbers in some tumours have been shown to correlate with poor prognosis following chemotherapy [88]. Conversely, recent studies indicate that TAM may be beneficial for rituximab-based immunochemotherapy regimes [89, 90]. However, these associations are far from clear and in fact the M2/TAM phenotype is associated with higher expression of FcγRIIB and reduced expression of activatory FcγR. Therefore, one strategy for augmenting mAb therapy is to manipulate the FcγR profile of associated effector populations (see below).

Removal of Target: mAb Conjugates by "Shaving"

An additional property of the effector phagocytic population, proposed to limit mAb efficacy, is its propensity to undertake "shaving". First described by Ron Taylor's group in 2006 [13], shaving describes a process whereby antibody:antigen complexes are effectively 'plucked' from the target cell surface by monocytes or macrophages in a reaction mediated by FcγR. It is proposed that the process is initiated when phagocytes become saturated and unable to engulf more opsonised target cells. Under these conditions, rather than fully engulfing target cells, the myeloid cells instead 'shave' them of the mAb-coated targets. This leaves the target cells viable but antigen negative and resistant to further antibody-mediated attack [91]. Such membrane capture is often called trogocytosis, and is not molecularly specific, since effector cells can remove a range of membrane molecules in addition to those engaged by the mAb [92]. This mechanism of mAb resistance may be doubly effective as, in addition to loss of the target antigen, the potency of the effector cells is reduced by removal and internalization of their FcγR [91, 93]. Although originally postulated to be largely dependent upon FcγRI [11], subsequent studies have shown that shaving can be triggered by multiple FcγRs, with clear redundancy. Furthermore, both activatory and inhibitory FcγRs, at least in the mouse, have been reported as capable of triggering shaving [94]. Hence, it is the proximity between effector and target that triggers shaving as opposed to specific activatory FcγR signalling.

It has previously been proposed that shaving/trogocytosis may be influenced by the anatomical location of the tumour and nature of the effector [94]. It would also be interesting to assess whether the M1:M2:TAM nature of effectors serves to influence the process. Importantly, with respect to CD20 mAb, shaving, like other modes of effector deficiency, targets both Type I and II anti-CD20 mAb equivalently [95] and so may require alternative means of intervention to prevent its occurrence. One potential solution is to prevent effector saturation by, for example, giving lower doses of mAbs more frequently [14, 96]. It should be noted that even when trogocytosis/shaving had occurred in vivo (in mice) these cells could still be killed ex vivo in ADCC but not CDC assays, which may indicate that under current treatment regimes, CDC but not ADCC is rendered redundant. This observation is consistent with the higher levels of cell surface IgG required to mediate CDC vs ADCC. The effects on ADCP remain to be determined. Currently, there is no suggestion that shaving is a dominant mechanism in vivo as clinical trials with either rituximab or ofatumumab suggest that higher doses are more efficacious than low doses [97, 98]. However, the mini-R phase II ARCTIC trial in CLL using only 100 mg Rituximab doses may help to specifically address these questions. One of the complications of assessing the importance of shaving as a resistance mechanism in this setting, is that it will occur at the same time that rituximab is being modulated. This will be a particular issue in the ARCTIC trial as CLL cells generally display a high level of FcγRIIB (albeit over a wide range), and it is likely that the promotion of modulation, which is apparently largely unaffected by mAb saturation (unpublished observations), predominates in this situation.

Strategies to Overcome FcγR-Mediated Resistance

It was demonstrated over a decade ago that genetic deletion of the inhibitory FcR, FcγRIIB, can improve cancer immunotherapy [17]. In xenograft models of breast or colorectal cancer, various therapeutic mAbs (4D5, trastuzumab and anti-E-cadherin) showed either great improvement in therapy or complete inhibition of tumour growth in FcγRIIB -/- mice compared with WT controls with similar results seen in the syngeneic B16 melanoma model (using TA99 mAb) [17, 40]. It has, therefore, been long proposed that preventing the interaction of FcγRIIB with therapeutic mAb, should augment mAb immunotherapy.

Other than ablating the expression of FcγRIIB through gene therapy, recapitulating the effects seen in the mouse experiments will require alternative approaches including; reducing its expression through immunomodulatory molecules (such as IFN-γ and TLR-agonists); blocking the interaction with FcγRIIB-specific mAb or manipulating the Fc region of the mAb to prevent binding (Fig. 3).

One clear direction of travel in the field to date has been to re-engineer the Fc portion of IgG to interact with greater affinity to activatory FcγRs and with lower affinity to inhibitory FcγRs and, consequently, enhance efficacy [99, 100]. This strategy has been developed in two parallel approaches—either through genetic modification of the Fc region to augment the A:I ratio [100–104] or post-translational glycomodification [105–107]. It is this latter approach that has been taken with GA101 (Obinutuzumab). Originally developed by GlycArt Biotechnology AG, GA101, is a Type II anti-CD20 mAb whose Fc region is glycoengineered by producing the antibody in CHO cells which overexpress β-1,4-N-acetyl-glucosaminyltransferase III and Golgi α-mannosidase II. This results in non-fucosylated sugars becoming attached to asparagine 297 in the Fc region [108], allowing tighter binding to FcγRIIIA and augmented ADCC. Importantly, it should be noted that binding to other FcγRs is largely unaffected by this approach and so whether further modifications (such as a reduction in FcγRIIB-engagement) would further benefit the activity of GA101 remains to be determined.

An alternative approach could be to block the immunosuppressive cytokines which help drive expression of the inhibitory receptor as discussed above. Similarly, immunomodulatory molecules (such as TLR-agonists) could be incorporated into antibody therapy regimes to drive down expression of FcγRIIB (and increase activatory FcγRs). Clearly, this approach will require careful development given the often highly pleiotropic nature of these reagents.

One area where we would anticipate reduced FcγRIIB-engagement to have a profound effect on therapeutic mAbs would be in reducing the FcγRIIB-dependent modulation observed with Type I anti-CD20 mAbs. Regardless of how this is achieved, through genetic engineering, receptor blockade with anti-FcγRIIB mAbs

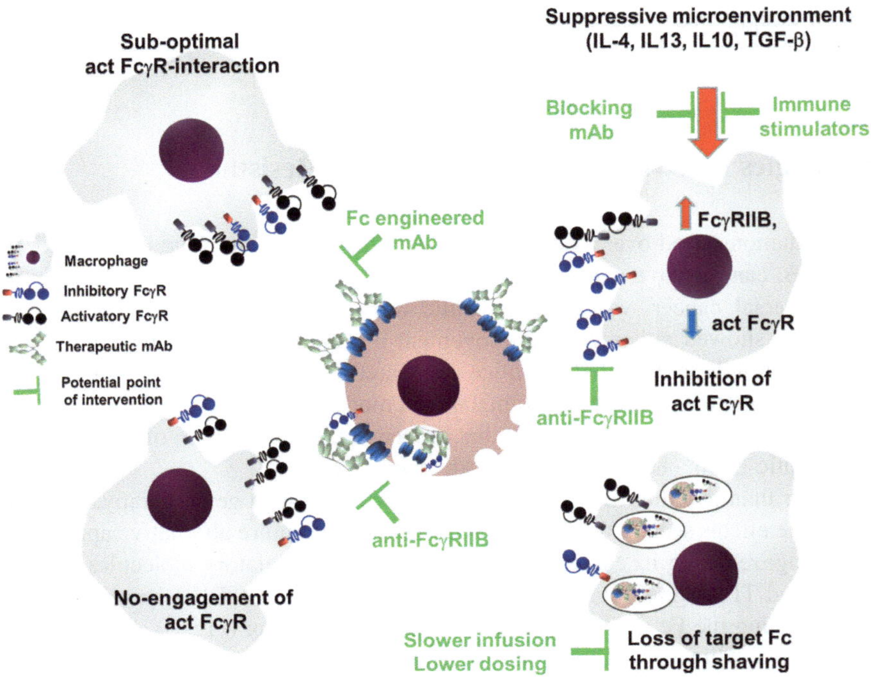

Fig. 3 Potential modulation of therapeutic mAb efficacy through FcγR manipulation. Various mechanisms can inhibit optimal FcγR-mediated mAb immunotherapy including (clockwise from *top right*) suppressive microenvironments, "shaving", FcγRIIB-mediated internalisation and sub-optimal FcγR engagement through incorrect isotype. Potential points of intervention are highlighted in *green* and include using immune stimulators, blockers of suppressive cytokines, anti-FcγRIIB mAb, altered infusion rates and doses, and Fc-engineering

or immunomodulation of the FcγRIIB receptor itself, it should augment Fc-dependent effector function and promote extended mAbs half-life.

An attractive approach is to target FcγRIIB directly using specific mAbs. One of the problems in generating specific anti-FcγRIIB mAbs is that activatory FcγRIIA shares greater than 95 % homology in the extracellular region of the receptor with FcγRIIB. However, anti-FcγRIIB mAbs capable of specifically binding FcγRIIB have been developed. At least one of these reagents (2B6) has been shown to be efficient at blocking endogenous IC binding, attenuating FcγRIIB activity and enhancing the result of activatory FcγR engagement in vitro [109]. Further to this, these human anti-FcγRIIB mAbs have been shown to have direct cytotoxic effects on the tumours themselves resulting in growth inhibition and increased survival in xenograft models [110]. This study also demonstrated that the FcγRIIB was able to direct FcR-dependent functions towards human B cell lymphomas in vitro and required intact Fc for its function in vivo [110].

We have recently developed similar specific tools for targeting FcγRII in the mouse which will enable us to further assess the potential of this approach and to dissect its key mechanisms of action. Interestingly, we were able to generate reagents which either caused phosphorylation and subsequent activation of FcγRIIB (agonists) or those which blocked receptor phosphorylation (antagonists) [111]. For target cells expressing FcγRIIB (such as CLL cells and certain other NHL) both antagonistic and agonistic mAbs may have useful anti-tumour activities: the agonistic mAbs to induce direct cell death in the target cells and the antagonistic mAbs to prevent negative signalling from FcγRIIB on effector cells. A further mode of action suggested by our recent findings [9] is that anti-FcγRII mAbs can block the internalization of certain mAbs specificities, such as the Type I anti-CD20 mAbs and, thereby, augment phagocytosis. Extrapolation from our CD20 Tg mouse studies indicates that blocking internalization will also enhance mAbs half-life and potentially allow less frequent dosing [16]. Our current laboratory focus is on discriminating which of these mechanisms is most critical.

Augmentation of FcγR for Non-conventional mAbs

It should be noted that all of the various facets discussed above largely relate to conventional direct targeting mAbs such as anti-CD20, -CD19 and -CD52. Certain mAbs do not, or only partially, work via recruitment of FcR-expressing effectors and promote direct or indirect killing of target cells. For example, trastuzumab is able to block survival and proliferation signals emanating from the Her-2Neu receptor aberrantly expressed on breast cancer cells and the importance of FcR engagement remains controversial. In addition, so-called immunomodulatory mAbs, such as anti-CD40 and anti-CTLA-4 reagents, appear to act independently of the conventional direct targeting effector mechanisms of CDC, ADCC and ADCP, to stimulate cells of the adaptive immune system to augment endogenous anti-tumour responses to bring about tumour deletion [112]. However, even these classes of mAbs may be dependent on FcγR binding, as demonstrated recently with anti-CD40 mAbs [113, 114] and for apoptosis-triggering anti-DR5 mAbs [115]. It is clear, therefore, that the nature of the target and mechanism of action of the mAb may result in an entirely opposing set of FcR requirements for optimal efficacy. Furthermore, these requirements may explain the wide disparity of activities observed with some of these reagents in man as they vary in their immunoglobulin subclass (IgG 1, 2, 3, 4) which have widely differing affinities for FcγR as discussed above. Clearly, this information will have significant implications for the future rational selection and engineering of the next generation of mAbs.

In addition, APC functions are also regulated by FcγR interactions [22, 23, 116, 117]. For example, incubation of human dendritic cells with an FcγRIIb blocking antibody was sufficient to induce DC maturation by immune complexes, as demonstrated by the upregulation of costimulatory molecules [116]. Alongside DC maturation, enhanced generation and activation of tumour specific T cells and enhanced immune responses were observed [118]. This suggests that in addition to augmenting direct targeting mAb efficacy, blocking FcγRIIb might also be a strategy for generation of stronger, targeted adaptive anti-tumour responses, potentially in combination with cancer vaccines.

Conclusion

In conclusion, it is clear that mAbs have transformed our ability to treat cancer and that they do this through interaction with Fc receptors. However, it is also clear that FcγR expression profiles on the tumour and surrounding effector cells may not always be optimal for successful tumour deletion. A number of strategies are available or under development to circumvent these problems and it will be interesting to see how these approaches serve to improve mAb immunotherapy in the coming years.

Acknowledgments The authors would like to thank all of the members of the Antibody and Vaccine Group, past and present and in particular the members of the CD20 and FcγR teams. We also apologise to those authors whose work has not been cited in this review due to space limitations.

Conflict Statements:

Prof Cragg serves as a consultant for Bioinvent International and has previously served as an ad hoc consultant for Roche. MJG acts as a consultant to a number of biotech companies to write general antibody expert reports; he receives institutional payments and royalties from antibody patents and licenses. PWJ acts as a consultant to Roche and Pfizer and has received payments for lectures from Millennium Takeda and Pfizer. JCS has acted as a consultant for oxford gene technologies and received research funding from Roche.

References

1. Glennie MJ, Johnson PW. Clinical trials of antibody therapy. Immunol Today. 2000;21:403–10.
2. Glennie MJ, van de Winkel JG. Renaissance of cancer therapeutic antibodies. Drug Discov Today. 2003;8:503–10.
3. Glennie MJ, French RR, Cragg MS, Taylor RP. Mechanisms of killing by anti-CD20 monoclonal antibodies. Mol Immunol. 2007;44:3823–37.
4. Reff ME, Carner K, Chambers KS, Chinn PC, Leonard JE, Raab R, Newman RA, Hanna N, Anderson DR. Depletion of B cells in vivo by a chimeric mouse human monoclonal antibody to CD20. Blood. 1994;83:435–45.
5. Pescovitz MD. Rituximab, an anti-cd20 monoclonal antibody: history and mechanism of action. Am J Transplant. 2006;6:859–66.
6. Fisher RI, Gaynor ER, Dahlberg S, Oken MM, Grogan TM, Mize EM, Glick JH, Coltman CA Jr, Miller TP. Comparison of a standard regimen (CHOP) with three intensive chemotherapy regimens for advanced non-Hodgkin's lymphoma. N Engl J Med. 1993;328:1002–6.
7. Sehn LH, Donaldson J, Chhanabhai M, Fitzgerald C, Gill K, Klasa R, MacPherson N, O'Reilly S, Spinelli JJ, Sutherland J, Wilson KS, Gascoyne RD, Connors JM. Introduction

of combined CHOP plus rituximab therapy dramatically improved outcome of diffuse large B-cell lymphoma in British Columbia. J Clin Oncol. 2005;23:5027–33.
8. Salles GA. Clinical features, prognosis and treatment of follicular lymphoma. Hematology Am Soc Hematol Educ Program. 2007;2007:216–25.
9. Lim SH, Vaughan AT, Ashton-Key M, Williams EL, Dixon SV, Chan CH, Beers SA, French RR, Cox KL, Davies AJ, Potter KN, Mockridge CI, Oscier DG, Johnson PW, Cragg MS, Glennie MJ. Fc gamma receptor IIb on target B cells promotes rituximab internalization and reduces clinical efficacy. Blood. 2011;118:2530–40.
10. Lim SH, Beers SA, French RR, Johnson PW, Glennie MJ, Cragg MS. Anti-CD20 monoclonal antibodies: historical and future perspectives. Haematologica. 2010;95:135–43.
11. Li Y, Williams ME, Cousar JB, Pawluczkowycz AW, Lindorfer MA, Taylor RP. Rituximab-CD20 complexes are shaved from Z138 mantle cell lymphoma cells in intravenous and subcutaneous SCID mouse models. J Immunol. 2007;179:4263–71.
12. Kennedy AD, Beum PV, Solga MD, DiLillo DJ, Lindorfer MA, Hess CE, Densmore JJ, Williams ME, Taylor RP. Rituximab infusion promotes rapid complement depletion and acute CD20 loss in chronic lymphocytic leukemia. J Immunol. 2004;172:3280–8.
13. Beum PV, Kennedy AD, Williams ME, Lindorfer MA, Taylor RP. The shaving reaction: rituximab/CD20 complexes are removed from mantle cell lymphoma and chronic lymphocytic leukemia cells by THP-1 monocytes. J Immunol. 2006;176:2600–9.
14. Williams ME, Densmore JJ, Pawluczkowycz AW, Beum PV, Kennedy AD, Lindorfer MA, Hamil SH, Eggleton JC, Taylor RP. Thrice-weekly low-dose rituximab decreases CD20 loss via shaving and promotes enhanced targeting in chronic lymphocytic leukemia. J Immunol. 2006;177:7435–43.
15. Wang SY, Racila E, Taylor RP, Weiner GJ. NK-cell activation and antibody-dependent cellular cytotoxicity induced by rituximab-coated target cells is inhibited by the C3b component of complement. Blood. 2008;111:1456–63.
16. Beers SA, French RR, Chan CH, Lim SH, Jarrett TC, Mora Vidal R, Wijayaweera SS, Dixon SV, Kim H, Cox KL, Kerr JP, Johnston DA, Johnson PW, Verbeek JS, Glennie MJ, Cragg MS. Antigenic modulation limits the efficacy of anti-CD20 antibodies: implications for antibody selection. Blood. 2010;115:5191–201.
17. Clynes RA, Towers TL, Presta LG, Ravetch JV. Inhibitory Fc receptors modulate in vivo cytoxicity against tumor targets. Nat Med. 2000;6:443–6.
18. Kaneko Y, Nimmerjahn F, Ravetch JV. Anti-inflammatory activity of immunoglobulin G resulting from Fc sialylation. Science. 2006;313:670–3.
19. Hamaguchi Y, Xiu Y, Komura K, Nimmerjahn F, Tedder TF. Antibody isotype-specific engagement of Fcgamma receptors regulates B lymphocyte depletion during CD20 immunotherapy. J Exp Med. 2006;203:743–53.
20. Nimmerjahn F, Ravetch JV. Antibodies, Fc receptors and cancer. Curr Opin Immunol. 2007;19:239–45.
21. Ravetch JV, Bolland S. IgG Fc receptors. Annu Rev Immunol. 2001;19:275–90.
22. Nimmerjahn F, Ravetch JV. Fcgamma receptors as regulators of immune responses. Nat Rev. 2008;8:34–47.
23. Bruhns P, Iannascoli B, England P, Mancardi DA, Fernandez N, Jorieux S, Daeron M. Specificity and affinity of human Fcgamma receptors and their polymorphic variants for human IgG subclasses. Blood. 2009;113:3716–25.
24. Ravetch JV, Luster AD, Weinshank R, Kochan J, Pavlovec A, Portnoy DA, Hulmes J, Pan YC, Unkeless JC. Structural heterogeneity and functional domains of murine immunoglobulin G Fc receptors. Science. 1986;234:718–25.
25. Hogarth PM, Witort E, Hulett MD, Bonnerot C, Even J, Fridman WH, McKenzie IF. Structure of the mouse beta Fc gamma receptor II gene. J Immunol. 1991;146:369–76.
26. Joshi T, Ganesan LP, Cao X, Tridandapani S. Molecular analysis of expression and function of hFcgammaRIIbl and b2 isoforms in myeloid cells. Mol Immunol. 2006;43:839–50.

27. Cassel DL, Keller MA, Surrey S, Schwartz E, Schreiber AD, Rappaport EF, McKenzie SE. Differential expression of Fc gamma RIIA, Fc gamma RIIB and Fc gamma RIIC in hematopoietic cells: analysis of transcripts. Mol Immunol. 1993;30:451–60.
28. Van Den Herik-Oudijk IE, Westerdaal NA, Henriquez NV, Capel PJ, Van De Winkel JG. Functional analysis of human Fc gamma RII (CD32) isoforms expressed in B lymphocytes. J Immunol. 1994;152:574–85.
29. Budde P, Bewarder N, Weinrich V, Schulzeck O, Frey J. Tyrosine-containing sequence motifs of the human immunoglobulin G receptors FcRIIb1 and FcRIIb2 essential for endocytosis and regulation of calcium flux in B cells. J Biol Chem. 1994;269:30636–44.
30. Cartron G, Dacheux L, Salles G, Solal-Celigny P, Bardos P, Colombat P, Watier H. Therapeutic activity of humanized anti-CD20 monoclonal antibody and polymorphism in IgG Fc receptor FcgammaRIIIa gene. Blood. 2002;99:754–8.
31. Weng WK, Levy R. Two immunoglobulin G fragment C receptor polymorphisms independently predict response to rituximab in patients with follicular lymphoma. J Clin Oncol. 2003;21:3940–7.
32. Nimmerjahn F, Ravetch JV. Divergent immunoglobulin g subclass activity through selective Fc receptor binding. Science New York 2005, 310:1510–1512.
33. Nimmerjahn F, Ravetch JV. Fcgamma receptors: old friends and new family members. Immunity. 2006;24:19–28.
34. Kaminski MS, Kitamura K, Maloney DG, Campbell MJ, Levy R. Importance of antibody isotype in monoclonal anti-idiotype therapy of a murine B cell lymphoma. A study of hybridoma class switch variants. J Immunol. 1986;136:1123–30.
35. Kipps TJ, Parham P, Punt J, Herzenberg LA. Importance of immunoglobulin isotype in human antibody-dependent, cell-mediated cytotoxicity directed by murine monoclonal antibodies. J Exp Med. 1985;161:1–17.
36. Uchida J, Hamaguchi Y, Oliver JA, Ravetch JV, Poe JC, Haas KM, Tedder TF. The innate mononuclear phagocyte network depletes B lymphocytes through Fc receptor-dependent mechanisms during anti-CD20 antibody immunotherapy. J Exp Med. 2004;199:1659–69.
37. Tedder TF, Baras A, Xiu Y. Fcgamma receptor-dependent effector mechanisms regulate CD19 and CD20 antibody immunotherapies for B lymphocyte malignancies and autoimmunity. Springer Semin Immunopathol. 2006;28:351–64.
38. Minard-Colin V, Xiu Y, Poe JC, Horikawa M, Magro CM, Hamaguchi Y, Haas KM, Tedder TF. Lymphoma depletion during CD20 immunotherapy in mice is mediated by macrophage FcgammaRI, FcgammaRIII, and FcgammaRIV. Blood. 2008;112:1205–13.
39. Gong Q, Ou Q, Ye S, Lee WP, Cornelius J, Diehl L, Lin WY, Nguyen K, Tran T, Zhang Y, Rosen H, Martin F. Importance of cellular microenvironment and circulatory dynamics in B cell immunotherapy. J Immunol. 2005;174:817–26.
40. Green SK, Karlsson MC, Ravetch JV, Kerbel RS. Disruption of cell-cell adhesion enhances antibody-dependent cellular cytotoxicity: implications for antibody-based therapeutics of cancer. Cancer Res. 2002;62:6891–900.
41. Fossati-Jimack L, Ioan-Facsinay A, Reininger L, Chicheportiche Y, Watanabe N, Saito T, Hofhuis FM, Gessner JE, Schiller C, Schmidt RE, Honjo T, Verbeek JS. Markedly different pathogenicity of four immunoglobulin G isotype-switch variants of an antierythrocyte autoantibody is based on their capacity to interact in vivo with the low-affinity Fcgamma receptor III. J Exp Med. 2000;191:1293–302.
42. Teeling JL, French RR, Cragg MS, van den Brakel J, Pluyter M, Huang H, Chan C, Parren PW, Hack CE, Dechant M, Valerius T, van de Winkel JG, Glennie MJ. Characterization of new human CD20 monoclonal antibodies with potent cytolytic activity against non-Hodgkin lymphomas. Blood. 2004;104:1793–800.
43. Golay J, Manganini M, Facchinetti V, Gramigna R, Broady R, Borleri G, Rambaldi A, Introna M. Rituximab-mediated antibody-dependent cellular cytotoxicity against neoplastic B cells is stimulated strongly by interleukin-2. Haematologica. 2003;88:1002–12.

44. Cartron G, Ohresser M, Salles G, Solal-Celigny P, Colombat P, Watier H. Neutrophil role in in vivo anti-lymphoma activity of rituximab: FCGR3B-NA1/NA2 polymorphism does not influence response and survival after rituximab treatment. Ann Oncol. 2008;19:1485–7.
45. Van Rooijen N, Sanders A. Liposome mediated depletion of macrophages: mechanism of action, preparation of liposomes and applications. J Immunol Methods. 1994;174:83–93.
46. Anolik JH, Campbell D, Felgar RE, Young F, Sanz I, Rosenblatt J, Looney RJ. The relationship of FcgammaRIIIa genotype to degree of B cell depletion by rituximab in the treatment of systemic lupus erythematosus. Arthritis Rheum. 2003;48:455–9.
47. Parren PW. Preparation of genetically engineered monoclonal antibodies for human immunotherapy. Hum Antibodies Hybridomas. 1992;3:137–45.
48. Hatjiharissi E, Xu L, Santos DD, Hunter ZR, Ciccarelli BT, Verselis S, Modica M, Cao Y, Manning RJ, Leleu X, Dimmock EA, Kortsaris A, Mitsiades C, Anderson KC, Fox EA, Treon SP. Increased natural killer cell expression of CD16, and augmented binding and ADCC activity to rituximab among individuals expressing the Fc{gamma}RIIIA-158 V/V and V/F polymorphism. Blood. 2007;110:2561–4.
49. Metes D, Ernst LK, Chambers WH, Sulica A, Herberman RB, Morel PA. Expression of functional CD32 molecules on human NK cells is determined by an allelic polymorphism of the FcgammaRIIC gene. Blood. 1998;91:2369–80.
50. Breunis WB, van Mirre E, Bruin M, Geissler J, de Boer M, Peters M, Roos D, de Haas M, Koene HR, Kuijpers TW. Copy number variation of the activating FCGR2C gene predisposes to idiopathic thrombocytopenic purpura. Blood. 2008;111:1029–38.
51. Floto RA, Clatworthy MR, Heilbronn KR, Rosner DR, MacAry PA, Rankin A, Lehner PJ, Ouwehand WH, Allen JM, Watkins NA, Smith KG. Loss of function of a lupus-associated FcgammaRIIb polymorphism through exclusion from lipid rafts. Nat Med. 2005;11:1056–8.
52. Kono H, Kyogoku C, Suzuki T, Tsuchiya N, Honda H, Yamamoto K, Tokunaga K, Zen-ichiro H. FcgammaRIIB Ile232Thr transmembrane polymorphism associated with human systemic lupus erythematosus decreases affinity to lipid rafts and attenuates inhibitory effects on B cell receptor signaling. Hum Mol Genet. 2005;14:2881–92.
53. Weng WK, Levy R. Genetic polymorphism of the inhibitory IgG Fc receptor FcgammaRIIb is not associated with clinical outcome in patients with follicular lymphoma treated with rituximab. Leuk Lymphoma. 2009;50:723–7.
54. Willcocks LC, Lyons PA, Clatworthy MR, Robinson JI, Yang W, Newland SA, Plagnol V, McGovern NN, Condliffe AM, Chilvers ER, Adu D, Jolly EC, Watts R, Lau YL, Morgan AW, Nash G, Smith KG. Copy number of FCGR3B, which is associated with systemic lupus erythematosus, correlates with protein expression and immune complex uptake. J Exp Med. 2008;205:1573–82.
55. Aitman TJ, Dong R, Vyse TJ, Norsworthy PJ, Johnson MD, Smith J, Mangion J, Roberton-Lowe C, Marshall AJ, Petretto E, Hodges MD, Bhangal G, Patel SG, Sheehan-Rooney K, Duda M, Cook PR, Evans DJ, Domin J, Flint J, Boyle JJ, Pusey CD, Cook HT. Copy number polymorphism in Fcgr3 predisposes to glomerulonephritis in rats and humans. Nature. 2006;439:851–5.
56. Fanciulli M, Norsworthy PJ, Petretto E, Dong R, Harper L, Kamesh L, Heward JM, Gough SC, de Smith A, Blakemore AI, Froguel P, Owen CJ, Pearce SH, Teixeira L, Guillevin L, Graham DS, Pusey CD, Cook HT, Vyse TJ, Aitman TJ. FCGR3B copy number variation is associated with susceptibility to systemic, but not organ-specific, autoimmunity. Nat Genet. 2007;39:721–3.
57. Breunis WB, van Mirre E, Geissler J, Laddach N, Wolbink G, van der Schoot E, de Haas M, de Boer M, Roos D, Kuijpers TW. Copy number variation at the FCGR locus includes FCGR3A, FCGR2C and FCGR3B but not FCGR2A and FCGR2B. Hum Mutat. 2009;30:E640–50.
58. Guyre PM, Morganelli PM, Miller R. Recombinant immune interferon increases immunoglobulin G Fc receptors on cultured human mononuclear phagocytes. J Clin Investig. 1983;72:393–7.

59. Sivo J, Politis AD, Vogel SN. Differential effects of interferon-gamma and glucocorticoids on Fc gamma R gene expression in murine macrophages. J Leukoc Biol. 1993;54:451–7.
60. Okayama Y, Kirshenbaum AS, Metcalfe DD. Expression of a functional high-affinity IgG receptor, Fc gamma RI, on human mast cells: Up-regulation by IFN-gamma. J Immunol. 2000;164:4332–9.
61. Yoshie O, Mellman IS, Broeze RJ, Garcia-Blanco M, Lengyel P. Interferon action: effects of mouse alpha and beta interferons on rosette formation, phagocytosis, and surface-antigen expression of cells of the macrophage-type line RAW 309Cr.1. Cell Immunol. 1982;73:128–40.
62. Shushakova N, Skokowa J, Schulman J, Baumann U, Zwirner J, Schmidt RE, Gessner JE. C5a anaphylatoxin is a major regulator of activating versus inhibitory FcgammaRs in immune complex-induced lung disease. J Clin Investig. 2002;110:1823–30.
63. Dovedi SJ, Melis MH, Wilkinson RW, Adlard AL, Stratford IJ, Honeychurch J, Illidge TM. Systemic delivery of a TLR7 agonist in combination with radiation primes durable anti-tumor immune responses in mouse models of lymphoma. Blood. 2012;121:251–9.
64. Tridandapani S, Wardrop R, Baran CP, Wang Y, Opalek JM, Caligiuri MA, Marsh CB. TGF-beta 1 suppresses [correction of supresses] myeloid Fc gamma receptor function by regulating the expression and function of the common gamma-subunit. J Immunol. 2003;170:4572–7.
65. Pricop L, Redecha P, Teillaud JL, Frey J, Fridman WH, Sautes-Fridman C, Salmon JE. Differential modulation of stimulatory and inhibitory Fc gamma receptors on human monocytes by Th1 and Th2 cytokines. J Immunol. 2001;166:531–7.
66. te Velde AA, Huijbens RJ, de Vries JE, Figdor CG. IL-4 decreases Fc gamma R membrane expression and Fc gamma R-mediated cytotoxic activity of human monocytes. J Immunol. 1990;144:3046–51.
67. Rudge EU, Cutler AJ, Pritchard NR, Smith KG. Interleukin 4 reduces expression of inhibitory receptors on B cells and abolishes CD22 and Fc gamma RII-mediated B cell suppression. J Exp Med. 2002;195:1079–85.
68. Witz IP, Ran M. FcR may function as a progression factor of nonlymphoid tumors. Immunol Res. 1992;11:283–95.
69. Ilfeld D, Barzilay J, Dux Z, Ran M. Correlation of Fc gamma receptors on peripheral blood mononuclear cells and survival in patients with metastatic breast cancer. Breast Cancer Res Treat. 1986;7:181–6.
70. Ran M, Teillaud JL, Fridman WH, Frenkel H, Halachmi E, Katz B, Gips M, Shlomo Y, Barzilay J, Witz IP. Increased expression of Fc gamma receptor in cancer patients and tumor bearing mice. Mol Immunol. 1988;25:1159–67.
71. Svennevig JL, Andersson TR. Cells bearing Fc receptors in human malignant solid tumours. Br J Cancer. 1982;45:201–8.
72. Ran M, Dux Z, Anavi R, Witz IP. Expression of Fc gamma receptors on a subpopulation of nonlymphoid tumor cells and its enrichment. J Natl Cancer Inst. 1984;73:437–46.
73. Callanan MB, Le Baccon P, Mossuz P, Duley S, Bastard C, Hamoudi R, Dyer MJ, Klobeck G, Rimokh R, Sotto JJ, Leroux D. The IgG Fc receptor, FcgammaRIIB, is a target for deregulation by chromosomal translocation in malignant lymphoma. Proc Natl Acad Sci USA. 2000;97:309–14.
74. Berko-Flint Y, Fridman WH, Grossman-Atlas E, Kimchi N, Ben-Baruch AL, Moss S, Teillaud JL, Witz IP, Ran M. Some cellular and molecular characteristics of high and low tumorigenicity variants of polyoma-virus transformed cells. Mol Immunol. 1990;27:1219–28.
75. Zusman T, Gohar O, Eliassi H, Avivi Y, Lisansky E, Sautes C, Even J, Bonnerot C, Fridman WH, Witz IP, Ran M. The murine Fc-gamma (Fc gamma) receptor type II B1 is a tumorigenicity-enhancing factor in polyoma-virus-transformed 3T3 cells. Int J Cancer. 1996;65:221–9.

76. Zusman T, Lisansky E, Arons E, Anavi R, Bonnerot C, Sautes C, Fridman WH, Witz IP, Ran M. Contribution of the intracellular domain of murine Fc-gamma receptor type IIB1 to its tumor-enhancing potential. Int J Cancer. 1996;68:219–27.
77. Langer AB, Emmanuel N, Even J, Fridman WH, Gohar O, Gonen B, Katz BZ, Ran M, Smorodinsky NI, Witz IP. Phenotypic properties of 3T3 cells transformed in vitro with polyoma virus and passaged once in syngeneic animals. Immunobiology. 1992;185:281–91.
78. Cassard L, Cohen-Solal JF, Fournier EM, Camilleri-Broët S, Spatz A, Chouaïb S, Badoual C, Varin A, Fisson S, Duvillard P, Boix C, Loncar SM, Sastre-Garau X, Houghton AN, Avril MF, Gresser I, Fridman WH, Sautès-Fridman C. Selective expression of inhibitory Fcgamma receptor by metastatic melanoma impairs tumor susceptibility to IgG-dependent cellular response. Int J Cancer. 2008;123:2832–9.
79. Camilleri-Broet S, Cassard L, Broet P, Delmer A, Le Touneau A, Diebold J, Fridman WH, Molina TJ, Sautès-Fridman C. FcgammaRIIB is differentially expressed during B cell maturation and in B-cell lymphomas. Br J Haematol. 2004;124:55–62.
80. Neauport-Sautes C, Daeron M, Teillaud JL, Blank U, Fridman WH. The occurrence, structural and functional properties of immunoglobulin Fc receptors on murine neoplastic cells. Int Rev Immunol. 1986;1:237–71.
81. Eshel R, Neumark E, Sagi-Assif O, Witz IP. Receptors involved in microenvironment-driven molecular evolution of cancer cells. Semin Cancer Biol. 2002;12:139–47.
82. Cassard L, Cohen-Solal JF, Galinha A, Sastre-Garau X, Mathiot C, Galon J, Dorval T, Bernheim A, Fridman WH, Sautès-Fridman C. Modulation of tumor growth by inhibitory Fc(gamma) receptor expressed by human melanoma cells. J Clin Investig. 2002;110:1549–57.
83. Ran M, Langer AB, Eliassi I, Gohar O, Gonen B, Gradsztajn S, Fridman WH, Teillaud JL, Witz IP. Possibilities of interference with the immune system of tumor bearers by non-lymphoid Fc gamma RII expressing tumor cells. Immunobiology. 1992;185:415–25.
84. Cragg MS, Morgan SM, Chan HT, Morgan BP, Filatov AV, Johnson PW, French RR, Glennie MJ. Complement-mediated lysis by anti-CD20 mAb correlates with segregation into lipid rafts. Blood. 2003;101:1045–52.
85. Lee CA-K, Margaret; Cogliatti S, Crowe S, Cragg MS, Schmitz S-FH, Ghielmini M, Johnson PW. Expression of inhibitory Fc receptor (Fc!RIIB) Is a marker of poor response to Rituximab monotherapy in follicular lymphoma (FL). ASH abstract 50396 2012.
86. Condeelis J, Pollard JW. Macrophages: obligate partners for tumor cell migration, invasion, and metastasis. Cell. 2006;124:263–6.
87. Mantovani A, Sica A, Allavena P, Garlanda C, Locati M. Tumor-associated macrophages and the related myeloid-derived suppressor cells as a paradigm of the diversity of macrophage activation. Hum Immunol. 2009;70:325–30.
88. Sica A, Schioppa T, Mantovani A, Allavena P. Tumour-associated macrophages are a distinct M2 polarised population promoting tumour progression: potential targets of anti-cancer therapy. Eur J Cancer. 2006;42:717–27.
89. Canioni D, Salles G, Mounier N, Brousse N, Keuppens M, Morchhauser F, Lamy T, Sonet A, Rousselet MC, Foussard C, Xerri L. High numbers of tumor-associated macrophages have an adverse prognostic value that can be circumvented by rituximab in patients with follicular lymphoma enrolled onto the GELA-GOELAMS FL-2000 trial. J Clin Oncol. 2008;26:440–6.
90. Edwards JP, Zhang X, Frauwirth KA, Mosser DM. Biochemical and functional characterization of three activated macrophage populations. J Leukoc Biol. 2006;80:1298–307.
91. Beum PV, Mack DA, Pawluczkowycz AW, Lindorfer MA, Taylor RP. Binding of rituximab, trastuzumab, cetuximab, or mAb T101 to cancer cells promotes trogocytosis mediated by THP-1 cells and monocytes. J Immunol. 2008;181:8120–32.
92. Jones JD, Hamilton BJ, Rigby WF. Rituximab mediates loss of CD19 on B cells in the absence of cell death. Arthritis Rheum. 2012;64:3111–8.

93. Beum PV, Lindorfer MA, Taylor RP. Within peripheral blood mononuclear cells, antibody-dependent cellular cytotoxicity of rituximab-opsonized Daudi cells is promoted by NK cells and inhibited by monocytes due to shaving. J Immunol. 2008;181:2916–24.
94. Boross P, Jansen JH, Pastula A, van der Poel CE, Leusen JH. Both activating and inhibitory Fc gamma receptors mediate rituximab-induced trogocytosis of CD20 in mice. Immunol Lett. 2012;143:44–52.
95. Pedersen AE, Jungersen MB, Pedersen CD. Monocytes mediate shaving of B-cell-bound anti-CD20 antibodies. Immunology. 2011;133:239–45.
96. Taylor RP, Lindorfer MA. Impact of low-dose rituximab on splenic B cells: evidence for the shaving reaction. Transpl Int. 2010;23:116–7.
97. O'Brien SM, Kantarjian H, Thomas DA, Giles FJ, Freireich EJ, Cortes J, Lerner S, Keating MJ. Rituximab dose-escalation trial in chronic lymphocytic leukemia. J Clin Oncol. 2001;19:2165–70.
98. Coiffier B, Lepretre S, Pedersen LM, Gadeberg O, Fredriksen H, van Oers MH, Wooldridge J, Kloczko J, Holowiecki J, Hellmann A, Walewski J, Flensburg M, Petersen J, Robak T. Safety and efficacy of ofatumumab, a fully human monoclonal anti-CD20 antibody, in patients with relapsed or refractory B-cell chronic lymphocytic leukemia: a phase 1–2 study. Blood. 2008;111:1094–100.
99. Stavenhagen JB, Gorlatov S, Tuaillon N, Rankin CT, Li H, Burke S, Huang L, Vijh S, Johnson S, Bonvini E, Koenig S. Fc optimization of therapeutic antibodies enhances their ability to kill tumor cells in vitro and controls tumor expansion in vivo via low-affinity activating Fcgamma receptors. Cancer Res. 2007;67:8882–90.
100. Stavenhagen JB, Gorlatov S, Tuaillon N, Rankin CT, Li H, Burke S, Huang L, Johnson S, Koenig S, Bonvini E. Enhancing the potency of therapeutic monoclonal antibodies via Fc optimization. Adv Enzyme Regul. 2008;48:152–64.
101. Shields RL, Namenuk AK, Hong K, Meng YG, Rae J, Briggs J, Xie D, Lai J, Stadlen A, Li B, Fox JA, Presta LG. High resolution mapping of the binding site on human IgG1 for Fc gamma RI, Fc gamma RII, Fc gamma RIII, and FcRn and design of IgG1 variants with improved binding to the Fc gamma R. J Biol Chem. 2001;276:6591–604.
102. Lazar GA, Dang W, Karki S, Vafa O, Peng JS, Hyun L, Chan C, Chung HS, Eivazi A, Yoder SC, Vielmetter J, Carmichael DF, Hayes RJ, Dahiyat BI. Engineered antibody Fc variants with enhanced effector function. Proc Natl Acad Sci USA. 2006;103:4005–10.
103. Horton HM, Bernett MJ, Pong E, Peipp M, Karki S, Chu SY, Richards JO, Vostiar I, Joyce PF, Repp R, Desjarlais JR, Zhukovsky EA. Potent in vitro and in vivo activity of an Fc-engineered anti-CD19 monoclonal antibody against lymphoma and leukemia. Cancer Res. 2008;68:8049–57.
104. Stavenhagen JB, Gorlatov S, Tuaillon N, Rankin CT, Li H, Burke S, Huang L, Vijh S, Johnson S, Bonvini E, Koenig S. Fc optimization of therapeutic antibodies enhances their ability to kill tumor cells in vitro and controls tumor expansion in vivo via low-affinity activating Fcgamma receptors. Cancer Res. 2007;67:8882–90.
105. Umana P, Jean-Mairet J, Moudry R, Amstutz H, Bailey JE. Engineered glycoforms of an antineuroblastoma IgG1 with optimized antibody-dependent cellular cytotoxic activity. Nat Biotechnol. 1999;17:176–80.
106. Shields RL, Lai J, Keck R, O'Connell LY, Hong K, Meng YG, Weikert SH, Presta LG. Lack of fucose on human IgG1 N-linked oligosaccharide improves binding to human Fcgamma RIII and antibody-dependent cellular toxicity. J Biol Chem. 2002;277:26733–40.
107. Shinkawa T, Nakamura K, Yamane N, Shoji-Hosaka E, Kanda Y, Sakurada M, Uchida K, Anazawa H, Satoh M, Yamasaki M, Hanai N, Shitara K. The absence of fucose but not the presence of galactose or bisecting N-acetylglucosamine of human IgG1 complex-type oligosaccharides shows the critical role of enhancing antibody-dependent cellular cytotoxicity. J Biol Chem. 2003;278:3466–73.
108. Mossner E, Brunker P, Moser S, Puntener U, Schmidt C, Herter S, Grau R, Gerdes C, Nopora A, van Puijenbroek E, Ferrara C, Sondermann P, Jäger C, Strein P, Fertig G, Friess T, Schüll C, Bauer S, Dal Porto J, Del Nagro C, Dabbagh K, Dyer MJ, Poppema S, Klein C,

Umaña P. Increasing the efficacy of CD20 antibody therapy through the engineering of a new type II anti-CD20 antibody with enhanced direct and immune effector cell-mediated B-cell cytotoxicity. Blood. 2010;115:4393–402.
109. Veri MC, Gorlatov S, Li H, Burke S, Johnson S, Stavenhagen J, Stein KE, Bonvini E, Koenig S. Monoclonal antibodies capable of discriminating the human inhibitory Fcgamma-receptor IIB (CD32B) from the activating Fcgamma-receptor IIA (CD32A): biochemical, biological and functional characterization. Immunology. 2007;121:392–404.
110. Rankin CT, Veri MC, Gorlatov S, Tuaillon N, Burke S, Huang L, Inzunza HD, Li H, Thomas S, Johnson S, Stavenhagen J, Koenig S, Bonvini E. CD32B, the human inhibitory Fc-gamma receptor IIB, as a target for monoclonal antibody therapy of B-cell lymphoma. Blood. 2006;108:2384–91.
111. Williams EL, Tutt AL, French RR, Chan HT, Lau B, Penfold CA, Mockridge CI, Roghanian A, Cox KL, Verbeek JS, Glennie MJ, Cragg MS. Development and characterisation of monoclonal antibodies specific for the murine inhibitory FcgammaRIIB (CD32B). Eur J Immunol. 2012;42:2109–20.
112. Lee CCM, Glennie M, Johnson P. Novel monoclonal antibody approaches to cancer immunotherapy. Br J Clinic Pharmacol, 2012.
113. White AL, Chan HT, Roghanian A, French RR, Mockridge CI, Tutt AL, Dixon SV, Ajona D, Verbeek JS, Al-Shamkhani A, Cragg MS, Beers SA, Glennie MJ. Interaction with FcgammaRIIB is critical for the agonistic activity of anti-CD40 monoclonal antibody. J Immunol. 2011;187:1754–63.
114. Li F, Ravetch JV. Inhibitory Fcgamma receptor engagement drives adjuvant and anti-tumor activities of agonistic CD40 antibodies. Science. 2011;333:1030–4.
115. Li F, Ravetch JV. Apoptotic and antitumor activity of death receptor antibodies require inhibitory Fcgamma receptor engagement. Proc Natl Acad Sci USA. 2012;109:10966–71.
116. Dhodapkar KM, Kaufman JL, Ehlers M, Banerjee DK, Bonvini E, Koenig S, Steinman RM, Ravetch JV, Dhodapkar MV. Selective blockade of inhibitory Fcgamma receptor enables human dendritic cell maturation with IL-12p70 production and immunity to antibody-coated tumor cells. Proc Natl Acad Sci USA. 2005;102:2910–5.
117. Desai DD, Harbers SO, Flores M, Colonna L, Downie MP, Bergtold A, Jung S, Clynes R. Fc{gamma} receptor IIB on dendritic cells enforces peripheral tolerance by inhibiting effector T cell responses. J Immunol. 2007;178:6217–26.
118. Dhodapkar KM, Banerjee D, Connolly J, Kukreja A, Matayeva E, Veri MC, Ravetch JV, Steinman RM, Dhodapkar MV. Selective blockade of the inhibitory Fcgamma receptor (FcgammaRIIB) in human dendritic cells and monocytes induces a type I interferon response program. J Exp Med. 2007;204:1359–69.

Understanding the Mechanisms of Resistance to Rituximab: Paving the Road for the Development of Therapeutic Strategies to Overcome Rituximab-Resistance

Francisco J. Hernandez-Ilizaliturri and Myron S. Czuczman

Abstract Rituximab-resistance is an emerging challenge for both the scientific community and the practicing oncologist. Parallel to the improvement clinic outcomes, the incorporation of rituximab into the management of patients with B-cell lymphoma appears to be changing the biology of relapsed/refractory disease. At least in the patients with diffuse large B-cell lymphoma (DLBCL), previously established salvage rituximab-chemotherapy-based treatments [including high dose chemotherapy and autologous stem cell support (HDC-ASCS)] are less effective in patients failing rituximab immunochemotherapy induction. The estimated 3-year failure free survival in previously treated R-CHOP DLBCL following HDC-ASCT is only 33 %, stressing the need to: (1) understand the mechanisms responsible for rituximab-resistance, (2) identify cellular pathways playing a pivotal role in acquired resistance and (3) develop novel therapeutic strategies to overcome or circumvent rituximab-resistance in B-cell lymphoma. Pre-clinical models to study rituximab-resistance have been generated and characterized. Moreover, repeated exposure of lymphoma cells to rituximab, not only results in a decrease in rituximab anti-tumor activity, but also cross-resistance to multiple chemotherapy agents (suggesting shared pathways of resistance). Insightful information regarding the biological basis for rituximab-resistance is paving the next generation of clinical trials evaluating novel monoclonal antibodies, immunoconjugates, and/or targeted agents aimed at blocking key-regulatory proteins associated with acquired resistance. Here, we provide a general overview of the mechanisms associated with rituximab-resistance that have been identified so far and review some of the early therapeutic interventions being tested in pre-clinical models and in early clinical trials for patients with rituximab-resistant B-cell lymphoma.

F. J. Hernandez-Ilizaliturri · M. S. Czuczman (✉)
Departments of Immunology and Medical Oncology, Roswell Park Cancer Institute,
Elm and Carlton Streets, Buffalo, NY 14263, USA
e-mail: myron.czuczman@roswellpark.org

B. Bonavida (ed.), *Resistance to Immunotherapeutic Antibodies in Cancer*,
Resistance to Targeted Anti-Cancer Therapeutics 2, DOI: 10.1007/978-1-4614-7654-2_4,

Keywords Rituximab-resistance · B-lymphoma · FcR polymorphism · Signal pathways · Ofatumumab

Abbreviations

ADCC	Antibody-dependent cellular cytotoxicity
BIR	Baculoviral IAP repeat
CARD	Caspase activating and recruitment domain
CMC	Complement-mediated cytotoxicity
DLBCL	Diffuse large B-cell lymphoma
ESHAP	Etoposide, methylprednisolone, cytarabine and cisplatin
FcγRIIA CD32	Fcγ receptor IIA
FcR	Fc receptors
GA101	Obinutuzumab
HDC-ASCS	High dose chemotherapy and autologous stem cell support
MCL	Mantle cell lymphomas
NHL	Non-Hodgkin lymphoma
R	Rituximab
RING zinc-finger	RING
RRCL	Rituximab-resistant cell lines

Introduction: Acknowledging that B-Cell Lymphoma Cells are Capable of Developing Rituximab Resistance

Acquirement of resistance by cancer cells hinders the clinical outcome in a significant number of patients with non-Hodgkin lymphoma (NHL). Approximately 66,360 new non-Hodgkin lymphoma (NHL) cases and 19,320 deaths were estimated in the United States last year [1]. The early use of rituximab (R) as a single agent or in combination with various systemic chemotherapy regimens [i.e. cyclophosphamide, vincristine and prednisone (CVP), or cyclophosphamide, doxorubicin, vincristine and prednisone (CHOP)] have resulted in improved response-rates, duration of remission and improved overall survival (OS) in patients with follicular lymphoma (FL) [2, 3] and (with R-CHOP) in diffuse large B-cell lymphoma (DLBCL) [4–12].

In an attempt to improve the clinical outcomes of patients with B-cell lymphoma, rituximab extended dose-schedule regimens (i.e. maintenance regimens) had been prospectively tested and reported in the following clinical scenarios: (a) following rituximab single agent therapy in upfront/relapsed low-grade lymphomas; (b) following systemic chemotherapy or chemo-immunotherapy in patients with relapsed/refractory B-cell indolent lymphoma; (c) previously untreated FL patients upon completion of systemic chemotherapy (CVP) therapy;

(d) previously untreated diffuse large B-cell lymphoma; and, in (e) relapsed/refractory mantle cell lymphomas (MCL) [11, 13–16]. The efficacy of rituximab maintenance varied within a given clinical trial. The general consensus is that the extended use of rituximab may produce some degree of clinical benefit (primarily improvement in response rates and time-to-progression), but its use has not been associated with an improved OS in patients with B-cell lymphoma treated with upfront rituximab-based immunochemotherapy. Moreover, the indiscriminate use of rituximab maintenance raises the potential risk for the development of rituximab-resistance [17–19].

Based on simple laws that govern evolutionary biology, the emergence of resistance was an anticipated concern early in the development of rituximab. However, it was not until recently that rituximab-resistance has become more clinically relevant. The development of the clinical consequences of rituximab-resistance varies depending on histological subtypes of B-cell lymphoma. Perhaps the growth rate associated with each specific subtype of B-cell lymphoma affects the "speed" in which rituximab-resistance is clinically manifested. In other words, the effects of acquired resistance to rituximab may be less obvious in patients with indolent subtypes (i.e. FL) than in patients with aggressive B-cell lymphoma (i.e. DLBCL or MCL).

As rituximab changed the treatment paradigm of patients with DLBCL, it has been postulated that the current subset of patients with refractory or relapsed DLBCL represents a different patient population to the one studied in pre-rituximab clinical trials. Several investigators questioned if the response to second line chemotherapy or the value of high dose chemotherapy and autologous stem cell support (HDC-ASCS) in patients with relapsed or primary refractory DLBCL previously treated with R-CHOP had decreased when compared to historical controls. Dr. Martin on behalf of the Grupo Espanol de Linfomas/Transplante Autologo de Medula Osea (GEL/TAMO) reported results from a retrospective analysis in the outcome of patients with DLBCL evaluating the influence of rituximab in response rate to rituximab in combination with etoposide, methylprednisolone, cytarabine and cisplatin (ESHAP) as salvage therapy [20]. Martin and colleagues studied 163 consecutive patients with relapsed/refractory DLBCL who received R-ESHAP as second line therapy, 94 patients were previously treated with rituximab-chemotherapy (R+ group) in the front line setting and 69 patients received only chemotherapy alone (R− group). The response rates were higher in patients who were not previously exposed to rituximab in a univariate analysis but not in a multivariate analysis. The overall response and complete rates to R-ESHAP were 67 and 37 % for DLBCL previously treated with rituximab-CHOP versus 81 and 56 % for patients previously treated with CHOP ($P = 0.045$, $P = 0.015$), respectively. In addition, the PFS and OS at 3 years were significantly higher for the patients in the R− group (57 and 64 %) when compared to those patients in the R+ group (38 and 17 %), respectively; ($P < 0.0001$ and $P = 0.0005$). Of note, the same percentage of patients in both groups subsequently underwent HDC-ASCS. In a multivariate analysis, prior exposure to rituximab was found to be a negative prognostic indicator for PFS and OS [20].

The need to develop novel salvage regimens following rituximab-CHOP failures was further confirmed prospectively by the results of the multicenter phase III Collaborative trial in Relapsed Aggressive Lymphoma (CORAL) study. The CORAL investigators demonstrated that prior rituximab exposure in the frontline setting negatively affected the event free survival (EFS) (34 vs. 66 %, $P < 0.001$) [21]. Moreover, the complete remission (CR) rate in R-CHOP pre-treated patients to either R-ICE or R-DHAP was only 38 % [21, 22].

Scientific efforts must now be focused not only in defining the pathways by which lymphoma cells evade immunochemotherapy, but also in developing novel therapeutic strategies to overcome it. In an attempt to define the mechanisms of rituximab-resistance and to develop strategies to overcome it, we developed a rituximab-resistant cell-line model and found that the acquirement of rituximab-resistance also leads to resistance to multiple chemotherapy agents commonly used to treat B-cell lymphoma [17, 18]. *Our preclinical data demonstrate the development of therapy resistance and simulate what was observed clinically in the CORAL study; it also suggests the possible existence of shared pathway(s) of resistance to both biological and chemotherapeutic agents.*

The emergence of rituximab-resistance is an anticipated clinical problem that will likely increase in incidence as a consequence from the repeated exposure of B-cell lymphoma patients to this mAb. A better understanding of the mechanisms responsible for acquired resistance to rituximab will most likely aid in the development of novel therapeutic strategies to improve clinical outcomes of relapsed/refractory B-cell lymphoma patients in the post-rituximab era. In this chapter, we present an overview of the mechanisms associated with rituximab-resistance and outline potential therapeutic targets/pathways for drug development in an attempt to overcome or circumvent rituximab- resistance.

Rituximab Mechanism(s)-of-Action

Rituximab was the first mAb approved for the treatment of B-cell lymphomas by the U.S. Federal Drug Administration (FDA). Rituximab is an IgG1 chimeric monoclonal antibody (mAb) composed of murine variable regions from the anti-CD20 antibody 2B8 that are linked to human constant regions (Fc) directed against the CD20 antigen. Several biological effects had been postulated to contribute to rituximab's primary mechanism(s)-of-action, including: antibody-dependent cellular cytotoxicity (ADCC), complement-mediated cytotoxicity (CMC), and induction of apoptosis/anti-proliferation. Recently, a "vaccinal" effect has been described as an additional potential mechanism of rituximab anti-tumor activity (especially in the re-treatment setting). It has been demonstrated that rituximab facilitates the uptake and presentation of antigens by dendritic cells to T-cells and elucidates an adaptive immune response against B-cell antigens [23]. Rituximab-associated biological activity is dependent on several factors: (1) CD20 antigen density expression; (2) cellular pathways driving the underlying lymphoma;

(3) pharmacokinetics/pharmacodynamics; (4) tumor burden; and (5) status of the host innate [i.e. complement system proteins, neutrophils, natural killer (NK) cells, and macrophages] or adaptive [i.e. antigen presenting cells (APCs) and T-cells] immune system.

A major area of research has been the study of intracellular signals that results in apoptosis of lymphoma cells following binding of rituximab to the CD20 antigen and factors associated with the activation of the innate immune system [24–35]. Exposure of lymphoma cells to rituximab results in the activation of Src-family protein tyrosine kinases, leading to phosphorylation of the PLCγ2 and increase in cytoplasmic Ca++ [25–31]. These early signal transduction events activate caspase 3 to promote apoptotic cell death of NHL B-cells [31]. In addition, in vitro exposure of lymphoma cell lines to rituximab is associated with a sustained phosphorylation of p-38-MAP, JNK, and ERK kinases [32]. Stabilization of CD20 into lipid rafts following rituximab exposure within the cell membrane plays an important role in signal transduction events leading to apoptosis in cancer cells (i.e. Ca++ influx) [36–38]. Additionally, several in vitro studies have demonstrated that rituximab can sensitize cells to the action of chemotherapeutic agents by affecting cellular signaling via down-regulation of Bcl-2, thus sensitizing cells to apoptotic stimuli [39].

Host-dependent factors influencing the anti-tumor activity of rituximab. In contrast to traditional chemotherapy agents, the biological activity of rituximab depends not only on the cancer cell, but also on the tumor microenvironment (e.g. immune-effector cells) [34, 35]. One of the most well characterized mechanisms-of-action of rituximab is ADCC. Once rituximab binds to its CD20 epitope, effector cells recognize the rituximab constant region (Fc) portion via the Fc receptors (FcR). FcR (CD16 and CD64 and to a lesser degree CD32) possesses several functions that affect rituximab activity observed in B-cell lymphoma. Monocytes, macrophages and NK cells kill target cells mainly by phagocytosis. In addition, NK-cells can also induce B-cell NHL cell lysis through the release of perforin and granzyme-B or by apoptosis after the induction of Fas Ligand signaling [40]. It has been demonstrated that FcγRIII receptor expression is necessary to eradicate NHL in a murine animal model [35].

Genetic polymorphisms in the *FCGR3A* gene which encodes FcγRIIIA with either a phenylalanine (F) or a valine (V) at amino acid position 158 or in the FCGR2A which encodes a Fcγ receptor IIA (FcγRIIA)(CD32) with either a histidine (H) 131 or arginine (R) at amino acid position 131 had been associated with differences in the anti-tumor activity of single-agent rituximab in patients with follicular cell lymphoma [41, 42]. Indolent B-cell lymphoma patients with the FCGR3A-158 V/V and/or FCGR2A-131 H/H appear to have higher responsiveness to single-agent rituximab [41, 42]. The differences in rituximab responses have been correlated to the binding affinity to IgG1 and the absolute number of CD16 receptors per effector cell (macrophages and NK cells) which ultimately influences the ability of effector cells to induce ADCC [43].

These data stress the importance of ADCC in rituximab anti-tumor activity as a single agent. The role of ADCC in regimens combining systemic chemotherapy and rituximab is less defined. The correlation between the FCGR3A polymorphism versus the therapeutic response to rituximab seems to be essentially lost when rituximab is combined with chemotherapy [44–46]. In contrast to what was observed by other investigators, Kim et al. demonstrated that gene polymorphisms in the *FCGR*3 gene correlated with higher complete response (CR) rates in patients with DLBCL treated with R-CHOP. The response rate for patients carrying the FCGR3-158 V/V or -158 V/F was higher (88 and 78 %, respectively) than seen in patients with the FCGR3-158 F/F genotype (50 %; $P = 0.002$), there were no differences in term of OS or EFS. Moreover, in this patient population genetic polymorphisms in the *FCGR*2 gene did not affect the outcome following treatment with R-CHOP or CHOP [47]. As noted with effector cells, host complement components may affect rituximab activity in pre-clinical models and in B-cell lymphoma patients [48, 49].

Definition and Incidence of Rituximab-Resistance

Data from early clinical studies evaluating the anti-tumor activity of single-agent rituximab in previously treated or untreated indolent lymphoma have demonstrated a response rate ranging from 46 to 67 % [14, 50, 51]. Re-treatment upon progression results in an overall response rate of 40 % by strict response criteria [51]. Based on this information, clinicians can estimate that ~30 % of previously untreated indolent lymphoma patients exhibit some degree of rituximab-resistance. However, the concurrent administration of systemic chemotherapy, the response criteria utilized to measure response (Cheson criteria versus Waterfall charts), and the utilization of extended schedules of rituximab introduce additional bias in determining whose patients are truly rituximab resistant.

> Adding to the complexity of the rituximab-resistance, B-cell lymphoma patients that exhibit innate rituximab-resistance may be different than rituximab-responding patients that eventually acquired rituximab-resistance over time at a cellular/molecular level.

The accurate incidence of rituximab-resistance is difficult to estimate as it is affected by: (1) the lack of an universally accepted definition of the term "rituximab-resistance"; (2) the diverse factors driving the proliferation rate and survival of various B-cell lymphoma subtypes; and (3) the concurrent administration of systemic chemotherapy, radiation or other biological agents (i.e. cytokines, immunomodulatory agents, etc.). In an attempt to better characterize the incidence and mechanism(s) of rituximab-resistance, scientists have accepted the definition of rituximab-resistance as "a lack of response to, progression during or within 6 months of treatment with a rituximab-containing regimen". Long-term follow-up data from prospective clinical trials evaluating the role of rituximab maintenance in the management of indolent [i.e. Primary Rituximab And Maintenance (PRIMA) and ECOG 4402: Rituximab Extended Schedule or Retreatment Trial (RESORT) studies] or relapsed/refractory aggressive lymphoma (e.g. rituximab maintenance in MCL patients) may aid in determining the actual incidence of rituximab-resistance in B-cell lymphoma patients.

Phenotypic Changes Associated with Rituximab-Resistance

A. *Changes in CD20 Antigen*:

Changes in CD20 antigen density or structure have been reported in rituximab-resistant cell lines and in a limited number of patients with rituximab-resistant B-cell NHL [48, 52, 53]. Initial reports of CD20 loss were based on primarily case reports [54, 55]. Down-regulation of CD20 has been observed in patients with relapsed/refractory B-cell lymphoma following prior rituximab therapy [56–58].

In an attempt to further define if acquired rituximab resistance affected CD20 expression, several investigators established rituximab-resistant cell lines (RRCL) [17, 59]. Similar to observations made by other investigators, we demonstrated that the repeated exposure of lymphoma cells to rituximab resulted in CD20 down-regulation and a decrease in rituximab-associated biological activity [17, 52, 53, 56, 60].

Based on initial studies, it appears that CD20 surface expression is a limiting step for rituximab activity. van Meerten et al. [61] demonstrated a linear correlation between rituximab-CMC and CD20 expression in CD20 transfected T-cells and in malignant cells isolated from patients with chronic lymphocytic leukemia (CLL). In contrast, no correlation was observed between CD20 levels and rituximab-associated ADCC in the same pre-clinical model [61]. Using RRCL we recently defined a CD20 surface expression "threshold" (i.e. 150 CD20-FITC per μm^2) necessary for effective rituximab-CMC [60]. However, this observation has not been validated in more clinically relevant models (e.g. primary tumor cells derived from lymphoma patients).

The mechanism(s) responsible for changes in CD20 expression observed in rituximab-resistant lymphomas are poorly defined. A limiting factor in understanding CD20 regulation in normal B-cells is the absence of immunological defects in CD20-knockout mouse models [62]. Recently, a group of investigators reported the case of a pediatric patient lacking CD20 expression in B-cells showing signs/symptoms compatible with immunodeficiency which has awakened the scientific community to study the function and regulation of CD20 in normal B-cell differentiation in more detail [63]. Several transcription factors regulating the CD20 promoter (and thereby CD20 expression) in B-cells have been identified [PU.1/Pip complex; other basic helix-loop-helix-zipper family of transcription factors (such as USF, TFE3, and octamer protein 2)] [64].

On the other hand, the mechanism(s) by which CD20 expression is altered in rituximab-resistant lymphomas are largely unknown. Taylor and colleagues demonstrated the concept of "CD20 shaving" by effector cells that expressed FcγR [65]; recent data from Beers and colleagues showed internalization of CD20 into lysosomes after rituximab binding [66]. Terui et al. [53] demonstrated that a subset of patients with rituximab-resistant B-cell lymphoma has a point mutation in the CD20 gene (leading to the formation of truncated forms of CD20 lacking the C-terminal region). In addition, Henry et al. [67] identified an alternative CD20 transcript variant in B-cell malignancies coding for a truncated protein associated with rituximab-resistance. This group of investigators initially identified an alternatively spliced CD20 mRNA coding for a truncated form of CD20 in primary tumor cells isolated from patients with DLBCL, FL, and marginal zone lymphoma (MZL) as well as in several B-cell lymphoma cell lines. Subsequently, they generated several rituximab-resistant cell lines by exposing Raji and Ramos cells to escalating doses of rituximab. The alternative spliced CD20 mRNA was not only present in the rituximab-resistant cells generated, but its expression correlated with rituximab exposure [67].

In contrast to what was reported by Terui et al. and Henry et al., we found a global downregulation in the CD20 mRNA and no CD20 gene mutations affecting the primary structure of CD20. Moreover, we could not find changes in the CD20 mRNA stability in our RRCL to explain the low CD20 mRNA levels observed. In contrast, we recently demonstrated that RRCL had a lower CD20 promoter activity and/or a defect impairing the transport of CD20 from the intracellular compartment to the cell surface membrane [60].

Therapeutic strategies to target B-cell lymphomas with altered CD20 structure/ expression levels can be divided in the following categories: (1) new generation of anti-CD20 mAbs antibodies with higher binding capacity and/or re-engineered FC regions facilitating a more efficient ADCC than rituximab (ofatumumab or GA-101) [68, 69]; or (2) re-expression of CD20 antigen by altering its epigenetic regulation using pharmacological inhibitors.

Novel mAbs targeting CD20 are currently being evaluated in pre-clinical models and clinical trials. Obinutuzumab (GA101) is a fully humanized type II anti-CD20 antibody that has been glyco-engineered to exhibit a 50-fold increase in binding affinity to the FcγRIII receptors of effector cells and inducing a higher degree of ADCC [69]. Ofatumumab is a fully human mAb targeting a unique CD20 epitope closer to the cell membrane and capable of more efficiently activating the complement cascade compared to rituximab. Our group demonstrated that ofatumumab was more effective in elucidating CMC than rituximab in vitro and was more effective in controlling in vivo lymphoma growth than rituximab [68]. Moreover, we demonstrated that ofatumumab activity was preserved even at low CD20 levels and thus may represent an attractive strategy to use in rituximab-resistant lymphoma patients.

Early clinical trials of ofatumumab and obinutuzumab (GA101) in relapsed/ refractory indolent lymphoma and CLL have demonstrated encouraging results and activity in patients with rituximab-resistant lymphoid malignancies (Table 1) [70–73]. Ofatumumab, a potent mAB approved by the FDA for the treatment of recurrent/refractory CLL, was also prospectively evaluated in rituximab-refractory indolent B-lymphoma. Czuczman et al., reported the results of 116 rituximab-refractory indolent lymphoma patients (27 patients were refractory to rituximab

Table 1 Clinical studies evaluating novel anti-CD20 monoclonal antibodies in relapsed/refractory B-cell lymphoid malignancies

Author	Design	Study schema	Population	ORR	TTP/PFS
Czuczman et al. [71]	Phase I	Ofatumumab weekly × 8	RR N = 116	11 % for all pts.	TTP = 5.8 months
		Initial dose 300 mg		22 % for rituximab single agent refractory	PFS = 9.1 months
		Cohorts: 500 and 1,000 mg			
Salles et al. [70]	Phase I	Obinutuzumab every 21 days for 8 cycles	Rel/ref B-cell NHL N = 21	33 % in all pts.	NR
		[a]Dose-escalation (range 100–2,000 mg)	RR = 9 (43 %)	22 % in RR pts.	
Sehn et al. [73]	Phase I	Obinutuzumab weekly × 4.	Rel/ref NHL or CLL	23 % in all pts.	3–21 months
		[a]Dose range (400–2,000 mg)	N = 22		
		Responding patients received ObM every 3 m for 8 infusions	RR = 13 (68 %)		
Ogura et al. [72]	Phase I	Obinutuzumab every 21 days for 8 cycles	Rel/ref B-cell NHL	58 %	NR
		[b]Dose escalation (400–2,000 mg)	N = 12		
			RR = 2/12		

[a] The first dose of obinutuzumab was reduced in each cohort. [b] The first cycle of obinutuzmab included a reduced dose on day +1 and a second full tested dose on day +8. *ORR* overall response rate, *CR* complete remission, *PR* partial remission, *TTP* time to progression, *PFS* progression free survival, *RR* rituximab-refractory, *Rel/ref* relapsed/refractory, *NHL* non-Hodgkin's lymphoma, *CLL* chronic lymphocytic leukemia, *ObM* obinutuzumab maintenance, *NR* not reported

monotherapy, 45 to rituximab maintenance therapy, and 44 were refractory to rituximab-chemotherapy combination therapy) treated with 8 weekly infusions of ofatumumab at two dose-groups (500 or 1,000 mg) (first dose was 300 mg in all patients). While the antibody was well tolerable, its activity was modest at best (11 %); the overall response rate (ORR) was 10 % in the 1,000 mg group (1 CR and 8 PR) and 13 % in the 500 mg group (2 CRu and 2 PR) and the progression free survival (PFS) was ~6 months [71].

Salles et al. conducted the first multicenter, phase I study evaluating the safety, tolerability, pharmacokinetics, and clinical activity of escalating doses of single-agent obinutuzumab in patients with relapsed/refractory B-cell NHL (indolent and aggressive subtypes were included). Eligible patients received a fix dose of o-binutuzumab every 21 days for 8 cycles (dose range 100, 200, 400, 800, 1,200 and 2,000 mg cohort groups). In each cohort, the first dose of obinutuzumab was reduced by 50 % (first 4 cohorts) or adjusted (reduced to 800 and 1,200 mg in the 1,200 mg and 2,000 mg cohort, respectively) to prevent infusion-related toxicities. Based on pharmacokinetic data generated, a 7th cohort was treated with a loading antibody dose of 1,600 mg followed by 7 weekly infusions of obinutuzumab at 800 mg [70]. While obinutuzumab was well tolerable, unexpected grade 3–4 neutropenia (33 %) was observed triggering the need for further studies to define the role of Fc receptors in anti-CD20 (rituximab or obinutuzumab)-mediated neutropenia. The response rate at the end of treatment was 33 % (all responses were FL patients). Two out of 9 rituximab-refractory patients responded to obinutuzumab [70].

Sehn et al. reported the results of a similar phase I study, evaluating obinutuzumab in refractory B-cell lymphoma and CLL (N = 22; 13 were considered rituximab-resistant). Obinutuzumab was administered as a four weekly intravenous infusions during induction therapy. Patients with a CR or PR at the end of induction were eligible to receive extended therapy with obinutuzumab every 3 months for a maximum of 8 infusions, until disease progression or unacceptable toxicity [73]. Objective responses were observed in 23 % of the patients (all PRs). Only 8 patients received maintenance therapy and the best response during this phase was 32 %. As previously observed, neutropenia was observed in 23 % of the patients [73]. Recently, a Japanese phase I clinical trial evaluated obinutuzumab in relapsed/refractory indolent B-cell lymphoma. Dose-escalation and design were similar to other obinutuzumab phase I studies without a maintenance phase [70]. In contrast, significant anti-tumor activity was observed in 58 % of the patients (CR 17 % and PR 42 %) [72]. While 100 % of the patients in this clinical trial had previously received rituximab, it is unclear how many patients were rituximab-refractory/resistant. Additional studies in indolent subtypes of B-cell lymphoma are necessary to further delineate the therapeutic effect of obinutuzumab in rituximab-resistant B-cell lymphoma.

An alternative to re-engineering anti-CD20 mAbs, the ability to increase surface CD20 antigen expression is a theoretically attractive strategy to overcome rituximab- resistance. Re-expressing CD20 antigen in rituximab-resistant cells has been a more challenging enterprise. A better understanding in the mechanisms that regulate CD20 antigen expression is likely to someday contribute to the eventual development of novel therapeutic strategies to overcome low CD20 surface antigen density someday. Several factors can affect CD20 promoter activity, such as the presence of regulatory transcription factors and their methylation/acetylation status. "Pharmacologic strategies" to increase CD20 promoter activity can potentially lead to clinically applicable strategies to restore rituximab-sensitivity in rituximab-resistant lymphomas. The use of IL-4 has been shown to modulate CD20 expression in various B-cell lymphoma cell lines [74]. In our RRCL, in vitro exposure to IL-4 increased CD20 promoter activity, CD20 antigen expression and enhanced rituximab activity. Similar findings were found in a subset of primary tumor cells isolated from patients with B-cell lymphoma [60]. IL-4-mediated increase in the CD20 promoter activity was observed in CD20 promoter fragments containing positive or negative regulatory binding sites, suggesting that IL-4 effects may be mediated by altering the expression or structure of regulatory transcription factors [60]. Epigenetic regulation of CD20 is another area of active research. Recently, Shimuzi et al. increased CD20 antigen levels by using two histone deactylase inhibitors (HDAC) (romidepsin and valproic acid) resulting in an improvement in rituximab activity both in vitro and in vivo [75].

B. *Changes in other surface antigens*: *Upregulation of complement inhibitory proteins* (*CIP*) *versus rituximab activity*. Given the multiple mechanism(s)-of-action of rituximab (i.e. CMC, ADCC and/or apoptosis), the overall clinical relevance of variable CD20 surface antigen expression on lymphoma cells in vivo is difficult to fully ascertain. We accomplished the forced expression of CD20 antigen without significantly improving the activity of rituximab in RRCL, suggesting the presence of additional factors influencing rituximab activity in rituximab-resistant models [60]. Surface levels of CIPs (CD46, CD55 and CD59) had been described to impact rituximab-mediated CMC [76]. Moreover, upregulation of CD55 and CD59 had been described in rituximab-resistant cell line models [17].
C. *Signaling pathways that play a role in the acquirement of rituximab-resistance*. Rituximab binding to CD20 results in several signaling events leading to programed cell death (PCD, apoptosis) in lymphoma cells. Apoptosis essential for the development and maintenance of the mammalian immune system [77] and is a tightly regulated cellular process that is often disrupted in neoplasms, including B-cell lymphoma. Bcl-2 was the first protein involved in regulating apoptosis that was determined to be an oncogene [78, 79]. Over the last two decades, scientists had identified and characterized the structure and/or function of several regulatory proteins of apoptosis, known as the Bcl-2 family proteins. Aberrant expression of Bcl-2 family members may lead to an increase in the apoptotic threshold of cancer cells and is associated with chemotherapy resistance which may explain limited rituximab anti-tumor activity seen in some subsets of refractory NHL [80–86]. Several groups of investigators, including our group, have demonstrated that the chronic exposure of B-cell

lymphoma cell lines to rituximab results in a deregulation of several members of the Bcl-2 family of proteins leading not only to rituximab-resistance, but also concomitant resistance to various chemotherapeutic agents [17, 18, 59].

These findings suggest the existence of common shared resistance pathways between chemotherapy agents and monoclonal antibodies targeting CD20, and strongly suggest the importance of Bcl-2 family members in the biology of relapsed/refractory B-cell lymphoma. Furthermore, these findings support our hypothesis that targeting Bcl-2 family members may prove to be a valuable strategy to overcome or circumvent rituximab-chemotherapy resistance. Almost a decade ago, the use of BCL-2 oligonucleotides targeting endogenous Bcl-2, G3139 (i.e. oblimersen sodium), was explored in pre-clinical lymphoma models [87, 88]. Our group of investigators demonstrated that in vitro or in vivo exposure of lymphoma cells to G3139 resulted in Bcl-2 down-regulation and potentiated the anti-tumor activity of rituximab [88]. Subsequently, clinical trials evaluated the anti-tumor activity of BCL-2 anti-sense oligonucleotides in patients with relapsed/refractory CLL or melanoma [89, 90]. The results from such trials were rather disappointing and led scientists to develop alternative ways to target Bcl-2 family members. Several compounds that mimic the binding site of the BH3 single domain proteins have been developed and had been evaluated in pre-clinical and clinical studies, particularly in the rituximab-refractory setting (i.e. ABT-269 and Obatoclax) [91, 92]. Despite evident anti-tumor activity in patients with hematological malignancies, the development of BH3-mimetics had been hindered by unanticipated CNS and/or hematological toxicities (e.g. thrombocytopenia) observed in clinical trials. This furthers the need to develop novel agents altering the apoptotic threshold of cancer cells. IAPs, a family of endogenous caspase inhibitors, are highly conserved throughout evolution and comprise the human analogues XIAP, cIAP1, cIAP2, survivin, apollon and livin (ML-IAP). The IAP family of proteins contains three conserved structural motifs, the baculoviral IAP repeat (BIR), the RING (RING zinc-finger) and the Caspase Activating and Recruitment Domain (CARD). Of the mammalian IAP proteins known to be involved in apoptosis, XIAP has been characterized most extensively, which contains three BIR domains and a C-terminal RING motif. The second and third BIR domains of XIAP are potent inhibitors of caspase-3/-7 and caspase-9, respectively, via distinct mechanisms. The linker segment preceding the BIR2 domain binds to the active site of effector caspase-3 or -7, thereby preventing substrate binding and subsequent catalysis. IAPs are expressed at high levels in many human cancers, which have been associated with treatment resistance and dismal prognosis. Since IAPs block apoptosis at the core of the apoptotic machinery by the activation of caspases, therapeutics targeting IAPs are an attractive choice in the treatment of resistant lymphomas and preliminary work utilizing IAP inhibitors appears promising.

Applying cDNA microarray technology, we screened a total of 11,519 genes for changes between rituximab-sensitive cell lines (RSCL) and RRCL. Our studies demonstrated that significant changes in expression of genes occur in rituximab-resistant cells when compared to their rituximab-sensitive parental cells. A total of 148 genes were found to be upregulated in Raji-2R cells and 365 genes in the Raji-4RH cells when compared to the Raji parental cell line. In addition, down-regulation of 10 genes (2R cells) and 23 genes (4RH) were detected in rituximab-resistant cells, respectively. Common genetic changes were observed between the 2R and 4RH cell lines. In addition to deregulation of the Bcl-2 family members, we observed that rituximab-resistant cell lines upregulated IAP genes as determined by gene expression profiling studies [17]. As aforementioned, IAP inhibitors may be potentially effective future agents used in rituximab-chemotherapy resistant lymphoma.

Contributing to the de-regulation of the Bcl-2 family members, an increase in components of the ubiquitin-proteasome system was associated with increased degradation of pro-apoptotic Bcl-2 family members (i.e. Bax); an increase in NF-κB activity was also observed in pre-clinical models of rituximab-resistance [18, 59]. Pharmacological inhibition of the proteasome results in: (1) decrease NF-κB activity and (2) accumulation of Bax, thus, decreasing the apoptotic threshold to chemotherapy drugs in rituximab-chemotherapy-resistant cell lines. While single-agent bortezomib has limited activity against aggressive B-cell lymphoma, meaningful clinical activity in relapsed/refractory DLBCL was seen when it was combined with systemic chemotherapy [93]. Ongoing clinical studies are testing if bortezomib or 2nd-generation proteasome inhibitors (e.g. carfilzomib) can re-sensitize resistant lymphomas to the cytotoxic effects of rituximab-chemotherapy regimens in the relapsed/refractory setting.

Concluding Remarks

While significant clinical improvements had been achieved by the introduction of mAbs in the management of B-cell lymphoma, this progress has also resulted in new challenges for scientists and practicing oncologists. Lymphoma cells are adapting to rituximab-based therapies and the acquirement of resistance is now an increasing clinical problem. Ongoing scientific translational research studies are providing some insightful information on potentially molecular mechanisms that may play a role in the development of rituximab-resistance. The identification of several key factors affecting rituximab activity (i.e. down-regulation of CD20, upregulation of CIPs, etc.) or de-regulation of intracellular signaling pathways regulatory proteins (i.e. ubiquitin-proteasome system, Bcl-2 family members, or IAPs) upon the development of rituximab-resistance is paving the road for the development of therapeutic strategies in an attempt to overcome or circumvent rituximab-resistance (see Fig. 1). It is important to continue the study of additional genetic/protein changes that translate into phenotypic variations associated with reduction/loss of rituximab-associated anti-tumor activity. The identification and functional characterization of such proteins is fundamental for the future design of effective therapeutic interventions for relapsed/refractory lymphoma patients. In

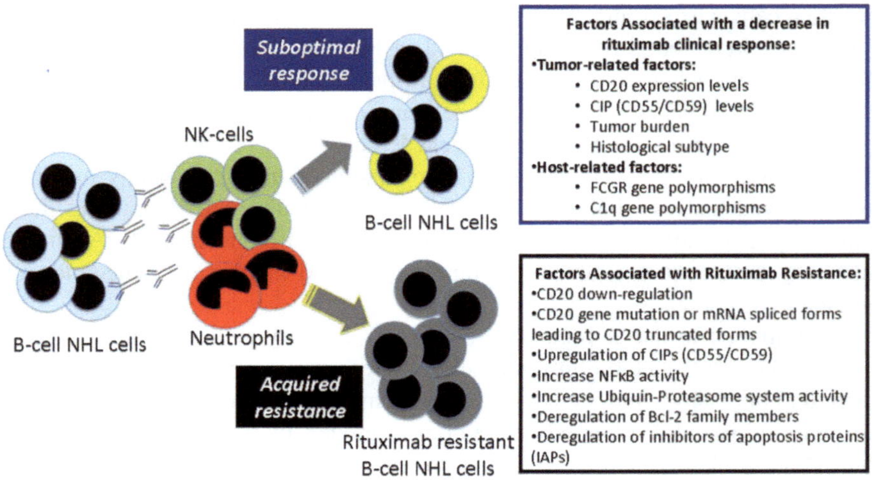

Fig. 1 Factors influencing rituximab activity and identified mechanisms of resistance to rituximab in pre-clinical models and/or lymphoma patients. *NHL* non-Hodgkin's lymphoma, *NK* natural killer, *CIPS* complement inhibitory proteins

addition, carefully planned clinical studies will be necessary to optimally evaluate novel therapeutic strategies against rituximab-resistant B-cell NHL.

Acknowledgments Supported by NIH grant R01 CA136907-01A1 awarded to Roswell Park Cancer Institute.

Conflict of Interest
No potential conflicts of interest were disclosed.

References

1. Siegel R, Ward E, Brawley O, Jemal A. Cancer statistics, 2011: the impact of eliminating socioeconomic and racial disparities on premature cancer deaths. CA Cancer J Clin. 2011;61:212–36.
2. Fisher RI, LeBlanc M, Press OW, Maloney DG, Unger JM, Miller TP. New treatment options have changed the survival of patients with follicular lymphoma. J Clin Oncol. 2005;23:8447–52.
3. Liu Q, Fayad L, Cabanillas F, Hagemeister FB, Ayers GD, Hess M, Romaguera J, Rodriguez MA, Tsimberidou AM, Verstovsek S, Younes A, Pro B, Lee MS, Ayala A, McLaughlin P. Improvement of overall and failure-free survival in stage IV follicular lymphoma: 25 years of treatment experience at The University of Texas M.D. Anderson Cancer Center. J Clin Oncol. 2006;24:1582–9.
4. Piro LD, White CA, Grillo-Lopez AJ, Janakiraman N, Saven A, Beck TM, Varns C, Shuey S, Czuczman M, Lynch JW, Kolitz JE, Jain V. Extended rituximab (anti-CD20 monoclonal antibody) therapy for relapsed or refractory low-grade or follicular non-Hodgkin's lymphoma. Ann Oncol: Official J Eur Soc Med Oncol/ESMO. 1999;10:655–61.

5. McLaughlin P, Grillo-Lopez AJ, Link BK, Levy R, Czuczman MS, Williams ME, Heyman MR, Bence-Bruckler I, White CA, Cabanillas F, Jain V, Ho AD, Lister J, Wey K, Shen D, Dallaire BK. Rituximab chimeric anti-CD20 monoclonal antibody therapy for relapsed indolent lymphoma: half of patients respond to a four-dose treatment program. J Clin Oncol. 1998;16:2825–33.
6. Leget GA, Czuczman MS. Use of rituximab, the new FDA-approved antibody. Curr Opin Oncol. 1998;10:548–51.
7. Czuczman MS, Grillo-Lopez AJ, White CA, Saleh M, Gordon L, LoBuglio AF, Jonas C, Klippenstein D, Dallaire B, Varns C. Treatment of patients with low-grade B-cell lymphoma with the combination of chimeric anti-CD20 monoclonal antibody and CHOP chemotherapy. J Clin Oncol. 1999;17:268–76.
8. Hiddemann W, Kneba M, Dreyling M, Schmitz N, Lengfelder E, Schmits R, Reiser M, Metzner B, Harder H, Hegewisch-Becker S, Fischer T, Kropff M, Reis HE, Freund M, Wörmann B, Fuchs R, Planker M, Schimke J, Eimermacher H, Trümper L, Aldaoud A, Parwaresch R, Unterhalt M. Frontline therapy with rituximab added to the combination of cyclophosphamide, doxorubicin, vincristine, and prednisone (CHOP) significantly improves the outcome for patients with advanced-stage follicular lymphoma compared with therapy with CHOP alone: results of a prospective randomized study of the German Low-Grade Lymphoma Study Group. Blood. 2005;106:3725–32.
9. Marcus R, Imrie K, Belch A, Cunningham D, Flores E, Catalano J, Solal-Celigny P, Offner F, Walewski J, Raposo J, Jack A, Smith P. CVP chemotherapy plus rituximab compared with CVP as first-line treatment for advanced follicular lymphoma. Blood. 2005;105:1417–23.
10. Coiffier B, Lepage E, Briere J, Herbrecht R, Tilly H, Bouabdallah R, Morel P, Van Den Neste E, Salles G, Gaulard P, Reyes F, Lederlin P, Gisselbrecht C. CHOP chemotherapy plus rituximab compared with CHOP alone in elderly patients with diffuse large-B-cell lymphoma. N Engl J Med. 2002;346:235–42.
11. Forstpointner R, Unterhalt M, Dreyling M, Böck HP, Repp R, Wandt H, Pott C, Seymour JF, Metzner B, Hänel A, Lehmann T, Hartmann F, Einsele H, Hiddemann W, German Low Grade Lymphoma Study Group (GLSG). Maintenance therapy with rituximab leads to a significant prolongation of response duration after salvage therapy with a combination of rituximab, fludarabine, cyclophosphamide, and mitoxantrone (R-FCM) in patients with recurring and refractory follicular and mantle cell lymphomas: results of a prospective randomized study of the German Low Grade Lymphoma Study Group (GLSG). Blood. 2006;108:4003–8.
12. Pfreundschuh M, Trümper L, Osterborg A, Pettengell R, Trneny M, Imrie K, Ma D, Gill D, Walewski J, Zinzani PL, Stahel R, Kvaloy S, Shpilberg O, Jaeger U, Hansen M, Lehtinen T, López-Guillermo A, Corrado C, Scheliga A, Milpied N, Mendila M, Rashford M, Kuhnt E, Loeffler M, MabThera International Trial Group. CHOP-like chemotherapy plus rituximab versus CHOP-like chemotherapy alone in young patients with good-prognosis diffuse large-B-cell lymphoma: a randomised controlled trial by the MabThera International Trial (MInT) Group. Lancet Oncol. 2006;7:379–91.
13. Hainsworth JD, Litchy S, Shaffer DW, Lackey VL, Grimaldi M, Greco FA. Maximizing therapeutic benefit of rituximab: maintenance therapy versus re-treatment at progression in patients with indolent non-Hodgkin's lymphoma—a randomized phase II trial of the Minnie Pearl Cancer Research Network. J Clin Oncol. 2005;23:1088–95.
14. Ghielmini M, Schmitz SF, Cogliatti SB, Pichert G, Hummerjohann J, Waltzer U, Fey MF, Betticher DC, Martinelli G, Peccatori F, Hess U, Zucca E, Stupp R, Kovacsovics T, Helg C, Lohri A, Bargetzi M, Vorobiof D, Cerny T. Prolonged treatment with rituximab in patients with follicular lymphoma significantly increases event-free survival and response duration compared with the standard weekly x4 schedule. Blood. 2004;103:4416–23.
15. Hochster H, Weller E, Gascoyne RD, Habermann TM, Gordon LI, Ryan T, Zhang L, Colocci N, Frankel S, Horning SJ. Maintenance rituximab after cyclophosphamide, vincristine, and prednisone prolongs progression-free survival in advanced indolent lymphoma: results of the randomized phase III ECOG1496 study. J Clin Oncol. 2009;27:1607–14.

16. van Oers MH, Klasa R, Marcus RE, Wolf M, Kimby E, Gascoyne RD, Jack A, Van't Veer M, Vranovsky A, Holte H, van Glabbeke M, Teodorovic I, Rozewicz C, Hagenbeek A. Rituximab maintenance improves clinical outcome of relapsed/resistant follicular non-Hodgkin lymphoma in patients both with and without rituximab during induction: results of a prospective randomized phase 3 intergroup trial. Blood. 2006;108:3295–301.
17. Czuczman MS, Olejniczak S, Gowda A, Kotowski A, Binder A, Kaur H, Knight J, Starostik P, Deans J, Hernandez-Ilizaliturri FJ. Acquirement of rituximab resistance in lymphoma cell lines is associated with both global CD20 gene and protein down-regulation regulated at the pretranscriptional and posttranscriptional levels. Clin Cancer Res. 2008;14:1561–70.
18. Olejniczak SH, Hernandez-Ilizaliturri FJ, Clements JL, Czuczman MS. Acquired resistance to rituximab is associated with chemotherapy resistance resulting from decreased Bax and Bak expression. Clin Cancer Res. 2008;14:1550–60.
19. Salles G, Seymour JF, Offner F, López-Guillermo A, Belada D, Xerri L, Feugier P, Bouabdallah R, Catalano JV, Brice P, Caballero D, Haioun C, Pedersen LM, Delmer A, Simpson D, Leppa S, Soubeyran P, Hagenbeek A, Casasnovas O, Intragumtornchai T, Fermé C, da Silva MG, Sebban C, Lister A, Estell JA, Milone G, Sonet A, Mendila M, Coiffier B, Tilly H. Rituximab maintenance for 2 years in patients with high tumour burden follicular lymphoma responding to rituximab plus chemotherapy (PRIMA): a phase 3, randomised controlled trial. Lancet. 2011;377:42–51.
20. Martín A, Conde E, Arnan M, Canales MA, Deben G, Sancho JM, Andreu R, Salar A, García-Sanchez P, Vázquez L, Nistal S, Requena MJ, Donato EM, González JA, León A, Ruiz C, Grande C, González-Barca E, Caballero MD, Grupo Español de Linfomas/Trasplante Autólogo de Médula Osea (GEL/TAMO Cooperative Group). R-ESHAP as salvage therapy for patients with relapsed or refractory diffuse large B-cell lymphoma: the influence of prior exposure to rituximab on outcome. A GEL/TAMO study. Haematologica. 2008;93:1829–36.
21. Thieblemont C, Briere J, Mounier N, Voelker HU, Cuccuini W, Hirchaud E, Rosenwald A, Jack A, Sundstrom C, Cogliatti S, Trougouboff P, Boudova L, Ysebaert L, Soulier J, Chevalier C, Bron D, Schmitz N, Gaulard P, Houlgatte R, Gisselbrecht C. The germinal center/activated B-cell subclassification has a prognostic impact for response to salvage therapy in relapsed/refractory diffuse large B-cell lymphoma: a Bio-CORAL study. J Clin Oncol. 2011;29:4079–87.
22. Gisselbrecht C, Glass B, Mounier N, Singh Gill D, Linch DC, Trneny M, Bosly A, Ketterer N, Shpilberg O, Hagberg H, Ma D, Brière J, Moskowitz CH, Schmitz N. Salvage regimens with autologous transplantation for relapsed large B-cell lymphoma in the rituximab era. J Clin Oncol. 2010;28:4184–90.
23. Selenko N, Majdic O, Jager U, Sillaber C, Stockl J, Knapp W. Cross-priming of cytotoxic T cells promoted by apoptosis-inducing tumor cell reactive antibodies? J Clin Immunol. 2002;22:124–30.
24. Deans JP, Schieven GL, Shu GL, Valentine MA, Gilliland LA, Aruffo A, Clark EA, Ledbetter JA. Association of tyrosine and serine kinases with the B cell surface antigen CD20. Induction via CD20 of tyrosine phosphorylation and activation of phospholipase C-gamma 1 and PLC phospholipase C-gamma 2. J Immunol. 1993;151:4494–504.
25. Shan D, Ledbetter JA, Press OW. Apoptosis of malignant human B cells by ligation of CD20 with monoclonal antibodies. Blood. 1998;91:1644–52.
26. Shan D, Ledbetter JA, Press OW. Signaling events involved in anti-CD20-induced apoptosis of malignant human B cells. Cancer Immunol Immunother. 2000;48:673–83.
27. Popoff IJ, Savage JA, Blake J, Johnson P, Deans JP. The association between CD20 and Src-family tyrosine kinases requires an additional factor. Mol Immunol. 1998;35:207–14.
28. Taji H, Kagami Y, Okada Y, Andou M, Nishi Y, Saito H, Seto M, Morishima Y. Growth inhibition of CD20-positive B lymphoma cell lines by IDEC-C2B8 anti-CD20 monoclonal antibody. Jpn J Cancer Res. 1998;89:748–56.
29. Holder M, Grafton G, MacDonald I, Finney M, Gordon J. Engagement of CD20 suppresses apoptosis in germinal center B cells. Eur J Immunol. 1995;25:3160–4.

30. Mathas S, Rickers A, Bommert K, Dorken B, Mapara MY. Anti-CD20- and B-cell receptor-mediated apoptosis: evidence for shared intracellular signaling pathways. Cancer Res. 2000;60:7170–6.
31. Hofmeister JK, Cooney D, Coggeshall KM. Clustered CD20 induced apoptosis: src-family kinase, the proximal regulator of tyrosine phosphorylation, calcium influx, and caspase 3-dependent apoptosis. Blood Cells Mol Dis. 2000;26:133–43.
32. Harjunpaa A, Junnikkala S, Meri S. Rituximab (anti-CD20) therapy of B-cell lymphomas: direct complement killing is superior to cellular effector mechanisms. Scand J Immunol. 2000;51:634–41.
33. Cragg MS, French RR, Glennie MJ. Signaling antibodies in cancer therapy. Curr Opin Immunol. 1999;11:541–7.
34. Hernandez-Ilizaliturri FJ, Jupudy V, Ostberg J, Oflazoglu E, Huberman A, Repasky E, Czuczman MS. Neutrophils contribute to the biological antitumor activity of rituximab in a non-Hodgkin's lymphoma severe combined immunodeficiency mouse model. Clin Cancer Res. 2003;9:5866–73.
35. Clynes RA, Towers TL, Presta LG, Ravetch JV. Inhibitory Fc receptors modulate in vivo cytotoxicity against tumor targets. Nat Med. 2000;6:443–6.
36. Deans JP, Robbins SM, Polyak MJ, Savage JA. Rapid redistribution of CD20 to a low density detergent-insoluble membrane compartment. J Biol Chem. 1998;273:344–8.
37. Polyak MJ, Tailor SH, Deans JP. Identification of a cytoplasmic region of CD20 required for its redistribution to a detergent-insoluble membrane compartment. J Immunol. 1998; 161:3242–8.
38. Semac I, Palomba C, Kulangara K, Klages N, van Echten-Deckert G, Borisch B, Hoessli DC. Anti-CD20 therapeutic antibody rituximab modifies the functional organization of rafts/microdomains of B lymphoma cells. Cancer Res. 2003;63:534–40.
39. Alas S, Bonavida B. Rituximab inactivates signal transducer and activation of transcription 3 (STAT3) activity in B-non-Hodgkin's lymphoma through inhibition of the interleukin 10 autocrine/paracrine loop and results in down-regulation of Bcl-2 and sensitization to cytotoxic drugs. Cancer Res. 2001;61:5137–44.
40. Maloney DG, Smith B, Rose A. Rituximab: mechanism of action and resistance. Semin Oncol. 2002;29:2–9.
41. Cartron G, Dacheux L, Salles G, Solal-Celigny P, Bardos P, Colombat P, Watier H. Therapeutic activity of humanized anti-CD20 monoclonal antibody and polymorphism in IgG Fc receptor FcgammaRIIIa gene. Blood. 2002;99:754–8.
42. Weng WK, Levy R. Two immunoglobulin G fragment C receptor polymorphisms independently predict response to rituximab in patients with follicular lymphoma. J Clin Oncol. 2003;21:3940–7.
43. Koene HR, Kleijer M, Algra J, Roos D, von dem Borne AE, de Haas M. Fc gammaRIIIa-158V/F polymorphism influences the binding of IgG by natural killer cell Fc gammaRIIIa, independently of the Fc gammaRIIIa-48L/R/H phenotype. Blood. 1997;90:1109–14.
44. Ghesquieres H, Cartron G, Seymour JF, Delfau-Larue MH, Offner F, Soubeyran P, Perrot A, Brice P, Bouabdallah R, Sonet A, Dupuis J, Casasnovas O, Catalano JV, Delmer A, Jardin F, Verney A, Dartigues P, Salles G. Clinical outcome of patients with follicular lymphoma receiving chemoimmunotherapy in the PRIMA study is not affected by FCGR3A and FCGR2A polymorphisms. Blood. 2012;120:2650–7.
45. Ahlgrimm M, Pfreundschuh M, Kreuz M, Regitz E, Preuss KD, Bittenbring J. The impact of Fc-gamma receptor polymorphisms in elderly patients with diffuse large B-cell lymphoma treated with CHOP with or without rituximab. Blood. 2011;118:4657–62.
46. Weng WK, Weng WK, Levy R. Immunoglobulin G Fc receptor polymorphisms do not correlate with response to chemotherapy or clinical course in patients with follicular lymphoma. Leuk Lymphoma. 2009;50:1494–500.
47. Kim DH, Jung HD, Kim JG, Lee JJ, Yang DH, Park YH, Do YR, Shin HJ, Kim MK, Hyun MS, Sohn SK. FCGR3A gene polymorphisms may correlate with response to frontline R-CHOP therapy for diffuse large B-cell lymphoma. Blood. 2006;108:2720–5.

48. Di Gaetano N, Cittera E, Nota R, Vecchi A, Grieco V, Scanziani E, Botto M, Introna M, Golay J. Complement activation determines the therapeutic activity of rituximab in vivo. J Immunol. 2003;171:1581–7.
49. Racila E, Link BK, Weng WK, Witzig TE, Ansell S, Maurer MJ, Huang J, Dahle C, Halwani A, Levy R, Weiner GJ. A polymorphism in the complement component C1qA correlates with prolonged response following rituximab therapy of follicular lymphoma. Clin Cancer Res. 2008;14:6697–703.
50. Maloney DG, Grillo-López AJ, White CA, Bodkin D, Schilder RJ, Neidhart JA, Janakiraman N, Foon KA, Liles TM, Dallaire BK, Wey K, Royston I, Davis T, Levy R. IDEC-C2B8 (Rituximab) anti-CD20 monoclonal antibody therapy in patients with relapsed low-grade non-Hodgkin's lymphoma. Blood. 1997;90:2188–95.
51. Davis TA, Grillo-López AJ, White CA, McLaughlin P, Czuczman MS, Link BK, Maloney DG, Weaver RL, Rosenberg J, Levy R. Rituximab anti-CD20 monoclonal antibody therapy in non-Hodgkin's lymphoma: safety and efficacy of re-treatment. J Clin Oncol. 2000;18:3135–43.
52. Hiraga J, Tomita A, Sugimoto T, Shimada K, Ito M, Nakamura S, Kiyoi H, Kinoshita T, Naoe T. Down-regulation of CD20 expression in B-cell lymphoma cells after treatment with rituximab-containing combination chemotherapies: its prevalence and clinical significance. Blood. 2009;113:4885–93.
53. Terui Y, Mishima Y, Sugimura N, Kojima K, Sakurai T, Mishima Y, Kuniyoshi R, Taniyama A, Yokoyama M, Sakajiri S, Takeuchi K, Watanabe C, Takahashi S, Ito Y, Hatake K. Identification of CD20 C-terminal deletion mutations associated with loss of CD20 expression in non-Hodgkin's lymphoma. Clin Cancer Res. 2009;15:2523–30.
54. Haidar JH, Shamseddine A, Salem Z, Mrad YA, Nasr MR, Zaatari G, Bazarbachi A. Loss of CD20 expression in relapsed lymphomas after rituximab therapy. Eur J Haematol. 2003;70:330–2.
55. Duman BB, Sahin B, Ergin M, Guvenc B. Loss of CD20 antigen expression after rituximab therapy of CD20 positive B cell lymphoma (diffuse large B cell extranodal marginal zone lymphoma combination): a case report and review of the literature. Med Oncol. 2012;29:1223–6.
56. Jilani I, O'Brien S, Manshuri T, Thomas DA, Thomazy VA, Imam M, Naeem S, Verstovsek S, Kantarjian H, Giles F, Keating M, Albitar M. Transient down-modulation of CD20 by rituximab in patients with chronic lymphocytic leukemia. Blood. 2003;102:3514–20.
57. Davis TA, Czerwinski DK, Levy R. Therapy of B-cell lymphoma with anti-CD20 antibodies can result in the loss of CD20 antigen expression. Clin Cancer Res. 1999;5:611–5.
58. Rawal YB, Nuovo GJ, Frambach GE, Porcu P, Baiocchi RA, Magro CM. The absence of CD20 messenger RNA in recurrent cutaneous B-cell lymphoma following rituximab therapy. J Cutan Pathol. 2005;32:616–21.
59. Jazirehi AR, Vega MI, Bonavida B. Development of rituximab-resistant lymphoma clones with altered cell signaling and cross-resistance to chemotherapy. Cancer Res. 2007;67:1270–81.
60. Tsai PC, Hernandez-Ilizaliturri FJ, Bangia N, Olejniczak SH, Czuczman MS. Regulation of CD20 in rituximab-resistant cell lines and B-cell non-Hodgkin lymphoma. Clin Cancer Res. 2012;18:1039–50.
61. van Meerten T, van Rijn RS, Hol S, Hagenbeek A, Ebeling SB. Complement-induced cell death by rituximab depends on CD20 expression level and acts complementary to antibody-dependent cellular cytotoxicity. Clin Cancer Res. 2006;12:4027–35.
62. Uchida J, Lee Y, Hasegawa M, Liang Y, Bradney A, Oliver JA, Bowen K, Steeber DA, Haas KM, Poe JC, Tedder TF. Mouse CD20 expression and function. Int Immunol. 2004;16:119–29.
63. Kuijpers TW, Bende RJ, Baars PA, Grummels A, Derks IA, Dolman KM, Beaumont T, Tedder TF, van Noesel CJ, Eldering E, van Lier RA. CD20 deficiency in humans results in impaired T cell-independent antibody responses. J Clin Investig. 2010;120:214–22.

64. Himmelmann A, Riva A, Wilson GL, Lucas BP, Thevenin C, Kehrl JH. PU.1/Pip and basic helix loop helix zipper transcription factors interact with binding sites in the CD20 promoter to help confer lineage- and stage-specific expression of CD20 in B lymphocytes. Blood. 1997;90:3984–95.
65. Beum PV, Kennedy AD, Williams ME, Lindorfer MA, Taylor RP. The shaving reaction: rituximab/CD20 complexes are removed from mantle cell lymphoma and chronic lymphocytic leukemia cells by THP-1 monocytes. J Immunol. 2006;176:2600–9.
66. Beers SA, French RR, Chan HT, Lim SH, Jarrett TC, Vidal RM, Wijayaweera SS, Dixon SV, Kim H, Cox KL, Kerr JP, Johnston DA, Johnson PW, Verbeek JS, Glennie MJ, Cragg MS. Antigenic modulation limits the efficacy of anti-CD20 antibodies: implications for antibody selection. Blood. 2010;115:5191–201.
67. Henry C, Deschamps M, Rohrlich PS, Pallandre JR, Rémy-Martin JP, Callanan M, Traverse-Glehen A, GrandClément C, Garnache-Ottou F, Gressin R, Deconinck E, Salles G, Robinet E, Tiberghien P, Borg C, Ferrand C. Identification of an alternative CD20 transcript variant in B-cell malignancies coding for a novel protein associated to rituximab resistance. Blood. 2010;115:2420–9.
68. Barth MJ, Hernandez-Ilizaliturri FJ, Mavis C, Tsai PC, Gibbs JF, Deeb G, Czuczman MS. Ofatumumab demonstrates activity against rituximab-sensitive and -resistant cell lines, lymphoma xenografts and primary tumour cells from patients with B-cell lymphoma. Br J Haematol. 2012;156:490–8.
69. Alduaij W, Ivanov A, Honeychurch J, Cheadle EJ, Potluri S, Lim SH, Shimada K, Chan CH, Tutt A, Beers SA, Glennie MJ, Cragg MS, Illidge TM. Novel type II anti-CD20 monoclonal antibody (GA101) evokes homotypic adhesion and actin-dependent, lysosome-mediated cell death in B-cell malignancies. Blood. 2011;117:4519–29.
70. Salles G, Morschhauser F, Lamy T, Milpied N, Thieblemont C, Tilly H, Bieska G, Asikanius E, Carlile D, Birkett J, Pisa P, Cartron G. Phase 1 study results of the type II glycoengineered humanized anti-CD20 monoclonal antibody obinutuzumab (GA101) in B-cell lymphoma patients. Blood. 2012;119:5126–32.
71. Czuczman MS, Fayad L, Delwail V, Cartron G, Jacobsen E, Kuliczkowski K, Link BK, Pinter-Brown L, Radford J, Hellmann A, Gallop-Evans E, DiRienzo CG, Goldstein N, Gupta I, Jewell RC, Lin TS, Lisby S, Schultz M, Russell CA, Hagenbeek A, 405 Study Investigators. Ofatumumab monotherapy in rituximab-refractory follicular lymphoma: results from a multicenter study. Blood. 2012;119:3698–704.
72. Ogura M, Tobinai K, Hatake K, Uchida T, Suzuki T, Kobayashi Y, Mori M, Terui Y, Yokoyama M, Hotta T. Phase I study of obinutuzumab (GA101) in Japanese patients with relapsed or refractory B-cell non-Hodgkin lymphoma. Cancer Sci. 2013;104:105–10.
73. Sehn LH, Assouline SE, Stewart DA, Mangel J, Gascoyne RD, Fine G, Frances-Lasserre S, Carlile DJ, Crump M. A phase 1 study of obinutuzumab induction followed by 2 years of maintenance in patients with relapsed CD20-positive B-cell malignancies. Blood. 2012;119:5118–25.
74. Venugopal P, Sivaraman S, Huang XK, Nayini J, Gregory SA, Preisler HD. Effects of cytokines on CD20 antigen expression on tumor cells from patients with chronic lymphocytic leukemia. Leuk Res. 2000;24:411–5.
75. Shimizu R, Kikuchi J, Wada T, Ozawa K, Kano Y, Furukawa Y. HDAC inhibitors augment cytotoxic activity of rituximab by upregulating CD20 expression on lymphoma cells. Leukemia. 2010;24:1760–8.
76. Golay J, Lazzari M, Facchinetti V, Bernasconi S, Borleri G, Barbui T, Rambaldi A, Introna M. CD20 levels determine the in vitro susceptibility to rituximab and complement of B-cell chronic lymphocytic leukemia: further regulation by CD55 and CD59. Blood. 2001;98:3383–9.
77. Opferman JT. Apoptosis in the development of the immune system. Cell Death Differ. 2008;15:234–42.
78. Tsujimoto Y, Cossman J, Jaffe E, Croce CM. Involvement of the bcl-2 gene in human follicular lymphoma. Science. 1985;228:1440–3.

79. Cleary ML, Smith SD, Sklar J. Cloning and structural analysis of cDNAs for bcl-2 and a hybrid bcl-2/immunoglobulin transcript resulting from the t(14;18) translocation. Cell. 1986;47:19–28.
80. Cory S, Adams JM. The Bcl2 family: regulators of the cellular life-or-death switch. Nat Rev Cancer. 2002;2:647–56.
81. Danial NN, Korsmeyer SJ. Cell death: critical control points. Cell. 2004;116:205–19.
82. Gulmann C, Espina V, Petricoin E 3rd, Longo DL, Santi M, Knutsen T, Raffeld M, Jaffe ES, Liotta LA, Feldman AL. Proteomic analysis of apoptotic pathways reveals prognostic factors in follicular lymphoma. Clin Cancer Res. 2005;11:5847–55.
83. Bannerji R, Kitada S, Flinn IW, Pearson M, Young D, Reed JC, Byrd JC. Apoptotic-regulatory and complement-protecting protein expression in chronic lymphocytic leukemia: relationship to in vivo rituximab resistance. J Clin Oncol. 2003;21:1466–71.
84. Agarwal B, Naresh KN. Bcl-2 family of proteins in indolent B-cell non-Hodgkin's lymphoma: study of 116 cases. Am J Hematol. 2002;70:278–82.
85. Sohn SK, Jung JT, Kim DH, Kim JG, Kwak EK, Park T, Shin DG, Sohn KR, Lee KB. Prognostic significance of bcl-2, bax, and p53 expression in diffuse large B-cell lymphoma. Am J Hematol. 2003;73:101–7.
86. Gascoyne RD, Adomat SA, Krajewski S, Krajewska M, Horsman DE, Tolcher AW, O'Reilly SE, Hoskins P, Coldman AJ, Reed JC, Connors JM. Prognostic significance of Bcl-2 protein expression and Bcl-2 gene rearrangement in diffuse aggressive non-Hodgkin's lymphoma. Blood. 1997;90:244–51.
87. Cotter FE, Waters J, Cunningham D. Human Bcl-2 antisense therapy for lymphomas. Biochim Biophys Acta. 1999;1489:97–106.
88. Ramanarayanan J, Hernandez-Ilizaliturri FJ, Chanan-Khan A, Czuczman MS. Pro-apoptotic therapy with the oligonucleotide Genasense (oblimersen sodium) targeting Bcl-2 protein expression enhances the biological anti-tumour activity of rituximab. Br J Haematol. 2004;127:519–30.
89. O'Brien S, Moore JO, Boyd TE, Larratt LM, Skotnicki A, Koziner B, Chanan-Khan AA, Seymour JF, Bociek RG, Pavletic S, Rai KR. Randomized phase III trial of fludarabine plus cyclophosphamide with or without oblimersen sodium (Bcl-2 antisense) in patients with relapsed or refractory chronic lymphocytic leukemia. J Clin Oncol. 2007;25:1114–20.
90. Bedikian AY, Millward M, Pehamberger H, Conry R, Gore M, Trefzer U, Pavlick AC, DeConti R, Hersh EM, Hersey P, Kirkwood JM, Haluska FG, Oblimersen Melanoma Study Group. Bcl-2 antisense (oblimersen sodium) plus dacarbazine in patients with advanced melanoma: the Oblimersen Melanoma Study Group. J Clin Oncol. 2006;24:4738–45.
91. Labi V, Grespi F, Baumgartner F, Villunger A. Targeting the Bcl-2-regulated apoptosis pathway by BH3 mimetics: a breakthrough in anticancer therapy? Cell Death Differ. 2008;15:977–87.
92. Brem EA, Thudium K, Khubchandani S, Tsai PC, Olejniczak SH, Bhat S, Riaz W, Gu J, Iqbal A, Campagna R, Knight J, Mavis C, Hoskin P, Deeb G, Gibbs JF, Fetterly G, Czuczman MS, Hernandez-Ilizaliturri FJ. Distinct cellular and therapeutic effects of obatoclax in rituximab-sensitive and -resistant lymphomas. Br J Haematol. 2011;153:599–611.
93. Dunleavy K, Pittaluga S, Czuczman MS, Dave SS, Wright G, Grant N, Shovlin M, Jaffe ES, Janik JE, Staudt LM, Wilson WH. Differential efficacy of bortezomib plus chemotherapy within molecular subtypes of diffuse large B-cell lymphoma. Blood. 2009;113:6069–76.

Tumor Resistance to Antibody-Mediated Immunotherapy and Reversal of Resistance: Rituximab as Prototype

Benjamin Bonavida

Abstract It took over a century to validate what Behring [153] and Ehrlich [154] have reasoned and predicted of the potential clinical use of antibody-mediated therapies against infectious diseases and cancer. However, the practical application of antibody-mediated therapies was only possible several decades later. Porter [155] and Edelman et al. [156] published the molecular structure of the immunoglobulin molecule and through the ingenuity of Kohler and Milstein they engineered the production of hybridoma cell lines capable of producing monoclonal antibodies (mAbs). Such mAbs are one of the most important and fastest growing classes of therapeutic drugs in the treatment of non-malignant and malignant diseases. The first FDA approved cancer therapeutic antibody was in 1997 for the treatment of B-Non-Hodgkin Lymphoma (B-NHL). The mAb is a chimeric anti-CD20 mAb, rituximab, which targets both non-malignant and malignant B cells. Rituximab is currently the standard therapy when used in combination with chemotherapy (CHOP). However, like other therapeutics, a subset of patients initially does not respond and a subset responding patients develops resistance to further treatments. Such patients are in an urgent need of novel therapies to reverse resistance. This review will cover rituximab as a therapeutic prototype mAb for analyses of its several modes of action on sensitive and resistant B-NHL tumor cells, its chemo-immuno-sensitizing effects and applications of various means to reverse resistance through the use of small molecule inhibitors targeting members of the constitutively overactivated survival/antiapoptotic pathways.

Keywords Rituximab · B-NHL · Rituximab-resistance · Signal transduction · Targeted inhibitors

B. Bonavida (✉)
Department of Microbiology, Immunology and Molecular Genetics, David Geffen School of Medicine, Jonsson Comprehensive Cancer Center at UCLA, University of California, Los Angeles, CA 90095, USA
e-mail: bbonavida@mednet.ucla.edu

B. Bonavida (ed.), *Resistance to Immunotherapeutic Antibodies in Cancer*,
Resistance to Targeted Anti-Cancer Therapeutics 2, DOI: 10.1007/978-1-4614-7654-2_5,

Abbreviations

ADCC	Antibody-dependent cell cytotoxicity
ARL	AIDS-related lymphoma
CDC	Complement-dependent cytotoxicity
CLL	Chronic lymphositic leukemia
CTL	Cytotoxic T lymphocyte
DLBCL	Diffused large B cell lymphoma
Fl	Follicular lymphoma
ITAM	Immunotyrosine activating motif
ITIM	Immunotyrosine inhibitory motif
NHL	Non-Hodgkin lymphoma
NK	Natural killer
TRAIL	Tumor necrosis-related apoptotic-inducing ligand
YY1	Yin Yang 1

Introduction

Since the introduction of various chemotherapeutic regimens in the treatment of cancer several decades ago, we have witnessed both the continuous development of novel drugs and several major advances made in deciphering the biochemical, molecular and genetic modifications that are responsible for cellular growth and resistance. There have been significant achievements in the early detection, treatment, and prolongation of survival for several cancers. However, a major limitation for the majority of current cancer therapeutics is their inability to target and kill resistant tumor cells. Both intrinsic and acquired drug resistance have been observed in many malignant cancers and these manifestations underlie the mechanisms of the observed failures of conventional therapeutics [1]. For instance, tumor cells develop mechanisms to inhibit drug-induced apoptosis through the constitutive activation of survival/anti-apoptotic pathways that are responsible for the transcription, expression, and activity of several members of the pro- and anti-apoptotic families. For example, the constitutive activation of the NF-κB and Raf-1/MEK1/2/ERK1/2 survival pathways have been associated with the development of drug resistant tumors [2, 3].

One of the objectives of cancer therapeutics (such as chemotherapy, immunotherapy, radiation, hormonal) is to inhibit cell proliferation and growth and to inflict a lethal damage. Although the initial development of many drugs was designed to interfere with DNA replication, it was found that many chemotherapeutic drugs (e.g. cisplatinum (CDDP), vincristine, paclitaxel, etoposide, etc.), radiation, hormonal, and immunotherapies exert their cytotoxic activities by killing tumor cells, primarily, through programmed cell death or apoptosis [4, 5]. Hence, it follows that tumor cell resistance is due, in large part, to the development in tumor cells of anti-apoptotic mechanisms. There exist primarily two types of apoptotic pathways, namely, the extrinsic (Type I) and intrinsic (Type II) pathways [6]. Several novel therapeutics that have been approved or in development are aimed at modifying and targeting the unbalanced anti-apoptotic pathways in order to preferentially potentiate the pro-apoptotic pathways that should lead to either spontaneous cancer cell death or to sensitization to apoptosis by conventional and novel therapeutics.

The introduction of immunotherapeutic approaches against cancer is based on the premise that the host immune system can fight the non-normal foreign cancer cells. Immunotherapy consists of innate immunity, cell-mediated immunity, and antibody-mediated immunity. Immunotherapy is a preferred choice, if successful, since it is targeted selectively against the cancer cell and not normal tissue and, therefore, it is less toxic than chemotherapy or radiation [7, 8]. In addition to the activation of host cell mediated anti-tumor immunity, antibody-mediated antitumor immunity has emerged as a very effective cancer therapeutic with high selectivity and minimal toxicity [9–11]. Currently, there are over thirty monoclonal antibodies (mAbs) approved clinically for various cancers and other diseases [12].

Exploration of immunotherapy for the treatment of malignancies using polyclonal antibody (Ab) preparations began in the 1950s. Major advances in Ab-mediated immunotherapy emerged in 1975 when techniques for producing mAbs were developed, making it feasible to produce large quantities of monoclonal Abs (mAbs) directed against specific antigenic eiptopes [13]. The first cancer therapeutic Abs studied were of murine, rabbit, or rat origins that were derived following immunization of the animal with an antigenic preparation. Treated patients with such antibodies often generated a humoral immune response against these xenogeneic therapeutic Abs referred to as human anti-mouse Ab (HAMA) or human anti-rabbit/rat Ab (HARA); these antibodies blocked the efficacy of the therapeutic Ab by prematurely clearing the Ab, thus, limiting the possibilities for an effective antitumor response to be manifested [14]. The host Ab responses, consequently, were mainly immune complex-related adverse events such as serum sickness and anaphylaxis. For example, HAMA rates as high as 41 % have been observed in previously untreated NHL patients receiving anti-B1 Ab [15].

In addition to HARA and HAMA, murine, rabbit, and rat Abs are poorly able to recruit human effector functions such as antibody-dependent cellular cytotoxicity (ADCC) and complement-dependent cytotoxicity (CDC), which facilitate the destruction of a tumor cell [14]. To overcome obstacles inherent in the first generation Abs, hybrids composed of mouse or primate Ab regions linked with a human backbone were constructed [15, 16]. These are referred to as chimeric, humanized or primatized Abs, depending on the exact Ab structure. For instance, humanized Ab is a human Ab containing the complementarity-determining regions (CDR) of non-human origin and human constant regions. These genetically engineered Abs are potent inducers of ADCC and CDC and also have an enhanced half-life which contributes to their efficacy. For instance, the half-life of the chimeric anti-CD20 Ab, rituximab, is 76 h after a single infusion and 206 h after four infusions [17] compared with 28 h for the murine counterpart, ibritumomab [18]. The incidence of immune responses with second-generation Abs is significantly lower than that seen with cross-species Abs.

Examples of early developed mAbs clinically used in the treatment of cancers are edrecolomab (Panorex®), which was approved in Europe in 1994 and trastuzumab (Herceptin®) that was approved in the US in 1998. These mAbs, in combination with chemotherapy, are effectively used in the treatment of patients with colorectal and breast cancer, respectively [14]. In February 2004, the Food and Drug Administration (FDA) approved bevacizumab, antivascular endothelial growth factor (VEGF) mAb, as a first-lime therapy for metastatic colorectal cancer, which is the first therapeutic to target tumor angiogenesis [19]. The anti-CD52 mAb, CAMPATH-1®, produces a combined response rate of 26 % in patients with chronic lymphocytic leukemia (CLL) given extensive prior therapy [20]. The anti-CD20 mAb rituximab (Rituxan®, IDEC-C2B8) is the first mAb for the treatment of low-grade and follicular NHL approved by the FDA in 1997. The followings will primarily elaborate on the functions of rituximab as a prototype for other therapeutic mAbs.

Rituximab in the Treatment of B-NHL

Rituximab is a chimeric anti-CD20 mAb and the first FDA-approved mAb for the treatment of B-NHL cancer. It is directed against the CD20 surface receptor expressed on cells of the B cell lineage. CD20 is a tetramembrane spanning protein (MW 33–37 kDa) located on chromosome 11q12-q13.1. CD20 is resident in lipid raft domains of the plasma membrane [21].

Non-Hodgkin Lymphoma

Non-Hodgkin's lymphomas (NHLs) are a heterogeneous group of malignancies that originate in the lymphoid system in which the cells usually express either B cell or T cell markers, or both, indicating a disruption of normal development at a precursor stage. Some cases of NHL are related to immune deficiency and chronic antigenic stimulation and particularly to Epstein–Barr virus (EBV) in the context of immune deficiency; however, the exact etiology of the majority of NHL cases remains elusive [22, 23]. NHL accounts for about 4 % of cancers in the US, ranks fifth in cancer mortality and is the leading cause of cancer-related deaths for people between 20 and 40 years of age. NHL is slightly more common in men and the median age at diagnosis is 65 years; the incidence increases with age and peaks in the 80–85 years age group [23, 24]. The incidence of NHL has been steadily increasing for the past 50 years. The largest increases are observed within patients with aggressive lymphoma. The incidence of extranodal lymphoma has increased more rapidly than the nodal form, whereas the incidence of primary central nervous system (CNS) lymphoma in the US has increased more than 10-folds between 1973 and 1992. This increase is partly due to the AIDS epidemic, although the incidence of CNS lymphoma has increased in non-AIDS populations as well. Thus, the observed increase in incidence of NHL is most likely multifactorial including chronic antigenic stimulation, reactivation of EBV infection, and severe immunodeficiency [23, 24].

Treatment of B-NHL

The major determinants for choosing the treatment options for NHL are the grade and the extent of the disease. Generally, low-grade (indolent) lymphomas are considered incurable with standard therapy when diagnosed at the advanced stages. Intermediate- and high-grade (aggressive) lymphomas are potentially curable with aggressive combination chemotherapy [25]. The two most common histologic forms of NHL are follicular lymphoma (FL) and diffuse large B cell lymphomas (DLBCL).

FLs serve as a paradigm for the management of all indolent lymphomas. Treatment options for patients with indolent lymphomas consist of a 'watch and wait' approach, single agent alkylators, nucleoside analogues, combination chemotherapy, immunotherapy with monoclonal antibodies (mAbs), radiolabeled mAbs, or interferon (IFN). Although up to 75 % of patients treated with conventional chemotherapy regimens exhibit sustained remissions, the vast majority eventually relapses. Thus, localized radiation therapy remains the treatment of choice, which is used for stages I and II disease, whereby 50–70 % of patients will show a sustained clinical remission that lasts >5 years. Chemotherapy with alkylating agents, immunotherapy, and radioimmunotherapy are most frequently used in stages III and IV of the disease. Most patients with FL enjoy prolonged survival but those with stages III and IV are potentially incurable [22, 24, 26–28].

DLBCL serves as a paradigm for the treatment and management of aggressive lymphomas. Combination chemotherapy with cyclophosphamide, doxorubicin, vincristine, and prednisone (CHOP) represents the treatment of choice, and may be restricted to 3–4 cycles in patients with limited-stage disease when followed by involved field radiotherapy. Even in advanced states of the disease, long-term remission and potential cure are achieved in 30–50 % of cases. Patients who fail initial management are treated with further chemotherapy. High-dose chemotherapy with stem cell rescue is effective as salvage treatment for DLBCL [22, 24–28], but relapse with the development of drug-resistance remains a major problem. In either case, intensification of therapy by myeloablative chemotherapy or combined chemoradiotherapy followed by autologous bone marrow transplantation (ABMT) or peripheral stem cell transplantation provides a promising and potentially curative prospective [26]. Eventually, most patients with low-grade (indolent) lymphoma will become refractory to treatment. Approximately

25–60 % of the cases will transform to aggressive lymphoma, usually diffuse large cell type [29, 30].

Relapsed or Refractory Lymphomas

In the past 10 years, high-dose chemotherapy and autologous stem cell reconstitution have become established parts of treatment for aggressive lymphomas. CHOP continues to hold ground as first-line therapy when compared to other regimens in aggressive lymphomas. Patients with chemosensitive relapse are suitable candidates for high-dose therapy. In relapsed or refractory disease, selective compounds appear to have activity as single agents and others have shown activity in combination therapy [31, 32]. Patients whose disease progresses after the initial administration of combination chemotherapy exhibit a poor prognosis. Retreatment with any of the first-line regimens usually does not result in sustained remission. Such patients are usually treated with one of several salvage regimens. These regimens, however, induce a response in 30–40 % of patients. The unresponsiveness in the majority of patients is due to the emergence and selective outgrowth of drug-resistant variants with a multidrug-resistant (MDR) phenotype that will eventually lead to the patient's demise [22, 24–28]. This pattern of inevitable failure of standard therapies highlights the importance of the design of new treatment modalities. A novel strategy that has attracted much attention within the past few years is the use of Ab-mediated immunotherapy targeted against specific surface markers, alone or in combination with chemotherapy. These modalities are less systematically toxic, less myelosuppressive and more specific. Rituximab in combination with CHOP is the current treatment choice for various B-NHLs and will be discussed below as a prototype mAb for its several mechanisms of action.

Postulated Mechanisms of Action by Rituximab

Several mechanisms have been proposed for the mechanisms of rituximab-mediated activities in vivo against B-NHL. These are briefly discussed below:

Rituximab-Mediated Antibody-Dependent Cellular Cytotoxicity

ADCC results from the ligation of the human Fc portion of rituximab to Fc receptors expressed by the effector cells and is considered as a major antitumor mechanism. Thus, studies were undertaken to assess the ability of rituximab to mediate ADCC. Highly purified normal peripheral blood $CD19^+$ B cells were minimally affected by rituximab in the presence of complement. In contrast, significant reduction in the number of Daudi and B-CLL cells was observed by the addition of mononuclear [NK ($CD56^+$) and monocytes ($CD14^+$)] cells. The depletion of B-CLL cells in patients-derived PBMCs (which contain circulating effector cells) was significantly increased in the presence of rituximab and was even more pronounced following the addition of granulocyte-macrophage colony stimulating factor (GM-CSF) [33]. Other cytokines also enhance ADCC. For instance, G-CSF-primed neutrophils (PMN) were efficient effector cells in mediating rituximab-mediated killing of Ramos and Raji cells [34]. Also, the combination of rituximab and low-dose IL-2 induced a response in 55 % of patients with relapsed and refractory FL. Immunophenotyping of the peripheral blood of all the evaluable patients showed significant increase in the levels of circulating $CD8^+$ and $CD56^+$ lymphocytes [35]. Another group showed that responses to rituximab, including ADCC and CDC, are associated with the Fcγ receptor polymorphism, as the human Fc region of rituximab is important in mobilizing ADCC and CDC effector functions [36]. Using multivariate analysis, a comparison between the expression of FcγRIIIa receptor 158V and 158F allotypes in 49 patients and controls who were treated with rituximab for the treatment of previously untreated FL was made. Noteworth, the homozygosity of the FcγRIIIa-158 V allotype was the single parameter associated with the clinical response rates at 2 and 12 months post treatment and molecular (disappearance of the *Bcl-2-JH* gene rearrangement in the peripheral blood and bone marrow) responses [37, 38]. Collectively, these results established ADCC as a potential in vivo antitumor mechanism of rituximab-mediated activity; however, the exact molecular determinants of ADCC resistance remain to be defined.

Rituximab-Mediated CDC

Rituximab is capable of binding to C1q [16], thus activating the complement cascade. The C1q-binding motif on human IgG1 is comprised of D270, K322, P329, and P331 residues. Substitution of these residues to alanine significantly reduces the binding of rituximab to C1q and its ability to activate complement. K326 and E333 are located at the extreme ends of the C1q-binding motif and mutation to tryptophan of K326 diminishes the ability of rituximab to mediate CDC [39]. Depending on their origin, lymphoma cells exhibit differential sensitivity to CDC. In a recent study, rituximab induced high CDC killing of FL cells, whereas MCL and DLBCL were moderately sensitive and small lymphocytic lymphoma (SLL) cells were almost resistant [40]. Rituximab also efficiently kills acquired immunodeficiency syndrome (AIDS)-related lymphoma (ARL) cell lines through ADCC and CDC. Despite the high expression of CD52 on ARL cells, rituximab was superior in activating CDC compared to Alemtuzumab (anti-CD52 mAb) [41]. Various agents have been shown to enhance CDC mediated by rituximab in vitro. For instance, dexamethasone enhances rituximab-mediated CDC, but has minimal and/or negative impact on ADCC. The 3E7 mAb directed against the C3b breakdown product [C3b(I)] increases C3b deposition on lymphoma cells and significantly enhances rituximab-mediated CDC in the presence of normal human serum [42].

The heterogeneity of the response to rituximab-mediated therapy led to the hypothesis that resistance to CDC may be linked to the expression of complement inhibitors. Support for this idea came from studies showing that BL and FL cells exhibit highly variable sensitivity to CDC (ranging from 100 % to complete resistance). The major contributors to CDC resistance were determined to be CD46 (MCP), CD55 (DAF), and CD59 as specific antagonistic Abs against these molecules significantly augmented killing in lymphoma and multiple myeloma cell lines [43–45]. Further, the levels of CD20 and complement inhibitors (CD46, CD55, CD59) were determinants in the clinical response of freshly isolated cells obtained from 33 patients with B-CLL, five with prolymphocytic leukemia (PLL), and six with MCL, where a functional block of CD55 and CD59 enhanced CDC [43]. Compared to rituximab, anti-B1 mAb (tositumomab) showed lower level of activity against CDC-sensitive Daudi and Ramos cells. A negative correlation was found between CD55 and CD59 expression and sensitivity to rituximab- and tositumomab-mediated CDC [46]. In the presence of human AB serum, rituximab induced significant CDC in cells from 55 patients with B cell lymphoproliferative disorders (B-CLL, MCL, FL, HCL). The efficiency of killing was directly related to the number of CD20 molecules per cell and preincubation with anti-CD59 increased the cytotoxic effects of rituximab [47]. Collectively, these studies support a role of complement inhibitors as a mechanism for lymphoma cells to escape CDC. Contrary to the aforementioned, the baseline expression of the Mcl-1/Bax ratio, not the expression of complement regulators (CD55, CD59), was predictive of the clinical response of a retrospective, single-agent rituximab trial on 21 CLL patients [48]. Further, analysis of tumor cells obtained from 29 rituximab-treated patients with FL showed no significant correlation between the expression of CD46, CD55, CD59, and rituximab-induced CDC [49]. Further studies are warranted to delineate the exact role of complement inhibitors in the ability of rituximab to exert its therapeutic activities in vivo.

Some investigators consider that both complement activation and cytokine accumulation are responsible for the infusion-related side effects of rituximab. Considerable release of cytokines (IL-6, -8, TNF-α) and accumulation of complement activation products (C3b/c, C4b/c) were observed during the first infusion of rituximab in five patients with relapsed low-grade NHL, which might contribute to the severity of side effects of rituximab therapy [34]. Complement activation was also noticed in the blood and cerebral spinal fluid in a patient with relapsing NHL with CNS involvement during the first infusion of rituximab [44]. Conversely, the limited number of cases makes the interpretation of data difficult. Collectively, these data support an effector function of CDC in the antitumor activity of rituximab. However, the role of complement inhibitors in conferring CDC-resistance is controversial and warrants further investigation.

Rituximab-Mediated Induction of Apoptosis

Studies were undertaken to investigate the apoptotic activity of rituximab in in vitro model systems. Initial studies demonstrated that rituximab is capable of inducing moderate levels of apoptosis in certain NHL cells [50]. The antitumor activity of mAbs that have little or no signaling activity (e.g. anti-CD19, -CD20, -CD21, -CD 22, and Her-2) is augmented when converted into IgG–IgG homodimers. Depending on the cell surface molecules they bind to, homodimers exert antitumor activity by exerting G0/G1 arrest or induction of apoptosis [51]. Thus, crosslinking rituximab became a new approach in eradicating NHL tumor cells. In a series of elegant studies it was shown that, compared to the monomeric form, homodimers [F(ab')2] of rituximab exhibit superior anti-growth activity and induce both apoptosis and necrosis in Raji, Daudi, Ramos and DHL-4 cells irrespective of the density of surface membrane CD20 or the presence of Fc receptors. Monomeric rituximab induced modest apoptosis in Ramos cells that was greatly enhanced upon clustering with a secondary Ab, which accompanied tyrosine kinase activation, PLC-2 phosphorylation, Ca^{2+} influx, and caspase-3 activation. These events were all inhibited by PP2, a selective inhibitor of the Src family kinases [52]. Another group compared the apoptotic activities of rituximab with anti-CD20 mAbs. They reported that anti-CD20 mAbs (1F5, anti-B1, and rituximab)) are capable of inducing modest apoptosis in various NHL cell lines. The magnitude of apoptosis induction was greater with rituximab than with the murine 1F5 and anti-B1. Crosslinking of the mAbs by secondary goat anti-mouse Ig Abs or Fc-receptor-bearing accessory cells significantly potentiated the rate of killing. The inhibitor of the protein tyrosine kinases Lck and Fyn (PP1), chelators of extracellular or intracellular Ca^{2+}, and caspase inhibitors attenuated the level of apoptosis. Also, varying the expression of Bcl-2 did not affect the magnitude of anti-B1-induced apoptosis, possibly due to the sequestering effects of other Bcl-2 family members, such as Bad [53]. Pedersen et al. [54]. showed that freshly isolated B-CLL cells cultured in the presence of rituximab and a crosslinking F(ab)2 fragment results in a concentration- and time-dependent induction of apoptosis independent of ADCC and CDC. Rituximab cross linking resulted in sustained and strong phosphorylation of MAPKs [(p38, JNK, ERK (extracellular signal-regulated kinase)], whereby the addition of SB203580 (p38MAPK specific inhibitor) significantly reduced the degree of apoptosis [54]). Additional studies were conducted to investigate the molecular mechanism of rituximab-mediated apoptosis upon crosslinking. In treated BL60-2 and SU-DHL-4 cell lines, there was a rapid upregulation of the proapoptotic Bax, as well as the activation of the extracellular-signal-regulated kinase 1/2 (ERK1/2) and increased DNA-binding activity of the activation protein 1 (AP-1) [55]. Also, the activation of caspase-9 and caspase-3 and PARP cleavage immediately following rituximab treatment was observed in patient-derived B-CLL cells, accompanied by significant downregulation of XIAP and Mcl-1 antiapoptotic proteins. In a separate study, CD20 crosslinking by rituximab induced apoptosis in Ramos cells via loss of the mitochondrial transmembrane potential, the release of cytochrome *c*, and caspase activation that occurred independent of the levels of Bcl-2 [34]. Collectively, the above data demonstrate the efficacy of rituximab in killing NHL cells upon cross linking.

CD20 and Lipid Rafts

Lipid rafts are heterogeneous lipid microdomains, relatively enriched in sphingomyelin, glycosphingolipids, and cholesterol that spontaneously form in cell membranes as a consequence of the biophysical properties of the different lipids that comprise the membrane and serve as a platform for the signaling molecules. The binding of CD20 Abs to B cells induces a rapid (as early as 15 s) redistribution of CD20 molecules (up to 95 %) to low-density, detergent-insoluble lipid rafts and induces the appearance of an approximately 50 kDa tyrosine phosphorylated protein in the same compartment. This is mediated through a membrane proximal sequence in the cytoplasmic carboxyl tail of CD20 corresponding to residues 219–252 [56]. The redistribution of CD20 into membrane lipid rafts appears to control the efficiency of anti-CD20 mAbs to mediate complement lysis of lymphoma cells [57]. In contrast, no association between CD20 redistribution to membrane lipid rafts and the induction of apoptosis has been demonstrated [58]. However, the coexistence of CD20 and Src family protein kinases in lipid rafts suggests a role of CD20 in cellular signaling. Redistribution of CD20 to lipid rafts depends on the nature of Abs used and its correlation with the ability to induce apoptosis warrants further scrutiny.

Rituximab-Mediated Cell Signaling and Chemo-Immuno Sensitizing Activities

Deans et al. [59] reported that CD20 was co-isolated with tyrosine and serine/threonine kinases following treatment of cells with anti-CD20 antibody and, thus, suggesting that CD20 may be involved in transmembrane signaling pathways. There does not appear the existence of a direct interaction of the CD20 cytoplasmic domain with cell signaling. Cell signaling results from the association of CD20 with raft signaling domains [60]. Rituximab induces redistribution of CD20 to lipid rafts and leads to decreased Lyn activity, depending on the presence of Cbp/PAG, with a decrease in the levels of activated phosphorylated Lyn and Cbp/PAG with no change in non-phosphorylated proteins [61]. These findings were corroborated by us and by the additional inhibition downstream of various survival pathways [62]. Bezombes et al. [63] reported that treatment with rituximab results in the rapid, but transient, increase in acid sphingomyelinase activity with concomitant accumulation of cellular ceramide in the raft microdomains. Deans et al. [64] reported that cell growth inhibited by rituximab was mediated through a ceramide-triggered signaling pathway via a mitogen-activated protein kinase (MAPK)-dependent mechanism.

An initial observation was made by Demidem et al. [65] who demonstrated that treatment of drug-resistant B-NHL cell lines with rituximab reversed the resistance to various chemotherapeutic drugs-induced cell death. This observation by our laboratory instigated our interest to further investigate the underlying molecular and biochemical mechanisms mediated by rituximab in the reversal of drug resistance. We hypothesized that rituximab may inhibit intracellular survival pathways and, thus, allowing the cytotoxic drugs to be effective. Indeed, our findings demonstrated that rituximab treatment inhibited several intracellular pathways including the p38 MAPK, NF-κB, ERK1/2, and AKT signaling pathways. Inhibition of these pathways resulted in the transcriptional inhibition of several members of the anti-apoptotic gene families such as the Bcl-2 family and, thus, reducing the threshold of resistance. Below, we briefly describe the various survival pathways inhibited by rituximab.

Cell Signaling Mediated by Rituximab and Chemosensitization

Inhibition by Rituximab of the p38 MAPK Pathway and Chemosensitization

We used a model of a diffuse large B cell Lymphoma (BLBCL) cell line whose cell growth was partially inhibited by rituximab. We hypothesized that inhibition of cell growth by rituximab may be mediated through blocking the activity of a growth factor(s), in either an autocrine or paracrine fashion. We demonstrated that rituximab inhibited the secretion of TNF-α and IL-10 growth factors and their neutralization inhibited tumor cell proliferation. We then examined the mechanism by which rituximab inhibited IL-10 secretion by examining its effect on the signaling pathway mediated by the interaction of IL-10 with its cognate IL-10 receptor. The constitutive activation of signal transducer and activator of transcription 3 (STAT3), phospho-STAT3, was inhibited by rituximab [66]. Rituximab inhibited the p38 MAPK pathway and resulted in the inhibition of STAT3 activity and the IL-10 transcription factor SP1. The inhibition of STAT3 activity by rituximab also resulted in downstream inhibition of the anti-apoptotic gene product Bcl-2 and, altogether, resulted in the sensitization of tumor cells to apoptosis by various chemotherapeutic drugs. The combination of rituximab and cis-platinum (CDDP) resulted in a synergistic apoptotic activity resulting from the activation of the type II mitochondrial apoptotic pathway [67]. The direct role of the p38 MAPK pathway in the regulation of Bcl-2 expression and reversal of drug resistance was corroborated by the use of specific chemical inhibitors of the p38 MAPK pathway [68, 69].

Inhibition by Rituximab of the Raf-1/MEK1/2/ERK1/2 Pathway and Chemisensitization

Using Burkitt lymphoma cell lines, treatment with rituximab reversed the drug resistance concomitant with the down regulation of the anti-apoptotic gene product Bcl_{xL} [70]. Since Bcl_{xL} is regulated by the Raf-1/MEK1/2/ERK1/2/AP-1 pathway, in part, we examined whether treatment with rituximab inhibited this pathway. The Raf-1/MEK1/2/ERK1/2 pathway was constitutively activated in the analyzed Burkitt lymphoma cell lines and treatment with rituximab inhibited the activation of this pathway as shown by inhibition of the phosphorylation, but not unphosphorylation, of those proteins regulated by the above pathway. The activity of the transcription factor AP-1 was inhibited by rituximab as assessed by inhibition of its DNA-binding activity. The role of rituximab-mediated inhibition of the Raf-1/Mek1/2/ERK1/2 pathway in the reversal of drug resistance was corroborated by the use of specific chemical inhibitors of this pathway and the use of an inhibitor of Bcl_{xL} [62].

Inhibition by Rituximab of the NF-κB Pathway and Chemosensitization

The above studies examined one pathway by which rituximab-mediated inhibition of Bcl_{xL} expression was regulated via the Raf-1/MEK1/2/ERK1/2 pathway. However, Bcl_{xL} gene expression is also regulated by another pathway, the NF-κB pathway [71, 72]. Therefore, we hypothesized the rituximab-mediated inhibition of Bcl_{xL} may also involve the inhibition of the constitutively active NF-κB pathway in the tested Burkitt lymphoma cell lines. Indeed, the findings demonstrated that rituximab treatment decreased the phosphorylation of the NF-κB pathway-inducing kinases (NIK, the IκB kinase, and the IκBα kinases); these inhibitions resulted in diminished IKK activity and decreased NF-κB DNA-binding activity. These various inhibitory activities of the NF-κB pathway by rituximab were corroborated with the inhibition of Bcl_{xL} expression as assessed by various chemical inhibitors of the NF-κB pathway [73]. The direct role of NF-κB-induced inhibition by rituximab and sensitization of drug-resistant B-NHL cell lines to chemotherapeutic drugs was corroborated by the use of specific NF-κB inhibitors (such as Bay11-7085 and DHMEQ) which mimicked rituximab in the inhibition of Bcl_{xL} and the reversal of drug resistance when combined with cytotoxic drugs [73].

Inhibition by Rituximab of the AKT Pathway and Chemosensitization

The PI3K/AKT pathway regulates the activity and expression of Bcl_{xL} [74]. Thus, like the above studies in (2) and (3) for the Raf-1/Mek1/2/ERK1/2 and NF-κB pathways, respectively, that regulate Bcl_{xL} and their inhibition by rituximab, we have also investigated the contribution of the PI3K pathway in the inhibition of

Bcl_{xL} by rituximab. Rituximab treatment inhibited the constitutively activated PI3K/AKT pathway through inhibition of phospho-PI3K, phospho-PDK-1, and phospho-AKT with no effect on the non-phosphorylated proteins. In addition, downstream of the PI3K/AKT pathway, we found that rituximab inhibited phospho-Bad which resulted in the augmented association of Bad with Bcl_{xL} to form complexes and, therefore, inhibiting Bcl_{xL} anti-apoptotic activity on the mitochondria The direct role of the PI3K/AKT pathway-induced inhibition of this pathway by rituximab in the reversal of drug resistance was corroborated by the use of both specific AKT chemical inhibitors and by transfection with small interference RNA (siRNA) AKT [75].

In conclusion, the above findings revealed, for the first time, a novel mechanism of action by a therapeutic anti-cancer antibody, like rituximab, and its multiple cell signaling inhibitory effects and its ability to modulate various anti-apoptotic pathways that result in the reversal of tumor cell resistance to chemotherapeutic drugs. This novel mechanism of cell signaling-mediated effects by rituximab adds to the commonly suggested mechanisms of action, described above, such as CDC, ADCC, and direct apoptosis. In addition, the findings reported with rituximab may be applicable to other anti-cancer therapeutic monoclonal antibodies currently in use.

Cell Signaling Mediated by Rituximab and Immunosensitization

The development of tumor cell resistance to chemotherapeutic drugs is the result, in large part, in the development in the tumor cells of anti-apoptotic mechanisms to maintain their survival. The cytotoxic immune system mediated by natural killer (NK) and cytotoxic T lymphocytes (CTL) mediate their killing by both necrotic and apoptotic mechanisms (e.g. FasL, TNF-α, TRAIL) [76–79]. These cytotoxic ligands are expressed on the cell membrane of NK, monocytes and CTL and can also be present in soluble secreted forms. These ligands bind to corresponding death receptors expressed on the surface of target cells. The interaction of death ligands with corresponding death receptors results in the activation of intrinsic and extrinsic apoptotic pathways in sensitive cells and leading to apoptosis. FasL interacts with Fas, TNF-α interacts with TNFR1 or TNFR2 and TRAIL interacts with DR4 and DR5 as well as with decoy receptors, DR1 and DR2 [80].

The fact that both chemotherapeutic and cytotoxic immunotherapeutics have in common a mechanism of apoptosis, we speculated that rituximab-induced reversal of chemoresistance, as described above, may also reverse immunoresistance to NK and CTL. We have used both FasL and TRAIL in recombinant soluble forms as models for NK and CTL-mediated cytotoxicities.

Rituximab-Induced Sensitization to FasL Apoptosis

In addition to rituximab-mediated inhibition of Bcl-2 and Bcl_{xL} and chemosensitization, described above, we also found that rituximab treatment sensitized B-NHL tumor cell lines to FasL-induced apoptosis. The underlying mechanism by which rituximab sensitized to Fas-ligand was examined. Previous findings with ovarian cancer cell lines demonstrated that treatment with interferon-γ or NO donors reverted their resistance to FasL apoptosis. The treatment also resulted in the upregulation of Fas expression which was found to be due to inhibition of the Fas transcription repressor Yin Yang 1 (YY1) [81]. Since YY1 is a target gene product of NF-κB, we reasoned that rituximab-mediated inhibition of NF-κB will also lead to YY1 inhibition, upregulation of Fas and sensitization of B-NHL to FasL apoptosis. We first demonstrated that inhibition of NF-κB by chemical inhibitors, like rituximab-induced inhibition of NF-κB, sensitized the cells to FasL apoptosis and was also concomitant with the inhibition of YY1 and upregulation of Fas expression. Similar to rituximab, the direct inhibition of YY1 by chemical inhibitors or YY1 siRNA resulted in upregulation of Fas and sensitization of FasL apoptosis. These findings established the potential in vivo role of rituximab recruitment of host FasL bearing effector cells to attack B-NHL cells that over express Fas and leading to their cell death [82]. It is not clear whether the observed upregulation of Fas by rituximab is essential and required for FasL apoptosis or is only a manifestation of rituximab-induced inhibition of resistance factors such as NF-κB and YY1. The role of rituximab-induced inhibition of the MAPK/NF-κB/YY1 signaling in FasL-induced apoptosis was corroborated by the use of chemical inhibitors (inhibition of Srs-kinases, p38 MAPK, NF-κB and YY1), all of which mimic rituximab in inducing Fas expression and sensitization to FasL.

The apoptotic pathway mediated by rituximab-induced sensitization to FasL apoptosis was examined. Treatment with rituximab or FasL alone had no effect on trigerring the apoptotic pathway, however, the combination resulted in the depolarization of the mitochondrial membrane potential, the release of cytochrome c and Smac/DIABLO, the activation of caspases 9 and 3, the cleavage of PARP, all of which led to apoptosis. Activation of the mitochondria was the result of rituximab-induced inhibition of Bcl-2 and Bcl_{xL} [82]. These findings established the type II apoptotic pathway activation in the sensitization by rituximab to FasL apoptosis.

Rituximab-Mediated TRAIL Sensitization

In addition to FasL, host effector cells (CTL, NK, macrophages) also express TRAIL and most tumor cells express corresponding death receptors (DR4 and DR5) [83]. Therefore, it was possible that rituximab will also sensitize the tumor cells to TRAIL-induced apoptosis. We examined this possibility both in vitro and in vivo. Both B-NHL cell lines and patient's B-NHL cells are generally resistant to TRAIL apoptosis [84]. However, resistance can be overcome by inhibition of anti-apoptotic survival pathways like NF-κB. Since rituximab inhibits NF-κB activity, therefore, we hypothesized that rituximab treatment may also sensitize B-NHL cells to TRAIL apoptosis. Our findings showed, indeed, that treatment of B-NHL cells with rituximab sensitized the cells to recombinant TRAIL-induced-apoptosis and to TRAIL expressing human-derived NK cells. The mechanism of sensitization to TRAIL revealed that rituximab-induced inhibition of YY1, as shown above. YY1 was demonstrated to be a transcription repressor for DR5 [85]. Hence, DR5 expression was overexpressed following treatment of B-NHL cells with rituximab. The sensitization to TRAIL apoptosis by rituximab was the result of activation of the mitochondrial type II apoptotic pathway. Like rituximab, treatment with YY1 siRNA resulted in the inhibition of YY1, upregulation of DR5, and sensitization to TRAIL, and, thus, mimicking rituximab. These findings with the cell lines were further validated with patient-derived B-NHL tumor samples in tissue microarrays (TMA) and showed that the tumors overexpressed YY1 and YY1 levels correlated with lower levels of DR5. These findings are in agreement with those of Daniels et al. [86] who demonstrated that the combination treatment of rituximab and TRAIL resulted in significant potentiation of apoptosis by rituximab described above and inhibition of tumor growth in vivo.

The sensitization to TRAIL apoptosis by rituximab is important for its potential implication for its antitumor activity in vivo in patients. Hence, in addition to the direct cytotoxic effect of rituximab used alone and/or in combination with drugs, it recruits host effector cells expressing Fas-L and TRAIL to mediate tumor cell killing independent of ADCC and CDC.

Rituximab Signaling is Independent of Fc

Our above findings demonstrated that treatment of various CD20+ B-NHL cell lines with rituximab resulted in significant inhibition of cell proliferation and several survival anti-apoptotic pathways and chemo-immunosensitization [87]. We assumed that these effects are the direct interaction of rituximab with CD20 and inhibiting survival cell signaling pathways. However, rituximab-induced cell signaling might have been, completely or partially, due to the participation of the interaction of the Fc fragment of rituximab with Fc receptors expressed on the membranes of tumor cells. Several Fc receptors when triggered may lead to either activation or inhibition of survival pathways. Four classes of Fc receptors have been identified, namely, FcγRI, FcγRII, FcγRIII, and FcγRIV. The activating receptors transmit their signals via immune-tyrosine based activating motifs (ITAM) and inhibitory receptors via immuno-tyrosine-based inhibitory motifs (ITIM), respectively [88, 89]. To investigate the role of Fc-FcR interactions on tumor cells signaling, we have selected to examine the effect of Fc devoid rituximab fragment (Fab')2 and compared the findings with wild type rituximab. Overall, we did not find any differences, qualitatively or quantitatively, between the effects of (Fab')2 or wild type rituximab in the various experimental designs examined. Briefly, the inhibition of cell proliferation, apoptosis-induced by cross linking with a secondary anti-IgG antibody, the inhibition of constitutively activated p38 MAPK and NF-κB signaling pathways and the sensitization to apoptosis by various drugs were achieved by (Fab')2 similar to findings achieved with rituximab. In addition to the in vitro findings, in vivo data with tumor xenografts correlated with the in vitro findings and demonstrated that inhibition of tumor growth following treatment with (Fab')2 and CDDP was comparable to the findings achieved with rituximab and CDDP [87]. Altogether, these findings establish a direct signaling by rituximab on CD20+ B-NHL cells leading inhibition of survival pathways. These findings suggest that the chemo and immuno-sensitization effects induced in patients by rituximab may be independent of the FcγR polymorphism [38].

Development of Resistance to Rituximab Treatment and Generation of Rituximab-Resistant Clones

It has been reported that deregulation of signal transduction pathways, such as the NF-κB, MAPKs, JAK/STAT, AKT/PI3, or aberrant expression of the signaling molecules, can contribute to the acquired chemoresistance [89, 90]. Since chemotherapeutic drugs utilize apoptosis as a mean of exerting their cytotoxic effects, drug-resistant tumor cells develop cross-resistance to apoptosis-induced by structurally and functionally distinct stimuli including immunotherapy and vice versa. Although rituximab therapy has significantly improved the treatment outcome of NHL patients, a subset of patients does not respond or relapses after the initial treatment. Selective outgrowth of the drug-resistant cells will complicate subsequent treatment regimens and will eventually lead to the patient's demise. It is, therefore, imperative to unravel the mechanisms of intrinsic or acquired resistance to rituximab treatment. Resistance acquired during the course of therapy, that is commonly seen in various cancers, appears to involve similar mechanisms of intrinsic resistance [89]. Thus, approaches that overcome intrinsic resistance should theoretically bypass the acquired resistance and vice versa. Various mechanisms have been postulated for rituximab resistance including transient CD20 downregulation [91–95], loss of CD20 [96, 97], circulating CD20 [98], and expression of complement inhibitors [45]. These issues have been elegantly reviewed [99–101].

Rituximab has been described as the most therapeutically effective antibody developed today. Its limitation is the development of resistance. Insights into rituximab resistance are relevant to other members of antitumor antibodies. The definition of rituximab resistance is lack of response to a rituximab-containing regimen within 6 months of treatment. Overt disease progression during treatment is the more defined form of rituximab resistance. 30–60 % of antibody naive patients with indolent NHL are resistant to the rituximab at baseline. This percentage is significantly lower with combination of rituximab and CHOP. Several mechanisms of resistance have been indentified such as resistance to CDC, resistance to ADCC, resistance to apoptosis, decrease expression and/or mutation of CD20, and dosing regimens. Several mechanisms have been suggested to circumvent resistance. These include administration of cytokines such as G-CSF, G-MCSF, IL-2, IL-15, CpG oligonucleotide. In addition, novel anti-CD20 antibodies have been developed such as Ofatumumab. See recent results on type 2 GA-101 antibody [102–104].

The role of ADCC and CDC in rituximab-mediated cytotoxicity and resistance has been examined by several investigators and reviewed by Taylor and Lindorfer [101]. Among the noted mechanisms of resistance to cytotoxic activity include inhibition of ADCC by deposition of C3 activation fragments [105] and polymorphism in FcγR in the cytotoxic cells [37, 49]. Also, inhibition of CDC through blocking the action of CD55 and CD59 [106]. Other mechanisms include the loss of CD20 on the surface of subclones [95, 107]. The tumor microenvironment may also affect the response [108].

In an attempt to recapitulate the non-responders and/or relapsed situations in the rituximab- treated patients, we have generated rituximab-refractory NHL clones by growing the cells in the presence of step-wise increasing concentrations of rituximab followed by multiple rounds of limiting dilution assays and rituximab-resistant (RR) clones were generated and assayed for alterations in the signal transduction pathways compared to the parental cell lines. In these rituximab-resistant clones, rituximab is incapable of either inhibition of cellular growth or induction of apoptosis (both in monomeric and crosslinked forms). Noteworthy, rituximab has lost its chemo or immunosensitizing effect on these CD20-expressing NHL B cell clones. Compared to the parental cells, the RR clones exhibited higher resistance to rituximab-mediated CDC (using human AB serum). There was a significantly higher overexpression of Bcl_{xL} and higher resistance to a wide array of antineopleastic agents in the RR clones [109], concordant with the protective role of Bcl_{xL} [110–114]. Therefore, as NHL cells develop resistance to rituximab, they may also develop crossresistance to the cytotoxic effects of the chemotherapeutic drugs and the immune system, consistent with our observation that the rituximab-resistant clones also exhibit higher resistance to TNF-related apoptosis-inducing ligand (TRAIL) and anti-Fas Ab. Thus, we hypothesized that pharmacological inhibition of these pathways could potentially avert the chemo- or immuno-resistant phenotype.

Comparing the RR clones to WT clones revealed that the RR clones expressed lower surface CD20, were unresponsive to ADCC, CDC, and cross-linking induced apoptosis. Further, there was no inhibition or alteration of intracellular survival pathways as shown in WT (such as inhibition of NF-κB, p38MAPK, Raf/ERK pathways). The lack of response of RR to rituximab was not due to the lower expression of CD20 as the activity by rituximab is autonomous of CD20 expression levels [95]. The RR clones exhibited hyperactivation of the NF-κB and ERK1/2 pathways compared to WT leading to overexpression of antiapoptotic gene products, targets of above pathways, Bcl-2, Bcl_{xL}, Mcl-1.

Reversal of Rituximab Resistance by the Use of Intracellular Target Inhibitors

NF-κB Inhibitors

We have reported that rituximab interferes and inhibits intracellular signal transduction pathways and sensitizes B-NHL cell lines to apoptosis by various chemo-immunotherapeutic drugs. The sensitization was the result of the selected inhibition of anti-apoptotic gene products, targets of upstream signaling pathways, such as Bcl-2 and Bcl_{xL} [70, 71, 73]. Bcl_{xL} and Bcl-2 exert their anti-apoptotic effects primarily on the membrane of the mitochondria preventing loss of cytochrome C and initiation of apoptosis [114]. The mechanism by which rituximab inhibits Bcl_{xL} expression may be the result of various mechanisms that have been implicated in the transcription of Bcl_{xL}. One of these mechanisms is via NF-κB which regulates Bcl_{xL} transcription [115].

The role of rituximab-induced inhibition of NF-κB and Bcl_{xL} and chemosensitization was corroborated by the use of various inhibitors, namely, functional blocking of NF-κB (ex: IκB mutant), physiological inhibitors of the NF-κB pathway (Bay-7805 and DMHEQ) or functional impairment of Bcl_{xL} (2MAM-A3), all of which have led to inhibition of Bcl_{xL} and chemosensitization [73].

We have reported the development in rituximab-RR clones and characterized their properties in comparison with parental wild type. In that study, we have demonstrated that treatment of RR with inhibitors of survival pathways can revert resistance to chemotherapy [116]. In a more detailed analysis, we have investigated the role of the FDA-approved proteasome inhibitor, Bortezomib, on the RR clones, following treatment with Bortezomib alone or in combination with chemotherapy. We initially focused on an AIDS-derived B-NHL cell line, 2F7, which was used to generate 2F7 RR clones. The rationale of this analysis was due, in part, to the fact that HIV-associated NHL remains a significant problem even in the era of retroactive therapy. Treatments of patients with rituximab in combination with chemotherapy resulted in improved complete response rates but was associated with increased incidence of infection in a subset of patients with low CD4 counts [117, 118]. A representative 2F7 RR1 clone was chosen as a prototype for analysis. Failure of the 2F7 RR1 clone to rituximab-induced inhibition of survival pathways and chemosensitization suggested that the use of inhibitors of intracellular survival pathways may reverse drug resistance. Hence, we used the proteasome inhibitor, Bortezomib, and the NF-κB inhibitor, DHMEQ. Following treatment of 2F7 RR1 with these inhibitors, Bcl-2 expression was down regulated as a result of NF-κB inhibition by these inhibitors. Such treatment sensitized the 2F7 RR1 clone to apoptosis by various drugs (ex. Taxol, VP-16, CDDP, vincristine)-induced apoptosis.

The overall response rate (ORR), time to progression (TTP), and duration of response (DOR) were determined in patients with relapsed and refractory CD20+ follicular lymphoma or marginal lymphoma following treatment by the combination of Bortezomib and rituximab. The findings demonstrated that the combination treatment had activity and the ORRs were 49 and 43 %, respectively, for two different regimens. The relationship between the response observed between the combination treatment and the treatment with rituximab alone is not clear and a randomized study comparing them should determine if Bortezomib added to the efficacy of rituximab [119].

HDAC Inhibitors and Rituximab

Rituximab resistance has emerged as an important clinical problem that needs remedy [99, 120]. The loss of CD20 expression is one of various mechanisms that is frequently associated with innate and adaptive immunity. For instance, several cases of $CD20^-$ lymphoma relapses were identified after treatment with rituximab-based regimens in DLBCL [95]. Hiraga et al. [121] reported that 30 % of patients with B cell lymphoma and treated with rituximab-containing chemotherapy their CD20 expression was lost. Of interest, DNA demethylating agents restored CD20 expression in those patients, hence, indicating underlying epigenetic mechanisms being involved. HDACs have been implicated in the drug resistance of B cell malignancies such as multiple myeloma (M/M) [122]. Therefore, HDAC inhibitors may restore the expression of genes that are apparently expressed in cancer such as CD20 in the present case. They examined the role of HDAC inhibitors on both CD20 expression and activity of rituximab. The HDAC inhibitors, Valproic acid (VA) and romidepsin were used on B cell lines and resulted in the potentiation of the cytotoxic effects of CDC by rituximab against resistant Burkitt's Lymphoma cell lines. In addition, the expression of CD20 was augmented following treatment in vitro and in vivo in mice-bearing tumor xenografts. In vivo, the authors demonstrated that there was synergy by the combination treatment of rituximab and HDAC inhibitors. It will be useful to study the role of HDAC inhibitors on RR clones and their chemo-immuno-sensitizing effects.

Combination Bcl-2 Inhibitor and Rituximab

Bcl-2 overexpression is common in NHL and has been associated with poor clinical response and shorter survival [123–125]. Oblimersen sodium (Bcl-2 antisense oligonucleotide, Genta Inc) is a single stranded 18 mer oligodeoxynucleotide complimentary to the first six codons of the human Bcl-2 reading frame. In a phase I study, oblimersen has been shown to modify Bcl-2 levels and induced objective responses in heavily-treated patients with NHL [126]. A phase II study was conducted in patients with B cell NHL to determine the efficacy and safety of the combination of oblimersen and rituximab. The findings demonstrated safety of administration by the combination. There was a modest activity in patients with recurrent disease. Also, there was a limited efficacy in patients with DLBCL. However, the highest response rate was observed in patients with follicular lymphoma. Seventy % of patients with follicular lymphoma had received prior treatment with rituximab and an encouraging response of 60 % was observed, suggesting synergy. Noteworthy, the combination of rituximab and oblimersen was effective in patients with rituximab-refractory disease suggesting that oblimersen could reverse the mechanism of resistance torituximab.

NO Donors

Among the many novel therapeutics that are currently in use or in development, nitric oxide (NO) has recently caught the attention for its potential use in cancer therapy. NO exerts many activities in the tested cell lines due to its pleiotropic effects. When used at low concentrations, NO exhibits its pro-inflammatory effects by inducing vasodilation and recruitment of neutrophils. The production of NO by nNOS and eNOS isoforms results in the regulation of the expression of adhesion molecules, cytokines and chemokines, and leading to migration/adhesion [127]. At high concentrations, however, NO down regulates the expression of adhesion molecules, suppresses the activation of inflammatory cells, and induces cell killing by apoptosis. NO has been shown to play a significant role in many diseases [128]. In cancer, NO has been shown to be involved in both the pathogenesis as well as in the protection of tumors. These contradictory effects are the result of both the source and concentration of NO, its sustenance in the tumor microenvironment and the tumor type. High levels of NO produced by iNOS have been reported to inhibit tumor cell proliferation and survival and can induce apoptosis in sensitive cancer cells. In addition, NO can sensitize resistant tumor cells to chemotherapy, radiation, and immunotherapy and can also inhibit metastasis [129–131].

There are several novel therapeutic agents under laboratory and clinical evaluations, several of which are directly targeting the cancer cell. Among these, attention has recently been given to the potential role of endogenous nitric oxide (NO) and exogenous NO donors. Due to the pleiotropic nature of NO and its various and contrasting activities, NO has emerged as a significant novel cancer therapeutic when used under appropriate conditions [85]. Below, I describe briefly the role of NO in cell signaling modification of survival/anti-apoptotic pathways and its ability to reverse resistance by sensitizing cancer cells to apoptotic stimuli.

NO is a highly inactive free radical, capable of mediating a variety of chemical reactions in the cell [127, 132, 133]. NO is a pleiotropic molecule that mediates a variety of cell signaling functions. It regulates mitochondrial respiration through binding to the cytochrome c-oxidase [134]. In addition, NO plays a role in cell death and apoptosis; sustained production of NO acts as a pro-apoptotic modulator by activating capases, whereas low or physiological levels of NO prevent cells from programmed cell death [135]. NO exerts many effects in a variety of physiological systems and diseases [136].

The rationale for considering NO as a cancer therapeutic emanated, in part, from the finding that NO inhibited the survival/anti-apoptotic NF-κB pathway via S-nitrosyliation of p50, [136] and, hence, inhibited downstream several anti-apoptotic gene products that regulate tumor resistance. This inhibitory effect by NO results in the reduction of the anti-apoptotic threshold and leading to the sensitization of resistant tumor cells to various apoptotic stimuli. This activity has been validated in various reports both in vitro and pre-clinically in vivo in animals. Wink et al. [137] were the first to report that NO reverses cancer cell resistance to chemotherapeutic drugs. Thereafter, other reports showed the chemosensitizing effects of NO [138]. Huerta-Yepez et al. [139] reported that the NO donor DETANONOate sensitizes prostate cancer cell lines to apoptosis by CDDP and NO inhibited the anti-apoptotic gene products Bcl_{xL} and XIAP. The in vitro findings were validated in vivo in mice bearing tumor xenografts that were treated with DETANONOate, CDDP and combination. The treatment by the combination, unlike single agents, resulted in significant tumor regression [139].

In addition to NO-mediated reversal of tumor cell resistance to chemotherapeutic drugs, NO also sensitized resistant tumor cells to immune therapy such as by FasL and TNF-α [81, 140–142]. In addition, NO sensitized tumor cells to TRAIL apoptosis. The sensitization was due in part to NO-mediated inhibition of NF-κB and YY1 and their nitrosylation and leading to upregulation of DR5. The in vitro findings were validated in vivo in mice bearing human tumor xenografts [143]. Further, NO donors were reported to sensitize tumor cells to radiation induced cell death [130, 144, 145].

The molecular mechanism mediated by NO in the reversal of resistance was briefly described above for immunotherapy and chemotherapy. Overall, NO inhibits NF-κB activity and downstream the resistant factors YY1 and Snail and resulting in the induction of the pro-apoptotic factor raft kinase inhibitor protein (RKIP). Thus, NO interferes with the dysregulated NF-κB/YY1/Snail/RKIP resistant loop and resulting in the reversal of tumor resistance to both chemo and immunotherapies [146]. Thus, RR clones may be treated with NO donors and resulting in the reversal of resistance to rituximab.

Combination of Anti-CD20 and Anti-CD22 for NHL

This study evaluated the effects of combining anti-CD20 (a new humanized, IMMU-106) and anti-CD22 (humanized Epratuzumab). CD22 functions as a adhesion receptor for B cells, T-cells, monocytes, neutrophils, and red blood cells. It is also involved in signal transduction and modulation of B cell antigen receptors-mediated signal transduction [147, 148]. Unlike other CD22 monoclonal antibodies studied, Epratuzumab does not block the ligand-binding site of CD22. However, ligation of CD22 with Epratuzumab causes rapid internalization of the monoclonal antibody and induces phosphorylation of the CD22 cytoplasmic tail [149]. In clinical studies, Epratuzumab has shown evidence of anti-tumor activity in patients with recurrent NHL and produced responses in patients with follicular lymphoma and DLBCL [150]. Thus, the combination of Epratuzumab with anti-CD20 monoclonal antibody may result in additive or synergistic activities. The overall response rate of Epratuzumab combined with rituximab in indolent follicular NHL was reported to be similar to rituximab alone but a higher complete response rate was found. These findings imply that the combination is synergistic in those patients having both target antigens and responding to either agent alone.

Combination of Rituximab and TRAIL or Anti-DR4/DR5 Antibody

Maddipatla et al. [151] examined the effect of the combination treatment with fully humanized Mapatumumab (anti-DR4) and Lexatumumab (anti-DR5) in combination with rituximab in studies done both in vitro and in vivo in mice bearing tumor xenografts. The advantages of using agonist monoclonal antibodies against death receptors of TRAIL over TRAIL ligand lies on the specificity for only functional TRAIL receptors (and not the non-functional decoy receptor) and the longer half life as compared to soluble TRAIL. The combination induced effective anti-lymphoma efficacy *in vitro* and *in vivo* [151, 152]. The potential clinical effects of anti-DR4 and anti-DR5 monoclonal antibodies may increase the

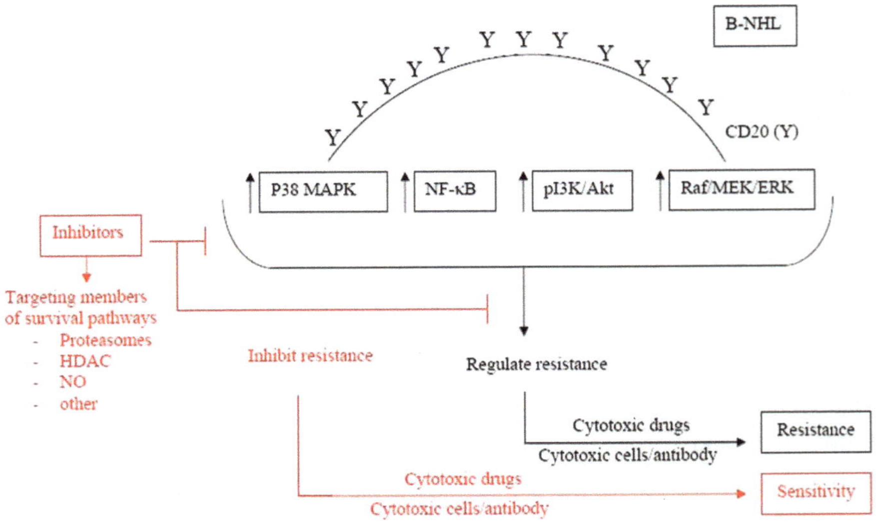

Fig. 1 Schematic diagram illustrating the constitutively activated survival pathways in B-NHL that regulate resistance to cytotoxic drugs, cells and antibodies. Treatment with various inhibitors directed against members of the activated survival pathways results in the inhibition of the activities of these pathways and rendering the cells sensitive to cytotoxic drugs, cells and antibodies

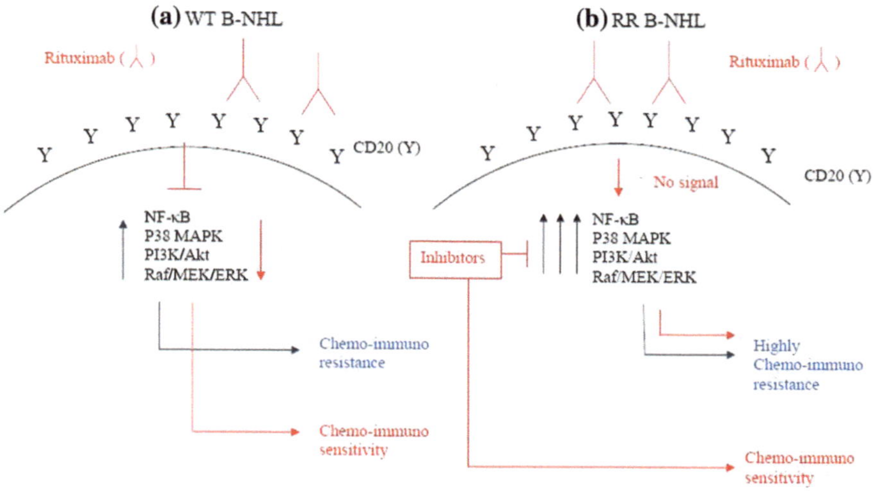

Fig. 2 Comparison between the responses of wildtype B-NHL and rituximab-resistant (*RR*) B-NHL following rituximab treatment. *A* Treatment of wild type (*WT*) B-NHL with rituximab results in inhibition of survival pathways and rendering the cells chemo- and immunosensitive to cytotoxic agents *B* Treatment of rituximab-resistant (*RR*) B-NHL cells with rituximab does not signal the cells and does not result in the inhibition of the survival pathways and, therefore, the cells remain highly resistant to cytotoxic agents. However, treatment with various inhibitors of the survival pathways results in the inhibition of these pathways and rendering the cells sensitive to cytotoxic agents

treatment options for many lymphoma patients. Using various B-NHL cell lines, it was found that Mapatumumab and not Lexatumumab induced cell growth inhibition and apoptosis in NHL cell lines in vitro and in xenografts. Mapatumumab also induced ADCC and CDC in sensitive B lymphoma cell lines. A phase II study with Mapatumumab showed 30 % of all the patients had diseased stabilization in patients with relapsed and refractory to rituximab. The combination of Mapatumumab and rituximab in vivo in mice bearing tumor xenografts showed that the survival of lymphoma bearing SCID mice was longest in mice receiving the combination compared to mice receiving a single treatment. In vitro, the combination showed additive effects in cell growth inhibition and ADCC activity.

Concluding Remarks

This review summarizes published reports on the underlying mechanisms responsible, in part, for the various functions and activities of the first FDA-approved anti cancer mAb, rituximab. The findings that have been obtained with rituximab, thus far, may serve as a backbone for the analyses and investigations for the functions of other therapeutic mAbs against cancer; these will determine both common and unique mechanisms of action (Fig. 1). The development of resistant mechanisms to antibody therapeutics are not clear in vivo and in vitro; however, the analysis of cell lines that have been developed for the resistance against a particular mAb, as discussed herein for the rituximab resistant (RR) clones, is an approach that is also applicable for other therapeutic antibodies as well (Fig. 2). The findings obtained with the RR clones have shed some insight into potential underlying mechanisms that regulate resistance that may also occur in vivo in patients. However, such studies must be undertaken for validation. Several approaches have been used to reverse the resistance to antibody therapeutics and some examples have been discussed in this review for the reversal of the rituximab-resistant clones and some of these approaches may be considered as novel strategies that can be translated in vivo. Since several examples of targeted inhibitors were shown in vitro to reverse resistance to both chemotherapeutic and immunotherapeutic drugs, it follows that such inhibitors and others may be tested clinically for their efficacies and synergies with conventional drugs [157]. Clearly, such strategies and novel ones are the means to proceed with further investigations to unravel additional mechanisms that regulate resistance and identify new targets of interest for both prognosis and new therapeutics.

Acknowledgments This work was supported by a gift from various donors and, in part, by the Jonsson Comprehensive Cancer Center at UCLA. The author acknowledges Drs. Ali R. Jazirehi, Mario I. Vega, and Stavroula Baritaki for their published research that forums and the basis of this review. The author also acknowledges the assistance of Daphne Liang, Melissa Cao, Kathy Nguyen, and Suzie Vardanyan for the preparation of the manuscript.

Conflicts of Interest No potential conflicts of interest were disclosed.

References

1. Lippert TH, Ruoff HJ, Volm M. Intrinsic and acquired drug resistance in malignant tumors. The main reason for therapeutic failure. Arzneimittelforschung. 2008;58:261–4.
2. Inoue J, Gohda J, Akiyama T, Semba K. NF-kappaB activation in development and progression of cancer. Cancer Sci. 2007;98:268–74.
3. McCubrey JA, Steelman LS, Chappell WH, Abrams SL, Wong EW, Chang F, Lehmann B, Terrian DM, Milella M, Tafuri A, Stivala F, Libra M, Basecke J, Evangelisti C, Martelli AM, Franklin RA. Roles of the Raf/MEK/ERK pathway in cell growth, malignant transformation and drug resistance. Biochim Biophys Acta. 2007;1773:1263–84.
4. MacKenzie SH, Clark AC. Targeting cell death in tumors by activating caspases. Curr Cancer Drug Targets. 2008;8:98–109.
5. Wu AA, Niparko KJ, Pai SI. Immunotherapy for head and neck cancer. J Biomed Sci. 2008;15:275–89.
6. Katsman A, Umezawa K, Bonavida B. Chemosensitization and immunosensitization of resistant cancer cells to apoptosis and inhibition of metastasis by the specific NF-κB inhibitor DHMEQ. Curr Pharm Des. 2009;15:792–808.
7. Ng CP, Bonavida B. A new challenge for successful immunotherapy by tumors that are resistant to apoptosis: two complementary signals to overcome cross-resistance. Adv Cancer Res. 2002;85:145–74.

8. Kipp RT, McNeel DG. Immunotherapy for prostate cancer—recent progress in clinical trials. Clin Adv Hematol Oncol. 2007;5:465–474, 477–479.
9. Strome SE, Sausville EA, Mann D. A mechanistic perspective of monoclonal antibodies in cancer therapy beyond target-related effects. Oncologist. 2007;12:1084–95.
10. Dalle S, Thieblemont C, Thomas L, Dumontet C. Monoclonal antibodies in clinical oncology. Anticancer Agents Med Chem. 2008;8:523–32.
11. Bonavida B. Rituximab-induced inhibition of antiapoptotic cell survival pathways: implications in chemo/immunoresistance, rituximab unresponsiveness, prognostic and novel therapeutic interventions. Oncogene. 2007;26:3629–36.
12. Firer MA, Gellerman G. Targeted drug delivery for cancer therapy: the other side of antibodies. J Hematol Oncol. 2012;5:70.
13. Kohler G, Milstein C. Continuous cultures of fused cells secreting antibody of predefined specificity. Nature 1975;256:495–7.
14. White DM, Jensen MA, Shi X, Qu Z, Arnason BG. Design and expression of polymeric immunoglobulin fusion proteins: a strategy for targeting low-affinity Fcgamma receptors. Protein Expr Purif. 2001;21:446–55.
15. Zelentez A. Presented at the international conference on malignant lymphoma. Switzerland: Lugano; 1999.
16. Reff ME, Carner K, Chambers KS, Chinn PC, Leonar JE, Raab R, Newman RA, Hanna N, Anderson DR. Depletion of B cells in vivo by a chimeric mouse human monoclonal antibody to CD20. Blood 1994;83:435–45.
17. Newman R, Alberts J, Anderson D, Carner K, Heard C, Norton F, Raab R, Reff M, Shuey S, Hanna N. "Primatization" of recombinant antibodies for immunotherapy of human diseases: a macaque/human chimeric antibody against human CD4. Biotechnology. 1992;10:1455–60.
18. McLaughlin P, Grillo-Lopez AJ, Link BK, Levy R, Czuczman MS, Williams ME, Heyman MR, Bence-Bruckler I, White CA, Cabanillas F, Jain V, Ho AD, Lister J, Wey K, Shen D, Dallaire BK. J Clin Oncol. 1998;16:2825–33.
19. Ferrara N, Hillan KJ, Gerber HP, Novotny W. Discovery and development of bevacizumab, an anti-VEGF antibody for treating cancer. Nat Rev Drug Discov. 2004;3:391–400.
20. Witzig TE, White CA, Wiseman GA, Gordon LI, Emmanouilides C, Raubitschek A, Janakiraman N, Gutheil J, Schilder RJ, Spies S, Silverman DH, Parker E, Grillo-Lopez AJ. J Clin Oncol. 1999;17:3793–803.
21. Cragg MS, Walshe CA, Ivanov AO, Glennie MJ. The biology of CD20 and its potential as a target for mAb therapy. Curr Dir Autoimmun. 2005;8:140–74.
22. Coffey J, Hodgson DC, Gospodarowicz MK. Eur J Nucl Med Mol Imaging. 2003; 30:S28–36.
23. Swerdlow AJ. Epidemiology of Hodgkin's disease and non-Hodgkin's lymphoma. Eur J Nucl Med Mol Imaging. 2003;30:S3–12.
24. Theodossiou C, Schwarzenberger P. Non-Hodgkin's lymphomas. Clin Obstet Gynecol. 2002;45:820–9.
25. Smith MR. Non-Hodgkin's lymphoma. Curr Probl Cancer. 1996;20:6–77.
26. Hiddemann W. Non-Hodgkin's lymphomas—current status of therapy and future perspectives. Eur J Cancer. 1995;31A:2141–5.
27. Tan BR, Bartlett NL. Treatment advances in non-Hodgkin's lymphoma. Expert Opin Pharmacother. 2000;1:451–66.
28. Fisher RI. Overview of non-Hodgkin's lymphoma: biology, staging, and treatment. Semin Oncol. 2003;30:3–9.
29. Acker B, Hoppe RT, Colby TV, Cox RS, Kaplan HS, Rosenberg SA. Histologic conversion in the non-Hodgkin's lymphomas. J Clin Oncol. 1983;1:11–6.
30. Horning SJ, Rosenberg SA. The natural history of initially untreated low-grade non-Hodgkin's lymphomas. N Engl J Med. 1984;311:1471–5.
31. Horning SJ, Negrin RS, Hoppe RT, Rosenberg SA, Chao NJ, Long GD, Brown BW, Blume KG. High-dose therapy and autologous bone marrow transplantation for follicular

lymphoma in first complete or partial remission: results of a phase II clinical trial. Blood. 2001;97:404–9.
32. Hennessy BT, Hanrahan EO, Daly PA. Non-Hodgkin lymphoma: an update. Lancet Oncol. 2004;5:341–53.
33. Vose JM. Antibody-targeted therapy for low-grade lymphoma. Semin Hematol. 1999; 36:15–20.
34. van der Kolk LE, de Haas M, Grillo-López AJ, Baars JW, van Oers MH. Analysis of CD20-dependent cellular cytotoxicity by G-CSF-stimulated neutrophils. Leukemia. 2002; 16:693–9.
35. Friedberg JW, Neuberg D, Gribben JG, Fisher DC, Canning C, Koval M, Poor CM, Green LM, Daley J, Soiffer R, Ritz J, Freedman AS. Combination immunotherapy with rituximab and interleukin 2 in patients with relapsed or refractory follicular non-Hodgkin's lymphoma. Br J Haematol. 2002;117:828–34.
36. Johnson P, Glennie M. The mechanisms of action of rituximab in the elimination of tumor cells. Semin Oncol. 2003;30:3–8.
37. Cartron G, Dacheux L, Salles G, Solal-Celigny P, Bardos P, Colombat P, Watier H. Therapeutic activity of humanized anti-CD20 monoclonal antibody and polymorphism in IgG Fc receptor FcgammaRIIIa gene. Blood. 2002;99:754–8.
38. Colombat P, Watier H. Therapeutic activity of humanized anti-CD20 monoclonal antibody and polymorphism in IgG Fc receptor FcgammaRIIIa gene. Blood. 2002;99:754–8.
39. Idusogie EE, Wong PY, Presta LG, Gazzano-Santoro H, Totpal K, Ultsch M, Mulkerrin MG. Engineered antibodies with increased activity to recruit complement. J Immunol. 2001;166:2571–5.
40. Manches O, Lui G, Chaperot L, Gressin R, Molens JP, Jacob MC, Sotto JJ, Leroux D, Bensa JC, Plumas J. In vitro mechanisms of action of rituximab on primary non-Hodgkin lymphomas. Blood. 2003;101:949–54.
41. Golay J, Gramigna R, Facchinetti V, Capello D, Gaidano G, Introna M. Acquired immunodeficiency syndrome-associated lymphomas are efficiently lysed through complement-dependent cytotoxicity and antibody-dependent cellular cytotoxicity by rituximab. Br J Haematol. 2002;119:923–9.
42. Kennedy AD, Solga MD, Shcuman TA, Chi AW, Lindorfer MA, Sutherland WM, Foley PL, Taylor RP. An anti-C3b(i) mAb enhances complement activation, C3b(i) deposition, and killing of CD20+ cells by rituximab. Blood. 2003;101:1071–9.
43. Golay J, Zaffaroni L, Vaccari T, Lazzari M, Borleri GM, Bernasconi S, Tedesco F, Rambaldi A, Introna M. Biologic response of B lymphoma cells to anti-CD20 monoclonal antibody rituximab in vitro: CD55 and CD59 regulate complement-mediated cell lysis. Blood. 2000;95:3900–8.
44. Harjunapaa A, Junnikkala S, Meri S. Rituximab (anti-CD20) therapy of B-cell lymphomas: direct complement killing is superior to cellular effector mechanisms. Scand J Immunol. 2000;51:634–41.
45. Treon SP, Mitsiades C, Mitsiades N, Young G, Doss D, Schlossman R, Anderson KC. Tumor cell expression of CD59 is associated with resistance to CD20 serotherapy in patients with B-cell malignancies. J Immunother. 2001;24:263–71.
46. Cardarelli PM, Quinn M, Buckman D, Fang Y, Colcher D, King DJ, Bebbington C, Yarranton G. Binding to CD20 by anti-B1 antibody or F(ab')(2) is sufficient for induction of apoptosis in B-cell lines. Cancer Immuno Immunother. 2002;51:15–24.
47. Bellosillo B, Villamor N, Lopez-Guillermo A, Marce S, Esteve J, Campo E, Colomer D, Montserrat E. Complement-mediated cell death induced by rituximab in B-cell lymphoproliferative disorders is mediated in vitro by a caspase-independent mechanism involving the generation of reactive oxygen species. Blood. 2001;98:2771–7.
48. Bannerji R, Kitada S, Flinn IW, Paerson M, Young D, Reed JC, Byrd JC. Apoptotic-regulatory and complement-protecting protein expression in chronic lymphocytic leukemia: relationship to in vivo rituximab resistance. J Clin Oncol. 2003;21:1466–71.

49. Weng WK, Levy R. Two immunoglobulin G fragment C receptor polymorphisms independently predict response to rituximab in patients with follicular lymphoma. J Clin Oncol. 2003;21:3940–7.
50. Demidem A, Hanna N, Hariharan H, Bonavida B. Chimeric anti-CD20 (IDEC-C2B8) monoclonal antibody sensitizes a B cell lymphoma cell line to cell killing by cytotoxic drugs. FASEB J. 1995;9:A206.
51. Ghetie MA, Podar EM, Ilgen A, Gordon BE, Uhr JW, Vivetta ES. Homodimerization of tumor-reactive monoclonal antibodies markedly increases their ability to induce growth arrest or apoptosis of tumor cells. Proc Natl Acad Sci USA. 1997;8:7509–14.
52. Hofmeister JK, Cooney D, Coggeshall KM. Clustered CD20 induced apoptosis: src-family kinase, the proximal regulator of tyrosine phosphorylation, calcium influx, and caspase 3-dependent apoptosis. Blood Cells Mol Dis. 2000;26:133–43.
53. Shan D, Ledbetter JA, Press OW. Signaling events involved in anti-CD20-induced apoptosis of malignant human B cells. Cancer Immunol Immunother. 2000;48:673–83.
54. Pedersen IM, Buhl AM, Klausen P, Geisler CH, Jurlander J. The chimeric anti-CD20 antibody rituximab induces apoptosis in B-cell chronic lymphocytic leukemia cells through a p38 mitogen activated protein-kinase-dependent mechanism. Blood. 2002;99:1314–9.
55. Mathas S, Rickers A, Bommert K, Dorken B, Mapara MY. Anti-CD20- and B-cell receptor-mediated apoptosis: evidence for shared intracellular signaling pathways. Cancer Res. 2000;60:7170–6.
56. Polyak MJ, Tailor SH, Deans JP. Identification of a cytoplasmic region of CD20 required for its redistribution to a detergent-insoluble membrane compartment. J Immunol. 1998;161:3242–8.
57. Cragg MS, Morgan SM, Chan HT, Morgan BP, Filatov AV, Johnson PW, French R, Glennie MJ. Complement-mediated lysis by anti-CD20 mAb correlates with segregation into lipid rafts. Blood. 2003;101:1045–52.
58. Claude Chan HT, Hughes D, French RR, Tutt AL, Walshe CA, Teeling JL, Glennie MJ, Cragg MS. CD20-induced lymphoma cell death is independent of both caspases and its redistribution into triton X-100 insoluble membrane rafts. Cancer Res. 2003;63:5480–9.
59. Deans JP, Kalt L, Ledbetter JA, Schieven GL, Bolen JB, Johnson P. Association of 75/80-kDa phosphoproteins and the tyrosine kinases Lyn, Fyn, and Lck with the B cell molecule CD20. Evidence against involvement of the cytoplasmic regions of CD20. J Biol Chem. 1995;270:22632–8.
60. Deans JP, Robbins SM, Polyak MJ, Savage JA. Rapid redistribution of CD20 to a low density detergent-insoluble. J Biol Chem. 1998;273:344–8.
61. Semac I, Palomba C, Kulangara K, Klages N, van Echten-Deckert G, Borisch B. Anti-CD20 therapeutic antibody rituximab modifies the functional organization of rafts/microdomains of B lymphoma cells. Cancer Res. 2003;63:534–40.
62. Jazirehi AR, Vega MI, Chatterjee D, Goodglick L, Bonavida B. Inhibition of the Raf-MEK1/2-ERK1/2 signaling pathway, Bcl_{xL} down-regulation, and chemosensitization of non-Hodgkin's lymphoma B cells by rituximab. Cancer Res. 2004;64:117–26.
63. Bezombes C, Grazide S, Garret C, Fabre C, Quillet-Mary A, Muller S, Jaffrezou JP, Laurent G. Rituximab antiproliferative effect in B-lymphoma cells is associated with acid-sphingomyelinase activation in raft microdomains. Blood. 2004;104:1166–73.
64. Deans JP, Li H, Polyak MJ. CD20-mediated apoptosis: signalling through lipid rafts. Immunology. 2002;107:176–82.
65. Demiden A, Lam T, Alas S, Hariharan K, Hanna N, Bonavida B. Chimeric Anti-CD20 (IDEC-c2B8) monoclonal antibody sensitizes a B-cell lymphoma cell line to cell killing by cytotoxic drugs. Cancer Biother Radiopharm. 1997;12:177–86.
66. Alas S, Bonavida B. Rituximab inactivates signal transducer and activation of transcription 3 (STAT3) activity in B-non-Hodgkin's lymphoma through inhibition of the interleukin 10 autocrine/paracrine loop and results in down-regulation of Bcl-2 and sensitization to cytotoxic drugs. Cancer Res. 2001;61:5137–44.

67. Alas S, Emmanouilides C, Bonavida B. Inhibition of interleukin 10 by rituximab results in down-regulation of bcl-2 and sensitization of B-cell non-Hodgkin's lymphoma to apoptosis. Clin Cancer Res. 2001;7:709–23.
68. Alas S, Bonavida B. Inhibition of constitutive STAT3 activity sensitizes resistant non-Hodgkin's lymphoma and multiple myeloma to chemotherapeutic drug-mediated apoptosis. Clin Cancer Res. 2003;9:316–26.
69. Vega MI, Huerta-Yepaz S, Garban H, Jazirehi A, Emmanouilides C, Bonavida B. Rituximab inhibits p38 MAPK activity in 2F7 B NHL and decreases IL-10 transcription: pivotal role of p38 MAPK in drug resistance. Oncogene. 2004;23:3530–40.
70. Jazirehi AR, Gan XH, De Vos S, Emmanouilides C, Bonavida B. Rituximab (anti-CD20) selectively modifies Bcl_{xL} and apoptosis protease activating factor-1 (Apaf-1) expression and sensitizes human non-Hodgkin's lymphoma B cell lines to paclitaxel-induced apoptosis. Mol Cancer Ther. 2003;2:1183–93.
71. Ghosh S, Karin M. Missing pieces in the NF-kappaB puzzle. Cell. 2002;109:S81–96.
72. Dixit V, Mak TW. NF-κB signaling. Many roads lead to Madrid. Cell. 2002;111:615–9.
73. Jazirehi AR, Huerta-Yepez S, Cheng G, Bonavida B. Rituximab (chimeric anti-CD20 monoclonal antibody) inhibits the constitutive nuclear factor-{kappa}B signaling pathway in non-Hodgkin's lymphoma B-cell lines: role in sensitization to chemotherapeutic drug-induced apoptosis. Cancer Res. 2005;65:264–76.
74. Vivanco I, Sawyers CL. The phosphatidylinositol 3-kinase AKT pathway in human cancer [review]. Nat Rev Cancer. 2002;2:489–501.
75. Suzuki E, Bonavida B. Rituximab inhibits the constitutively activated PI3K-Akt pathway in B-NHL cell lines: involvement in chemosensitization to drug-induced apoptosis. Oncogene. 2007;26:6184–93.
76. Arancia G, Malorni W, Donelli G. Cellular mechanisms of lymphocyte-mediated lysis of tumor cells. Ann Ist Super Sanita. 1990;26:369–84.
77. Goust JM. Cell-mediated immunity. Immunol Ser. 1990;50:195–215.
78. Shresta S, Pham CT, Thomas DA, Graubert TA, Ley TJ. How do cytotoxic lymphocytes kill their targets? Curr Opin Immunol. 1998;10:581–7.
79. Wilson NS, Dixit V, Ashkenazi A. Death receptor signal transducers: nodes of coordination in immune signaling networks. Nat Immunol. 2009;10:348–55.
80. Baritaki S, Bonavida B. Inhibition of snail-induced epithelial-mesenchymal transition and induction of the tumor metastasis suppressor gene raf-1 kinase inhibitor protein (RKIP) by DETANONOate. Forum Immunopathological Dis Ther. 2010;1:219–30.
81. Garban HJ, Bonavida B. Nitric oxide inhibits the transcription repressor Yin-Yang 1 binding activity at the silencer region of the Fas promoter: a pivotal role for nitric oxide in the up-regulation of Fas gene expression in human tumor cells. J Immunol. 2001;167:75–81.
82. Vega MI, Jazirehi AR, Huerta-Yepez S, Bonavida B. Rituximab-induced inhibition of YY1 and Bcl_{xL} expression in Ramos non-Hodgkin's lymphoma cell line via inhibition of NF-kappa B activity: role of YY1 and Bcl_{xL} in Fas resistance and chemoresistance, respectively. J Immunol. 2005;175:2174–83.
83. Vega MI, Baritaki S, Huerta-Yepez S, Martinez-Paniagua MA, Bonavida B. A potential mechanism of rituximab-induced inhibition of tumor growth through its sensitization to tumor necrosis factor-related apoptosis-inducing ligand-expressing host cytotoxic cells. Leuk Lymphoma. 2011;52:108–21.
84. MacFarlane M, Harper N, Snowden RT, et al. Mechanisms of resistance to TRAIL-induced apoptosis in primary B cell chronic lymphocytic leukaemia. Oncogene. 2002;21:6809–18.
85. Huerta S, Baay-Guzman G, Gonzalez-Bonilla CR, Livingston EH, Huerta-Yepez S, Bonavida B. In vitro and in vivo sensitization of SW620 metastatic colon cancer cells to CDDP-induced apoptosis by the nitric oxide donor DETANONOate: involvement of AIF. Nitric Oxide. 2009;20:182–94.
86. Daniel D, Yang B, Lawrence DA, Totpal K, Balter I, Lee WP, Gogineni A, Cole MJ, Yee SF, Ross S, Ashkenazi A. Cooperation of the proapoptotic receptor agonist

rhApo2L/TRAIL with the CD20 antibody rituximab against non-Hodgkin lymphoma xenografts. Blood. 2007;110:4037–46.
87. Vega MI, Huerta-Yepez S, Martinez-Paniagua M, Martinez-Miguel B, Hernandez-Pando R, Gonzalez-Bonilla CR, Chinn P, Hanna N, Hariharan K, Jazirehi AR, Bonavida B. Rituximab-mediated cell signalling and chem./immuno-sensitization of drug-resistant B-NHL is independent of its Fc functions. Clin Cancer Res. 2009;15:6582–94.
88. Daëron M, Malbec O, Latour S, Espinosa E, Pina P, Fridman WH. Regulation of tyrosine-containing activation motif-dependent cell signalling by Fc gamma RII. Immunol Lett. 1995;44:119–23.
89. Pommier Y, Sordet O, Antony S, Hayward RL, Kohn KW. Apoptosis defects and chemotherapy resistance: molecular interaction maps and networks. Oncogene. 2004;23:2934–49.
90. Wada T, Penninger JM. Mitogen-activated protein kinases in apoptosis regulation. Oncogene. 2004;23:2838–49.
91. Foran JM, Norton AJ, Micallef IN, Taussig DC, Amess JA, Rohatiner AZ, Lister TA. Br J Haematol. 2001;114:881–3.
92. Pickartz T, Ringel F, Wedde M, Renz H, Klein A, von Neuhoff N, Dreger P, Kreuzer KA, Schmidt CA, Srock S, Schoeler D, Schriever F. Exp Hematol. 2001;29:1410–6.
93. Alvaro-Naranjo T, Jaen-Martinez J, Guma-Padro J, Bosch-Princep R, Salvado-Usach MT. Ann Hematol. 2003;82:585–8.
94. Jilani I, O'Brien S, Manshuri T, Thomas DA, Thomazy VA, Imam M, Naeem S, Verstovsek S, Kantarjian H, Giles F, Keating M, Albitar M. Blood. 2003;102:3514–20.
95. Kennedy GA, Tey SK, Cobcroft R, Marlton P, Cull G, Grimmett K, Thomson D, Gill D. Incidence and nature of CD20-negative relapses following rituximab therapy in aggressive B-cell non-Hodgkin's lymphoma: a retrospective review. Br J Haematol. 2002;119:412–6.
96. Davis TA, Czerwinski DK, Levy R. Clin Cancer Res. 1999;5:611–5.
97. Haidar JH, Shamseddine A, Salem Z, Mrad YA, Nasr MR, Zaatari G, Bazarbachi A. Loss of CD20 expression in relapsed lymphomas after rituximab therapy. Eur J Haematol. 2003;70:330–2.
98. Manshouri T, Do KA, Wang X, Giles FJ, O'Brien SM, Saffer H, Thomas D, Jilani I, Kantarjian HM, Keating MJ, Albitar M. Circulating CD20 is detectable in the plasma of patients with chronic lymphocytic leukemia and is of prognostic significance. Leuk Lymphoma. 2003;44:S15–27.
99. Smith MR. Rituximab (monoclonal anti-CD20 antibody): mechanisms of action and resistance. Oncogene. 2003;22:7359–68.
100. Rezvani AR, Maloney DG. Rituximab resistance. Best Pract Res Clin Haematol. 2011;24:203–16.
101. Taylor RP, Lindorfer MA. Antigenic modulation and rituximab resistance. Semin Hematol. 2010;47:124–32.
102. Ghesquières H, Cartron G, Seymour JF, Delfau-Larue MH, Offner F, Soubeyran P, Perrot A, Brice P, Bouabdallah R, Sonet A, Dupuis J, Casasnovas O, Catalano JV, Delmer A, Jardin F, Verney A, Dartigues P, Salles G. Clinical outcome of patients with follicular lymphoma receiving chemoimmunotherapy in the PRIMA study is not affected by FCGR3A and FCGR2A polymorphisms. Blood. 2012;120:2650–7.
103. Gisselbrecht C, Schmitz N, Mounier N, Singh GD, Linch DC, Trneny M, Bosly A, Milpied NJ, Radford J, Ketterer N, Shpilberg O, Dührsen U, Hagberg H, Ma DD, Viardot A, Lowenthal R, Brière J, Salles G, Moskowitz CH, Glass B. Rituximab maintenance therapy after autologous stem-cell transplantation in patients with relapsed CD20+ diffuse large B-cell lymphoma: final analysis of the collaborative trial in relapsed aggressive lymphoma. J Clin Oncol. 2012;30:4462–9.
104. Motta G, Cea M, Moran E, Carbone F, Augusti V, Patrone F, Nencioni A. Monoclonal antibodies for non-Hodgkin's lymphoma: state of the art and perspectives. Clin Dev Immunol. 2010;2010:428253.

105. Wang SY, Racila E, Taylor RP, Weiner GJ. NK-cell activation and antibody-dependent cellular cytotoxicity induced by rituximab-coated target cells is inhibited by the C3b component of complement. Blood. 2008;111:1456–63.
106. Macor P, Tripodo C, Zorzet S, Piovan E, Bossi F, Marzari R, Amadori A, Tedesco F. In vivo targeting of human neutralizing antibodies against CD55 and CD59 to lymphoma cells increases the antitumor activity of rituximab. Cancer Res. 2007;67:10556–63.
107. Davis TA, Grillo-López AJ, White CA, McLaughlin P, Czuczman MS, Link BK, Maloney DG, Weaver RL, Rosenberg J, Levy R. Rituximab anti-CD20 monoclonal antibody therapy in non-Hodgkin's lymphoma: safety and efficacy of re-treatment. J Clin Oncol. 2000;18:3135–43.
108. Burger JA, Gandhi V. The lymphatic tissue microenvironments in chronic lymphocytic leukemia: in vitro models and the significance of CD40-CD154 interactions. Blood. 2009;114:2560–1.
109. Jazirehi AR, Bonavida B. Resveratrol modifies the expression of apoptotic regulatory proteins and sensitizes non-Hodgkin's lymphoma and multiple myeloma cell lines to paclitaxel-induced apoptosis. Mol Cancer Ther. 2004;3:71–84.
110. Minn AJ, Rudin CM, Boise LH, Thompson CB. Expression of bcl_{xL} can confer a multidrug resistance phenotype. Blood. 1995;86:1903–10.
111. Reed JC. Bcl-2 family proteins: regulators of chemoresistance in cancer. Toxicol Lett. 1995;82:155–8.
112. Xerri L, Parc P, Brousset P, Schlaifer D, Hassoun J, Reed JC, Krajewski S, Birnbaum D. Predominant expression of the long isoform of Bcl-x (Bcl_{xL}) in human lymphomas. Br J Haematol. 1996;92:900–6.
113. Amundson SA, Myers TG, Scudiero D, Kitada S, Reed JC, Fornace A Jr. An informatics approach identifying markers of chemosensitivity in human lymphomas. Cancer Res. 2000;60:6101–10.
114. Tudor G, Aguilera A, Halverson DO, Laing ND, Sauville EA. Susceptibility to drug-induced apoptosis correlates with differential modulation of Bad, Bcl-2 and Bcl_{xL} protein levels. Cell Death Differ. 2000;7:574–86.
115. Cheng J, Yang J, Xia Y, Karin M, Su B. Synergistic interaction of MEK kinase 2, c-Jun N-terminal kinase (JNK) kinase 2, and JNK1 results in efficient and specific JNK1 activation. Mol Cell Biol. 2000;20:2334–42.
116. Jazirehi AR, Vega MI, Bonavida B. Development of rituximab-resistant lymphoma clones with altered cell signaling and cross resistance to chemotherapy. Cancer Res. 2007;67:1270–81.
117. Spina M, Tirelli U. Rituximab for HIV-associated lymphoma: weighing the benefits and risks. Curr Opin Oncol. 2005;17:462–5.
118. Mounier N, Spina M, Gisselbrecht C. Modern management of non-Hodgkin lymphoma in HIV-infected patients. Br J Haematol. 2007;136:685–98.
119. de Vos S, Goy A, Dakhil SR, Saleh MN, McLaughlin P, Belt R, Flowers CR, Knapp M, Hart L, Patel-Donnelly D, Glenn M, Gregory SA, Holladay C, Zhang T, Boral AL. Multicenter randomized phase II study of weekly or twice-weekly bortezomib plus rituximab in patients with relapsed or refractory follicular or marginal-zone B-cell lymphoma. J Clin Oncol. 2009;27:5023–30.
120. Shimizu R, Kikuchi J, Wada T, Ozawa K, Kano Y, Furukawa Y. HDAC inhibitors augment cytotoxic activity of rituximab by upregulating CD20 expression on lymphoma cells. Leukemia. 2010;24:1760–8.
121. Hiraga J, Tomita A, Sugimoto T, Shimada K, Ito M, Nakamura S, Kiyoi H, Kinoshita T, Naoe T. Down-regulation of CD20 expression in B-cell lymphoma cells after treatment with rituximab-containing combination chemotherapies: its prevalence and clinical significance. Blood 2009; 14;113:4885–4893.
122. Maiso P, Carvajal-Vergara X, Ocio EM, López-Pérez R, Mateo G, Gutiérrez N, Atadja P, Pandiella A. San Miguel JF. The histone deacetylase inhibitor LBH589 is a potent antimyeloma agent that overcomes drug resistance. Cancer Res. 2006;66:5781–9.

123. Pro B, Leber B, Smith M, Fayad L, Romaguera J, Hagemeister F, Rodriguez A, McLaughlin P, Samaniego F, Zwiebel J, Lopez A, Kwak L, Younes A. Phase II multicenter study of oblimersen sodium, a Bcl-2 antisense oligonucleotide, in combination with rituximab in patients with recurrent B-cell non-Hodgkin lymphoma. Br J Haematol. 2008;143:355–60.
124. Hermine O, Haioun C, Lepage E, d'Agay MF, Briere J, Lavignac C, Fillet G, Salles G, Marolleau JP, Diebold J, Reyas F, Gaulard P. Prognostic significance of bcl-2 protein expression in aggressive non-Hodgkin's lymphoma. Groupe d'Etude des Lymphomes de l'Adulte (GELA). Blood. 1996;87:265–72.
125. Gascoyne RD, Adomat SA, Krajewski S, Krajewska M, Horsman DE, Tolcher AW, O'Reilly SE, Hoskins P, Coldman AJ, Reed JC, Connors JM. Prognostic significance of Bcl-2 protein expression and Bcl-2 gene rearrangement in diffuse aggressive non-Hodgkin's lymphoma. Blood. 1997;90:244–51.
126. Waters JS, Webb A, Cunningham D, Clarke PA, Raynaud F, di Stefano F, Cotter FE. Phase I clinical and pharmacokinetic study of bcl-2 antisense oligonucleotide therapy in patients with non-Hodgkin's lymphoma. J Clin Oncol. 2000;18:1812–23.
127. Bogdan C. Nitric oxide and the immune response. Nat Immunol. 2001;2:907–16.
128. Bonavida B. Novel therapeutic applications of nitric oxide in the inhibition of tumor malignancy and reversal of resistance. In: Ignarro LJ, editor. Nitric oxide: biology and pathobiology. 2nd ed. San Diego: Elsevier; 2010.
129. Wink DA, Ridnour LA, Hussain SP, Harris CC. The reemergence of nitric oxide and cancer. Nitric Oxide. 2008;19:65–7.
130. Ridnour LA, Thomas DD, Switzer C, Flores-Santana W, Isenberg JS, Ambs S, Roberts DD, Wink DA. Molecular mechanisms for discrete nitric oxide levels in cancer. Nitric Oxide. 2008;19:73–6.
131. Bonavida B, Baritaki S, Huerta-Yepez S, Vega MI, Chatterjee D, Yeung K. Novel therapeutic applications of nitric oxide donors in cancer: roles in chemo- and immunosensitization to apoptosis and inhibition of metastases. Nitric Oxide. 2008;19:152–7.
132. Blaise GA, Gauvin D, Gangal M, Authier S. Nitric oxide, cell signaling and cell death. Toxicology. 2005;208:177–92.
133. Tuteja N, Chandra M, Tuteja R, Misra MK. Nitric oxide as a unique bioactive signaling messenger in physiology and pathophysiology. J Biomed Biotechnol. 2004;4:227–37.
134. Moncada S, Erusalimsky JD. Does nitric oxide modulate mitochondrial energy generation and apoptosis? Nat Rev Mol Cell Biol. 2002;3:214–20.
135. Brune B. The intimate relation between nitric oxide and superoxide in apoptosis and cell survival. Antioxid Redox Signal. 2005;7:497–507.
136. Marshall HE, Stamler JS. Inhibition of NF-kappa B by S-nitrosylation. Biochemistry. 2001;40:1688–93.
137. Wink DA, Cook JA, Christodoulou D, Krishna MC, Pacelli R, Kim S, DeGraff W, Gamson J, Vodovotz Y, Russo A, Mitchell JB. Nitric oxide and some nitric oxide donor compounds enhance the cytotoxicity of cisplatin. Nitric Oxide. 1997;1:88–94.
138. Evig CB, Kelley EE, Weydert CJ, Chu Y, Buettner GR, Burns CP. Endogenous production and exogenous exposure to nitric oxide augment doxorubicin cytotoxicity for breast cancer cells but not cardiac myoblasts. Nitric Oxide. 2004;10:119–29.
139. Huerta-Yepez S, Baritaki S, Baay-Guzman G, Hernandez-Luna MA, Hernandez-Cueto A, Vega MI, Bonavida B. Contribution of either YY1 or Bcl(XL)-induced inhibition by the NO-donor DETANONOate in the reversal of drug resistance, both in vitro and in vivo. YY1 and Bcl(XL) are overexpressed in prostate cancer. Nitric Oxide. 2012;29C:17–24.
140. Fukuo K, Hata S, Suhara T, Nakahashi T, Shinto Y, Tsujimoto Y, Morimoto S, Ogihara T. Nitric oxide induces upregulation of Fas and apoptosis in vascular smooth muscle. Hypertension. 1996;27:823–6.
141. Garban HJ, Bonavida B. Nitric oxide sensitizes ovarian tumor cells to Fas-induced apoptosis. Gynecol Oncol. 1999;73:257–64.

142. Garban HJ, Bonavida B. Nitric oxide disrupts H2O2-dependent activation of nuclear factor kappa B. Role in sensitization of human tumor cells to tumor necrosis factor-alpha-induced cytotoxicity. J Biol Chem. 2001;276:8918–23.
143. Huerta-Yepez S, Vega M, Escoto-Chavez SE, Murdock B, Sakai T, Baritaki S, Bonavida B. Nitric oxide sensitizes tumor cells to TRAIL-induced apoptosis via inhibition of the DR5 transcription repressor Yin Yang 1. Nitric Oxide. 2009;20:39–52.
144. Worthington J, McCarthy HO, Barrett E, Adams C, Robson T, Hirst DG. Use of the radiation-inducible WAF1 promoter to drive iNOS gene therapy as a novel anti-cancer treatment. J Gene Med. 2004;6:673–80.
145. Jeannin JF, Leon L, Cortier M, Sassi N, Paul C, Bettaieb A. Nitric oxide-induced resistance or sensitization to death in tumor cells. Nitric Oxide. 2008;19:158–63.
146. Baritaki S, Suzuki E, Umezawa K, Spandidos DA, Berenson J, Daniels TR, Penichet ML, Jazirehi AR, Palladino M, Bonavida B. Inhibition of Yin Yang 1-dependent repressor activity of DR5 transcription and expression by the novel proteasome inhibitor NPI-0052 contributes to its TRAIL-enhanced apoptosis in cancer cells. J Immunol. 2008; 180:6199–210.
147. Stein R, Qu Z, Chen S, Rosario A, Shi V, Hayes M, Horak ID, Hansen HJ, Goldenberg DM. Characterization of a new humanized anti-CD20 monoclonal antibody, IMMU-106, and Its use in combination with the humanized anti-CD22 antibody, epratuzumab, for the therapy of non-Hodgkin's lymphoma. Clin Cancer Res. 2004;10:2868–78.
148. Peaker CJ, Neuberger MS. Association of CD22 with the B cell antigen receptor. Eur J Immunol. 1993;23:1358–63.
149. Carnahan J, Wang P, Kendall R, Chen C, Hu S, Boone T, Juan T, Talvenheimo J, Montestruque S, Sun J, Elliott G, Thomas J, Ferbas J, Kern B, Briddell R, Leonard JP, Cesano A. Epratuzumab, a humanized monoclonal antibody targeting CD22: characterization of in vitro properties. Clin Cancer Res. 2003;9:3982S–90S.
150. Leonard JP, Coleman M, Ketas JC, Chadburn A, Ely S, Furman RR, Wegener WA, Hansen HJ, Ziccardi H, Eschenberg M, Gayko U, Cesano A, Goldenberg DM. Phase I/II trial of epratuzumab (humanized anti-CD22 antibody) in indolent non-Hodgkin's lymphoma. J Clin Oncol. 2003;21:3051–9.
151. Maddipatla S, Hernandez-Ilizaliturri FJ, Knight J, Czuczman MS. Augmented antitumor activity against B-cell lymphoma by a combination of monoclonal antibodies targeting TRAIL-R1 and CD20. Clin Cancer Res. 2007;13:4556–64.
152. Shen J, Vil MD, Jimenez X, Zhang H, Iacolina M, Mangalampalli V, Balderes P, Ludwig DL, Zhu Z. Single variable domain antibody as a versatile building block for the construction of IgG-like bispecific antibodies. J Immunol Methods. 2007;318:65–74.
153. Behring E. Uber das zustandekommen der diphterie-immunitat und der tetanus-immunitat bei theiren. Deut Med Wochenschr. 1890;14:1113–4.
154. Ehrlich P. On immunity with special reference to cell life. Proc Roy Soc. 1900;66:424–48.
155. Porter RR. The structure of antibodies. The basic pattern of the principal class of molecules that neutralize antigens (foreign substances in the body) is four cross-linked chains. This pattern is modified so that antibodies can fit different antigens. Sci Am. 1967;217:81–7.
156. Edelman GM, Gall WE, Waxdal MJ, Konigsberg WH. The covalent structure of a human gamma G-immunoglobulin. I. Isolation and characterization of the whole molecule, the polypeptide chains, and the tryptic fragments. Biochemistry. 1968;7:1950–8.
157. Marcus R. Current treatment options in aggressive lymphoma. Leuk Lymphoma. 2003;44:S15–27.

Resistance to the Anti-EGFR Therapy, Beyond KRAS, in Patients with Metastatic Colorectal Cancer

Zacharenia Saridaki and John Souglakos

Abstract Several studies have shown that mutation profiles could influence the treatment decisions in patients with metastatic colorectal cancer (mCRC). It has been proven that patients with mutations in exon 2 of the *KRAS* ongogene gain no benefit from treatment with the monoclonal antibodies (moAbs) against Epidermal Growth Factor Receptor (EGFR), cetuximab and panitumumab. Currently, the determination of *KRAS* mutational status represents a paradigm for biomarkers development in the era of molecular targeted therapies. The current manuscript is an overview, which summarizes and critically reviews the clinical relevance of the proposed mechanism of resistance to beyond the *KRAS* exon 2 mutations, such as: *KRAS* outside codon 12 and 13, *NRAS*, *BRAF* V600E, *PIK3CA* exon 9 and 20 mutations, PTEN loss, EGFR ligands *AREG*, *EREG* mRNA expression and EGFR amplification. The aim is to identify molecular markers that might be used to select patients with the higher probability of response to anti-EGFR moAbs. Overall, the accumulating evidence of molecular biology of CRC has, substantially, changed the approach to mCRC and has given the clinicians more rational options for treating this illness.

Keywords Anti-EGFR monoclonal antibodies · Biomarkers · Colorectal cancer

Abbreviations

AREG	Affimetrix, Amphiregulin
EGFR	Epidermal growth factor receptor
EREG	Epiregulin
mCRC	Metastatic colorectal cancer
moAbs	Monoclonal antibodies

Z. Saridaki · J. Souglakos (✉)
Department of Medical Oncology, University Hospital of Heraklion and Laboratory of Tumor Cell Biology, Medical School, University of Crete, Voutes and Stavrakia, 1352 71110 Heraklion, Crete, Greece
e-mail: georgsec@med.uoc.gr

B. Bonavida (ed.), *Resistance to Immunotherapeutic Antibodies in Cancer*, Resistance to Targeted Anti-Cancer Therapeutics 2, DOI: 10.1007/978-1-4614-7654-2_6,

Introduction

Colorectal cancer (CRC) accounts for 8 % of all malignant tumors in adults and is considered as a major cause of cancer morbidity and mortality worldwide [1]. Although curative surgical resection is possible in 70–80 % of patients at diagnosis, almost half of them will develop local or/and metastatic recurrence and will die of the disease [2].

Combinations of infusional administrated 5-fluorouracil/Leucovorin with irinotecan or oxaliplatin are accepted as the mainstay of first-line treatment and have increased the median overall survival of patients with advanced CRC from 12 months to about 21–22 months [3]. In addition, resection for colorectal metastases (mainly in lung and liver), has become the standard of care, for patients with limited metastatic disease and currently remains the only potentially curative therapy [4]. The advent of targeted therapy further expanded treatment options for patients with mCRC. In particular, inhibition of the Epidermal Growth Factor Receptor (EGFR) using the moAbs, led to further improvement in the outcome of patients with mCRC [5, 6].

Indeed, two moAbs targeting EGFR have entered clinical practice in the metastatic colorectal cancer setting: cetuximab, a chimeric IgG1 moAb and panitumumab, a fully humanized IgG2 moAb. Both of them bind to the extracellular domain of the EGFR, thus leading to inhibition of its downstream signaling and have proven to provide a modest clinical benefit in pretreated patients [6–9]. Although they were initially registered for patients whose tumors were found to express the EGFR protein with immunohistochemistry, subsequently, it was clearly demonstrated that this methodology was neither enough, nor adequate to predict treatment efficacy [10]. Only the development of severe (grade 2 or 3) skin rash was constantly correlated with improved treatment outcome of patients treated with anti-EGFR moAbs [5, 6, 11].

However, several lines of evidence have proved that specific *KRAS* mutations in hotspots located in codons 12 and 13 are predictors of resistance to anti-EGFR moAbs therapy and are associated with diminished efficacy and shorter progression free and overall survival [5, 11, 12]. The analysis of the *KRAS* mutational status in codon 12 and 13 is now mandatory at the presentation of metastatic disease in CRC patients, since it is a strong predictor of resistance to anti-EGFR moAbs. Despite that, not all patients with *KRAS* wild type (wt) primary tumor present substantial benefit for the administration of cetuximab or panitumumab. In fact, the response rate of anti-EGFR moAbs is less than 25 % when they are administered as salvage monotherapy [11, 12] and indicating that other mechanisms of resistance may be implicated in the process.

Since clinical parameters seem to be inadequate for selection, a major challenge is the identification of specific biomarkers that are likely to predict which patients will achieve the best response to such a treatment. In CRC, despite the fact that the underpinning genetic alterations are well characterized [13, 14], this knowledge in the biology of the disease has limited application in the daily clinical practice.

The aim of the present report is to summarize and critically review the clinical relevance of the proposed mechanisms of resistance to anti-EGFR moAbs beyond the *KRAS* exon 2 mutations, such as: *KRAS* outside codon 12 and 13, mutations in other RAS family member, *BRAF* V600E, *PIK3CA* exon 9 and 20 mutational status in conjunction with PTEN loss, EGFR ligands *AREG*, *EREG* mRNA expression, protein overexpression, EGFR amplification, etc. Since most available data come from retrospective studies, validation in prospective trials is imperative.

KRAS Mutations Outside Hotspots in Codons 12 and 13

The *KRAS* proto-oncogene encodes K-ras, a G protein which has a key role in the Ras/MAPK signaling pathway. K-ras is located downstream of many growth factor receptors, including EGFR, that are involved in CRC carcinogenesis. The activation of a growth factor receptor induces the recruitment of K-ras which initiates the activation of a cascade of serine-threonine kinases leading to the signal transduction from the cell surface to the nucleus. *KRAS* mutations are present in more than one-third of CRC and lead to the activation of one of the most important pathways for cell proliferation, the Ras/MAPK pathway, by inducing cyclin D1 synthesis. Consequently, in the presence of a *KRAS* mutation, this pathway activation cannot be significantly inhibited by an anti-EGFR moAb (cetuximab or panitumumab) which acts upstream of the K-ras protein [15]. The *KRAS* mutations in CRC are located in exon 2, (codons 12 and 13) in more than 90 % of the cases while the rest are found mainly in exon 3 (codon 61) and 4 (codon) 146 [16]. Preclinical data indicate that the mutation in codon 61 [17] and the A to C change (Lys to Asn substitution) at codon 117, and G to A change (Ala to Thr substitution) at codon 146 [18] had phenotypes similar to the hotspot mutations leading to activation of the RAS-RAF-MAPK kinase pathway. In contrast, other *KRAS* mutations outside "hotspots" such as the G to T change (Leu to Phe substitution) at codon 19 had an attenuated phenotype while the G to A change (Arg to Gln substitution) at codon 164, and the 'silent' C to T nucleotide substitution, which did not alter the aspartic acid residue at codon 173, were phenotypically equivalent to wt *KRAS* [18].

The clinical relevance of *KRAS* mutations in codons 61 and 146 has been investigated in a retrospective analysis in small cohort of patients [19]. In 87 patients with codon 12 or 13 wt *KRAS* tumors, treated with anti-EGFR moAbs, mutations of codons 61 and 146 were found in 7 (8 %) and 1 (1 %) cases, respectively. None of these 8 patients harboring KRAS 61 or 146 mutated disease responded to the treatment, whereas the objective response rate for the *KRAS* wt patients was 32 % ($p = 0.096$). In addition, mutations in codon 61 or 146 were associated with shorter progression-free survival (PFS, HR: 0.46, $p = 0.028$). Moreover, in a retrospective consortium analysis, patients with the more rare codon 61 mutant tumors had a significantly lower response rate than did wild types (0/13 [0.0 %] vs. 123/345 [35.7 %]; $p = 0$ 0055), but this was not the case for patients with codon 146 mutant tumors (2/11 [18.2 %] vs. 101/274 [36.9 %]; $p = 0.34$) [20].

The impact of codon 61 *KRAS* mutation has been, retrospectively, investigated in the registration trial (Study 408) of panitumumab versus best supportive care [9, 12]. In this retrospective analysis of 288 tumor blocks from the patients enrolled in the trial, the frequency of the codon 61 *KRAS* mutation was 2.5 % [21]. Patients with exon 2 and 3 WT *KRAS* treated with panitumumab presented a 61 % decrease [Hazard Ratio (HR): 0.39; 95 % Confidence Interval (CI): 0.28–0.56] in the risk of disease progression in comparison with patients harboring a *KRAS* mutation in codon 12, 13 or 61 [21]. In comparison, when only exon 2 *KRAS* status were analyzed [12] in the same study the risk of recurrence was reduced by 55 % (95 % CI: 0.34–0.59) with the treatment of panitumumab, indicating that the analysis of the codon 61 *KRAS* mutation may slightly improve the patients' selection for the anti-EGFR moAbs administration.

In summary, despite the strong biologic rational, the analysis of *KRAS* mutation outside exon 2 hotspots is not recommended for use in the daily clinical practice, due to the limit and retrospective data regarding their clinical relevance. Prospective validation of the codon 61 and 146 *KRAS* mutations is warranted since the initial preclinical and clinical data indicate that they may improve the selection of patients with higher probability of response to anti-EGFR moAbs.

NRAS Mutation Status

The protein encoded by the *NRAS* gene is a member of the RAS superfamily of GTPases. The other RAS proteins play a key role in the MAPK signaling pathway, a critical pathway involved in cell growth, differentiation and survival. *NRAS* mutations are found in solid tumor malignancies including melanoma, colorectal cancer and thyroid cancer. Approximately 80 % of the mutations reported in the *NRAS* gene are located in codon 61, with Q61R and Q61 K substitutions being the most frequently reported in the literature (16). Recent data have shown that the *NRAS* mutation status may be predictive for the BRAF inhibitor response in metastatic melanoma patients and the anti-EGFR therapy response in metastatic CRC.

The clinical relevance of the *NRAS* mutation detection has been evaluated in a retrospective consortium analysis of patients treated with cetuximab as salvage treatment with or without chmeotherapy [20]. In this study, the frequency of *NRAS* mutations in *KRAS* and *BRAF* wt tumors studies was 4.8 %. *NRAS* mutations were mutually exclusive with *KRAS* or *BRAF* mutations and in only one case a *NRAS* mutation was found simultaneously with a *PIK3CA* mutation. Patients with *NRAS* mutants tumors presented a significantly lower response rate (OR 0.14, 95 % CI 0.007–0.70; $p = 0.013$) in comparison with those with wt tumors. Also, a no significant trend for increase median PFS (HR 1.82, 1.04–3.18; $p = 0.055$) and median overall survival (HR 1.89, 1.05–3.39; $p = 0.051$) was observed between

NRAS wild types and mutants. The investigators calculated that the analysis of *NRAS* mutations in *KRAS/BRAF* wt patients may increase the probability of response by 2.1 % (36.3–38.4 %) [20].

The impact of *NRAS* mutations in the resistance to anti-EGFR moAbs has been also questioned in the 408 study of panitumumab versus best supportive care [21]. *NRAS* mutations were detected in 5.0 % of the cases and were mutually exclusive with *KRAS* or *BRAF* mutations. In wt *KRAS* patients, treatment with panitumumab was found to reduce the risk of disease progression by 61 % (HR: 0.39; 95 % CI: 0.28–0.56) in case of *NRAS* wt tumors, while had no effect (HR: 1.94; 95 % CI: 0.44–8.44) in case of *NRAS* mutants.

In summary, the analysis of codon 61 *NRAS* mutations is not recommended for use in the daily clinical practice, due to the lack of prospective validation in a clinical trial. Despite that, the strong biologic rationale and the clinical data from large retrospective cohorts indicate that they may be helpful for the improvement of outcome of patients treated with anti-EGFR moAbs.

BRAF Mutations

One major effector of RAS is the RAF family of serine/threonine kinases, which comprises A-RAF, BRAF and C-RAF [13]. The RAS-RAF-MEK-ERK pathway normally connects extracellular signals, such as growth factors and hormones, to the nucleus, leading to the expression of genes that regulate cell proliferation, differentiation, and survival [22]. The RAS-RAF-MEK-ERK pathway may be constitutively activated in human cancers through mutations in RAS or RAF. Mutations in *BRAF* have been found in approximately 8 % of human cancers, including 50–60 % of melanomas, 30–70 % of thyroid cancers, 30 % of serous low-grade ovarian cancers and 10 % of colorectal cancers [23]. The single substitution missense mutation V600E, located within the kinase domain of *BRAF*, is the most common oncogenic mutation in cancer accounting for more than 80 % of all *BRAF* mutations and accounts for more than 95 % of *BRAF* mutations in CRC [16]. The V600E aminoacid change results in constitutive activation of the BRAF kinase and promotes cell transformation [23, 24]. *KRAS* and *BRAF* mutations are mutually exclusive in CRC [25–27].

Several studies have reported that *BRAF* mutation in the primary tumor marks patients who carry an especially poor prognosis, regardless of the specific treatment regimen. The presence of *BRAF* mutations in primary CRC has been associated with limited survival in early-operable stages [28] as well as in advanced/metastatic disease [27, 29]. In CRC tumors, *BRAF* mutations are reported to occur more frequently in those cases characterized by the presence of defective DNA mismatch repair (dMMR) [25, 29, 30], while the detection of *BRAF* mutations was also associated with cyclin D1 overexpression [29]. *BRAF* V600E is tightly associated with dMMR due to the hMLH1 promoter hypermethylation and not with dMMR due to the germ-line alterations [31, 32].

Furthermore, several retrospective studies have shown that patients with tumors harboring *BRAF*^{V600E} mutation didn't benefit for treatment with anti-EGFR moAbs. Initially, Di Nicolantonio et al. [24] analyzed retrospectively 113 mCRC tumors from cetuximab or panitumumab-treated patients for *KRAS* and *BRAF* mutations. The *BRAF* V600E mutation was detected in 11 of 79 *KRAS* WT patients. None of the *BRAF*-mutated patients responded to treatment, while *BRAF*-mutated patients had significantly shorter PFS ($P = 0.011$) and OS ($P < 0.0001$) than WT patients, indicating that the *BRAF* V600E mutation was inversely correlated with response to anti-EGFR MoAbs therapy. Moreover, the presence of or the transformation with the *BRAF* V600E mutant allele, in CRC cell lines, diminished the therapeutic potential of cetuximab or panitumumab [24].

Another retrospective study sought to determine, retrospectively, the predictive value of the *BRAF*$^{\text{V600E}}$, *KRAS* (exon 2) and *PIK3CA* (exons 9 and 20) point mutations with respect to clinical outcomes in 168 mCRC patients treated in the USA and Greece with 5-FU-based first-line chemotherapy [27]. In this study population, *KRAS*, *BRAF* and *PIK3CA* mutations were present in 62 (37 %), 13 (8 %) and 26 (15 %) cases, respectively. *BRAF* mutation was revealed as an independent prognostic factor for decreased survival (HR: 3.6, 95 % CI: 1.7–7.3) and PFS (HR: 1.9, 95 % CI: 1.03–3.5; $P < 0.0001$) than those whose primary tumors carried only wild-type *BRAF*. Among 100 patients treated with cetuximab *BRAF* mutations correlated with reduced Objective Response Rate (ORR) and PFS ($P < 0.001$). The likelihood of response between patients with *BRAF*-mutant or *BRAF* WT tumors was 0 versus 17 %, while *BRAF* mutations conferred higher risk of relapse (HR: 3.9, $P = 0.0005$) after treatment with cetuximab-containing salvage combinations. At least four studies [19–21, 26] have shown that *BRAF*$^{\text{V600E}}$ mCRC tumors do not respond to anti-EGFR moAbs and have lower progression free survival and lower overall survival as compared with *BRAF* wild type patients. Finaly, the posthoc subgroup analysis in two first line randomized trials (CAIRO2 and CRYSTAL) confirmed the adverse prognostic significance of *BRAF*$^{\text{V600E}}$ mutations [33, 34]. The results from the CRYSTAL trial [34] showed a trend in favor of the addition of cetuximab to chemotherapy and should be interpreted with caution since the p values for the interaction test were not reported in this subgroup analysis. This highlights, at the moment, the need of further investigations and validation for the impact of BRAF mutation in prospective randomized trials.

The above-mentioned data underscore the lack of cetuximab response observed with *KRAS*-mutant tumors and that may extend to other oncogene mutations, especially *BRAF*. The adverse significance of *BRAF* mutations should inform patient selection and stratification in future clinical trials [27]. Moreover, the available data support that the natural history and treatment response of *BRAF*-mutant CRC tumors differ markedly from all others CRC tumors. The mutant BRAF does not simply substitute for K-ras activation in a linear signaling pathway but likely confers additional and distinct properties, with ominous consequences.

PIK3CA Mutations and PTEN Expression

Besides the Ras/Raf MAPK pathway, EGFR also activates the PI3 K/AKT signaling pathway which can be deregulated, either by activating mutations of the PIK3CA p110 subunit or by, usually epigenetic, inactivation of the PTEN phosphatase. The *PIK3CA* gene encodes for a lipid kinase that regulates alongside KRAS signaling pathways downstream the EGFR. The p110α subunit of PI3 K which is encoded by *PIK3CA*, can be activated by interactions with the RAS proteins [35]. The *PIK3CA* gene is one of the most frequently mutated oncogenes in human tumors. The vast majority of its reported mutations cluster in the conserved regions within the helical and kinase domains of p110α, resulting in constitutive kinase activity and making this enzyme an ideal target for drug development [36]. In CRCs it is found mutated in approximately 20 % of the cases, and, as previously described, the majority of the relevant mutations are located in the "hotspots" of exon 9 (E542 K, E545 K) and exon 20 (H1047R) [37].

From the beginning it was evident that the role of *PIK3CA* mutations was not an easy matter to approach. Initially, regarding the outcome after cetuximab treatment, data were conflicting, with some groups reporting association with resistance and some others association with response [20, 26, 38–41]. Moreover, the role of *PIK3CA* mutations became more complicated due to the fact that in many cases they were present alongside *KRAS* or *BRAF* mutations. In an analyses of 110 mCRC patients treated with anti-EGFR moAbs by Sartore-Bianchi et al. [41], for mutations in *PIK3CA* and *KRAS* genes alongside PTEN expression, *PIK3CA* mutations were significantly associated with clinical resistance to panitumumab or cetuximab. None of the mutated patients achieved an objective response ($p = 0.038$), and, in the subgroup analysis of *KRAS* wt tumors the statistical correlation was even stronger ($p = 0.016$). *PIK3CA* mutated patients were characterized by a worse clinical outcome in terms of PFS as well ($p = 0.035$). In their conclusion, the authors state that their results support the notion that *PIK3CA* mutations can independently hamper the therapeutic response to panitumumab or cetuximab in mCRC. When the molecular status of the PIK3CA/PTEN and KRAS pathways are concomitantly ascertained, up to 70 % of mCRC patients who are unlikely to respond to anti-EGFR moAbs can be identified [41]. In another study by Souglakos et al. [27], *PIK3CA* mutations were also found to correlate with reduced PFS ($p = 0.06$) in response to second-line use of cetuximab. In the study by Saridaki et al. [26], *PIK3CA* mutations were identified in 11 tumors (9.8 %) predominantly in exon 9 than in exon 20, an observation in contrast with Sartore-Bianchi's et al. [41] but in agreement with Prenen's et al. [40]. A significant negative correlation between *PIK3CA* mutations and response to anti-EGFR moAbs has been documented in the Sartore-Bianchi's et al. [41] and the Perone's et al. [39] reports, whereas, Prenen et al. [40] could not find a clear association between the presence of *PIK3CA* mutation status and an impaired efficacy of anti-EGFR moAbs. Saridaki et al. [26], did not demonstrate a significant correlation between time to tumor progression (TTP) and OS and *PIK3CA* mutational status when the analysis was performed in the whole patients' group. However, in the KRAS wt patients' group, *PIK3CA* mutational status was correlated with a significantly lower TTP but not OS, as previously described as well [27]. In the recent study by De Roock et al. [20], where a large cohort of patients was evaluated, the role of *PIK3CA* mutations was more clearly revealed. Exon 9 and exon 20 *PIK3CA* mutations were analyzed separately and, indeed, only exon 20 mutations were found to be associated with a worse outcome after cetuximab administration. This could be a possible explanation for the conflicting results published in the literature, since there could be more than one interpretation when two events (exon 9 and exon 20 mutations) have different or opposite effects. Even before De Roock et al. [20], managed to show it in patients, it was postulated that *PIK3CA* mutations located in exon 9 and 20 hotspots exert different biochemical and oncogenic properties. It has been convincingly shown that the gain of function induced by exon 20 mutations (located in the kinase domain) is independent of Ras binding *in vitro*, whereas, exon 9 mutations (helical domain) require Ras–GTP interaction [42]. Thus, the codon-specific role of *PIK3CA* mutations in predicting cetuximab efficacy provides further evidence that individual mutations within a single cancer gene might have distinct roles on the response to a given therapeutic regimen [43].

Phosphate and tensin homologue deleted on chromosome ten (PTEN) normally inhibits PI3 K-initiated signaling. It has been shown *in vitro* that cell lines with activating *PIK3CA* mutations or loss of PTEN expression (PTEN null) were more resistant to cetuximab than wt *PIK3CA*/PTEN-expressing cell lines (14 ± 5.0 % vs. 38.5 ± 6.4 % growth inhibition, mean $\pm$ SE; $p = 0.008$). Furthermore, *PIK3CA* mutant isogenic HCT116 cells showed increased resistance to cetuximab compared with wt *PIK3CA* controls. Consistently, cell lines that were *PIK3CA* mutant/PTEN null and RAS/BRAF mutant were highly resistant to cetuximab compared with those without dual mutations/PTEN loss (10.8 ± 4.3 % vs. 38.8 ± 5.9 % growth inhibition, respectively; $p = 0.002$), indicating that constitutive and simultaneous activation of the RAS and PIK3CA pathways confer maximal resistance to this agent [44].

The role of PTEN loss and the evaluation of the consecutive over-activation of the AKT pathway are still under investigation, as far as response to anti-EGFR moAbs is concerned. *In vivo*, loss of PTEN expression, occurring in approximately 30 % of sporadic CRCs, has been elaborated in a number of studies regarding its association with cetuximab response [26, 39–41, 45, 46]. Four relatively small retrospective studies [39, 40, 45, 46] have provided evidence that PTEN status is associated with objective responses in cetuximab-treated mCRC patients suggesting that PTEN-positive tumors tend to have a better outcome than negative ones. However, two other studies failed to confirm this observation [26, 41]; in the Saridaki et al. [26] study, the significantly lower TTP which was observed in patients with wt KRAS and PIK3CA according to the down- and up-regulation of PTEN could not be translated into differences in OS. The reasons of discordance between published studies could probably be attributed to several methodological differences, such as the anti-PTEN antibodies used, the IHC scoring algorithms and cut-off criteria [47], further highlighting that the above mentioned results should be studied with caution. Since PTEN IHC is not yet adequately validated, it cannot be considered for immediate routine clinical use, but, it should be kept in mind in the planning process of prospective biomarkers' studies.

EGFR Ligands AREG and EREG mRNA Expression

Although we are not yet in the position to affirm the existence of predictive markers capturing the responding population to anti-EGFR treatments, with high specificity and sensitivity, nevertheless, some evidence towards this direction exists. EGFR epiregulin (EREG) and ampiregulin (AREG) ligands' expression in primary CRC tumors have been shown to significantly predict clinical outcome in *KRAS* wt mCRC patients treated with cetuximab, indicating a ligand-driven autocrine oncogenic EGFR signaling [26, 48, 49].

Khambata-Ford et al. [49] were the first to indentify, by biomarker exploratory analysis using Affimetrix, Amphiregulin (AREG) and Epiregulin (EREG), two EGFR ligands, to be among the top genes predicting cetuximab response. This gene signature was obtained from snap-frozen liver metastasis from mCRC patients uniformly treated with cetuximab monotherapy [49]. Later, these data were confirmed by Jacobs et al. [48] where the analysis of primary CRC formalin-fixed-paraffin embedded (FFPE) tumors from refractory metastatic patients treated with cetuximab-based therapy revealed AREG and EREG to predict cetuximab sensitivity [48]. In line with these results, in a cohort of 106 mCRC patients who received first line cetuximab/irinotecan combination the analyses revealed AREG and EREG overexpression in the *KRAS* wt subgroup that achieved clinical benefit [50]. Similar results were obtained by Saridaki et al. [26] in a total of 112 mCRC patients treated with salvage cetuximab-based combination chemotherapy. In this report [26] and in the group of *KRAS* wt patients, a statistically significant correlation of AREG and especially EREG mRNA overexpression with increased TTP and OS was observed in accordance with previous reports [48]. The authors concluded that their data seem to identify a subgroup of *KRAS* wt patients who could be considered more EGFR-dependent and, thus, have a higher probability of responding to EGFR inhibition, as it has also been reported by others [26, 48]. Patients whose tumors were characterized by ligands' downregulation behaved like *KRAS* mutants upon treatment with anti-EGFR moAbs [26].

Based on the above mentioned data we could conclude that AREG and EREG could be considered as markers of sensitivity of anti-EGFR moAbs therapy, and therefore, markers of EGFR dependency in CRC tumors [51]. In reality, this is not completely true since there are also some wt *KRAS* tumors with low ligands' expression that seem to respond to cetuximab [50]. Thus, the model of EGFR addiction has to be improved and additional markers need to be found [52].

In line with this hypothesis, Baker et al. [53], with the use of high-throughput RT–PCR, analyzed the mRNA expression of 110 candidate genes in a total of 144 *KRAS* wt mCRC patients treated with cetuximab monotherapy. The majority of these genes were found to be strongly associated with all evaluated clinical outcome variables (like disease control, RR, PFS) and a number of them were compatible with EGFR biology in CRC development. Activators of the EGFR signaling pathway, like AREG, EREG and VAV3 were found to be associated positively with clinical benefit, whereas DUSP6, a phosphatase feed-back inhibitor of the MAPK pathway was found to be associated negatively with clinical benefit. From the multivariate analysis, a four–gene classifier compiled from *EREG, AREG, DUSP6* and *SCL26A3* was generated. The four-gene classifier, alongside *KRAS* status, significantly improved the specificity and the positive predictive value of cetuximab benefit, as measured by disease control and RR compared to the use *KRAS* status alone. Furthermore, the model performed better than *AREG, EREG* or *KRAS* status alone when the parameter measured was PFS [53]. Apparently, with the use of one single marker we cannot adequately define EGFR-dependency in CRC tumors. A group of relevant markers, genes and proteins, will be needed to better identify the EGFR addicted/cetuximab sensitive CRC tumors and patients [26, 51].

EGFR Gene Copy Numbers

The tumoral EGFR gene copy number (GCN) measured by FISH and found increased in a fraction of mCRC patients of a cohort study was initially correlated with objective tumor response after treatment with the anti-EGFR moAbs cetuximab and panitumumab [54]. Subsequently, in following studies the predictive role of EGFR GCN was evaluated and an association with objective tumor response [15] and OS [55] was demonstrated.

In particular, Lievre et al. [15], using CISH instead of FISH, confirmed the results of Moroni et al. [54], but in both studies a limited number of patients was included and treatments were non-homogeneous. In the study by Lenz et al. [55], EGFR GCN was evaluated with polymerase chain reaction (PCR) and although no association was detected with objective responses and PFS, increased GCN was significantly positively correlated with OS. The discrepancies between these studies could be a result of different techniques or sample limitations, but the association of EGFR GCN with OS could also reflect its role as an independent prognostic variable [15, 54, 55].

Sartore-Bianchi et al. [56] tested the EGFR GCN parameter in a larger and more homogeneous patients' population, the registration panitumumab trial [9], in an attempt to clarify its predictive role in terms of OR, PFS and OS tumors. In this study, EGFR GCN was assessed by FISH and its status was evaluated as the mean value of EGFR gene copies/nucleus, as the mean value of EGFR gene/CEP7 (á-centromeric probe of chromosome 7) and as the percentage of chromosome 7 polysomy ($\geq$3 signals per nucleus) scoring 200 tumor cells. A statistically significant positive correlation between an increased mean EGFR GCN and probability of response to panitumumab (odds ratio = 5.62; 95 % CI, 1.506–20.974) was found with 98.1 % specificity (95 % CI, 78.5–96 %). Additionally, the best cut-off value of mean EGFR GCN to discriminate responders from non-responders was set at ≥2.47 EGFR gene copies/nucleous by ROC analysis and had a sensitivity of 100 % (95 % CI, 54.1–100 %), since no OR was observed when the EGFR GCN was less than this value. Because of the non-homogeneous pattern of EGFR GCN in the tumors, the percentage of cells displaying chromosome 7 polysomy and/or EGFR gene amplification was also calculated. In line with the above mentioned results, an increase in the percentage of chromosome 7 polysomy was also significantly associated with the probability of objective response (odds ratio = 1.04; 95 % CI, 1.007–1.074), with a specificity of 100 % (95 % CI, 93.2–100 %) and a negative predictive value of 89.7 % (95 % CI, 78.8–96.1 %). In other words, in patients treated with panitumumab, a mean EGFR GCN of less than 2.5/nucleus or less than 40 % of tumor cells displaying chromosome 7 polysomy within the tumor predicted for shorter PFS (PFS; $p = 0.039$ and $p = 0.029$, respectively) and OS ($p = 0.015$ and $p = 0.014$, respectively), thus generating the hypothesis that these tumors were probably not driven by the EGFR pathway. None of the treated patients with mean EGFR GCN of less than 2.47/nucleus or less than 43 % of tumor cells displaying chromosome 7 polysomy obtained objective response compared with six of 20 and six of 19 patients with values greater than these cut-off limits, respectively ($P = 0.0009$ and $P = 0.0007$, respectively). The evaluation of best supported care-treated patients showed no correlation between EGFR GCN and PFS, probably indicating more its predictive, rather than its prognostic role [56]. Lastly, in the exploratory clinical trial conducted by Khambata-Ford et al. [49], a large prospective human cohort uniformly treated with cetuximab was exploited in an attempt to systematically identify biomarkers associated with disease control after anti-EGFR moAbs treatment. Transcriptional profiling was conducted on RNA from tumor cells in order to identify genes whose expression correlates with best clinical response. EGFR GCN was detected at a frequency of 6 % by quantitative PCR but its increase within the disease control group was not statistically significant [49].

Mechanism of Acquired Resistance to Anti-EGFR moAbs

After an initial response to anti-EGFR moAbs, secondary resistance invariably arises, thereby limiting the clinical benefit of this type of treatment. In general, very little is known about the mechanisms of acquired drug resistance in patients who initially benefit from the therapy with EGFR moAbs. The most accepted hypothesis for the development of resistance to EGFR blockade is that rare cells with *KRAS* mutations preexist at low percentage in the primary tumors with supposedly wild-type KRAS cells. This assumption had limited evidence in support from either pre-clinical models or data from patients. In order to test this hypothesis, Diaz et al. [57] developed a sensitive method which was able to detect mutant KRAS DNA in the circulation of 28 patients receiving monotherapy with panitumumab. They detected 9 out of 24 (38 %) patients whose tumors were initially *KRAS* wild type developed detectable mutations in *KRAS* in their sera. More impressively, three of them developed multiple different *KRAS* mutations while the emergence of these mutations was very consistent, occurring between 5 and 6 months following the initiation of the treatment. With the use of bio-infomatics methods, they found that the mutations were present in expanded subclones before the initiation of panitumumab treatment.

Another group has shown that point mutations and other molecular alterations of *KRAS* are associated with the onset of acquired resistance to anti-EGFR treatment [58]. Analysis of metastases from patients who developed resistance to cetuximab or panitumumab showed the emergence of KRAS amplification in one sample and acquisition of secondary *KRAS* mutations in 6 out of 10 of the cases. Once again, *KRAS* mutant alleles were detectable in the blood of cetuximab-treated patients as early as 10 months before radiographic documentation of disease progression. In summary, the results identify *KRAS* genetic alterations as frequent drivers of acquired resistance to moAbs [58]. More importantly, expression of mutant *KRAS* under the control of its endogenous gene promoter was sufficient to confer resistance to cetuximab, but the resistant clones were sensitive to combinatorial inhibition of EGFR and mitogen-activated protein-kinase kinase (MEK) [58]. These results suggest that the emergence of KRAS mutations is a mediator of acquired resistance to EGFR blockade and that these mutations can be detected in a non-invasive manner.

In a different approach, Yonesaka et al. [59] have shown that cetuximab-resistant cancer cells, both in culture and in patients' samples, can up-regulate signaling through the ERBB2 growth factor receptor. This upregulation of ERBB2 permanently turning on extracellular signal resulting in activated ERK1/2-mediated growth, differentiation, and survival. Moreover, down-regulation of ERBB2 with a small interfering RNA or antibody restored sensitivity. Finally, in several patients' groups with colorectal cancer, they saw decreased survival after treatment with cetuximab in those who exhibited the amplified *ERBB2* gene.

These studies add to other knowledge for the mechanisms of acquired resistance to anti-EGFR moAbs and indicate that re-biopsy approaches with a standardized protocol, at the time of disease progression, would be an important tool for the treatment planning. In addition, promising data for the detection of important markers in the blood may revolutionize the field from both the scientific and clinical aspects.

Conclusion

The CRC mutation profiles should influence patient selection and/or stratification in prospective trials. The *KRAS* mutational status represents a paradigm for biomarkers development in the era of molecular targeted therapies. As a result of that, *KRAS* testing is now mandatory at the presentation of metastatic disease in patients with CRC. In total, almost 50–60 % of mCRC patients' tumors harbor a mutation in the RAS-RAF-MEPK-ERK pathway (exon 2 *KRAS* 40 %, exon 3 *KRAS* 3 %, *NRAS* 5 %, *BRAF*^{V600E} 10 %) and are resistant to anti-EGFR moAbs therapy. In addition, *PIK3CA* mutations appear to be useful predictors for response to anti-EGFR moAbs, but definitive conclusions should be based on the analysis of larger patients' cohorts in randomized trials that have included patients who have not been exposed to anti-EGFR targeted therapies. Also, the expression of AREG and EREG was consistently associated with the outcome to cetuximab and panitumumab combination chemotherapy. The data from the study of acquired resistance are interesting and provide a rationale for the design of the therapeutic plan in subsequent treatment lines. The results of GCN are premature and controversial, and thus need to be explored in a more systematic approach. The development of biomarkers for the optimization of anti-EGFR treatment in mCRC, beyond *KRAS* mutations, is a work in progress. The aim will be to identify molecular markers that might be used to select patients with the higher probability of response to anti-EGFR moAbs.

In summary, the multigene models seem to be more effective than single-gene analysis for the selection of patients who could gain the maximum benefit from the administration of anti-EGFR moAbs. The key issue of cost for the molecular analysis and the limited amount of tumor cells available in FFPE specimens for all potential biomarkers testing could be tackled with the development of multiplex assays [60].

Conflicts of Interest
No potential conflicts of interest were disclosed.

References

1. Jemal A, Bray F, Center MM, Ferlay J, Ward E, Forman D. Global cancer statistics. CA Cancer J Clin. 2011;61:69–90.
2. Köhne CH, Schöffski P, Wilke H, Käufer C, Andreesen R, Ohl U, Klaasen U, Westerhausen M, Hiddemann W, Schott G, Harstick A, Bade J, Horster A, Schubert U, Hecker H, Dörken B, Schmoll HJ. Effective biomodulation by leucovorin of high-dose infusion fluorouracil given as a weekly 24-hour infusion: results of a randomized trial in patients with advanced colorectal cancer. J Clin Oncol. 1998;16:418–26.
3. Tournigand C, André T, Achille E, Lledo G, Flesh M, Mery-Mignard D, Quinaux E, Couteau C, Buyse M, Ganem G, Landi B, Colin P, Louvet C, de Gramont A. FOLFIRI followed by FOLFOX6 or the reverse sequence in advanced colorectal cancer: a randomized GERCOR study. J Clin Oncol. 2004;22:229–37.
4. Adam R, Wicherts DA, de Haas RJ, Ciacio O, Lévi F, Paule B, Ducreux M, Azoulay D, Bismuth H, Castaing D. Patients with initially unresectable colorectal liver metastases: is there a possibility of cure? J Clin Oncol. 2009;27:1829–35.
5. Douillard J, Siena S, Cassidy J, Tabernero J, Burkes R, Barugel M, Humblet Y, Bodoky G, Cunningham D, Jassem J, Rivera F, Kocákova I, Ruff P, Błasińska-Morawiec M, Šmakal M, Canon JL, Rother M, Oliner KS, Wolf M, Gansert J (2009) Randomized phase 3 study of

panitumumab with FOLFOX4 compared to FOLFOX4 alone as 1st-line treatment (tx) for metastatic colorectal cancer (mCRC): the PRIME trial. AnnOncol supp. (Abstract).
6. Van Cutsem E, Köhne CH, Hitre E, Zaluski J, Chang Chien CR, Makhson A, D'Haens G, Pintér T, Lim R, Bodoky G, Roh JK, Folprecht G, Ruff P, Stroh C, Tejpar S, Schlichting M, Nippgen J, Rougier P. Cetuximab and chemotherapy as initial treatment for metastatic colorectal cancer. N Engl J Med. 2009;360:1408–17.
7. Cunningham D, Humblet Y, Siena S, Khayat D, Bleiberg H, Santoro A, Bets D, Mueser M, Harstrick A, Verslype C, Chau I, Van Cutsem E. Cetuximab monotherapy and cetuximab plus irinotecan in irinotecan-refractory metastatic colorectal cancer. N Engl J Med. 2004;351:337–45.
8. Saltz LB, Meropol NJ, Loehrer PJ Sr, Needle MN, Kopit J, Mayer RJ. Phase II trial of cetuximab in patients with refractory colorectal cancer that expresses the epidermal growth factor receptor. J Clin Oncol. 2004;22:1201–8.
9. Van Cutsem E, Peeters M, Siena S, Humblet Y, Hendlisz A, Neyns B, Canon JL, Van Laethem JL, Maurel J, Richardson G, Wolf M, Amado RG. Open-label phase III trial of panitumumab plus best supportive care compared with best supportive care alone in patients with chemotherapy-refractory metastatic colorectal cancer. J Clin Oncol. 2007;25:1658–64.
10. Chung KY, Shia J, Kemeny NE, Shah M, Schwartz GK, Tse A, Hamilton A, Pan D, Schrag D, Schwartz L, Klimstra DS, Fridman D, Kelsen DP, Saltz LB. Cetuximab shows activity in colorectal cancer patients with tumors that do not express the epidermal growth factor receptor by immunohistochemistry. J Clin Oncol. 2005;23:1803–10.
11. Karapetis CS, Khambata-Ford S, Jonker DJ, O'Callaghan CJ, Tu D, Tebbutt NC, Simes RJ, Chalchal H, Shapiro JD, Robitaille S, Price TJ, Shepherd L, Au HJ, Langer C, Moore MJ, Zalcberg JR. K-ras mutations and benefit from cetuximab in advanced colorectal cancer. N Engl J Med. 2008;359:1757–65.
12. Amado RG, Wolf M, Peeters M, Van Cutsem E, Siena S, Freeman DJ, Juan T, Sikorski R, Suggs S, Radinsky R, Patterson SD, Chang DD. Wild-type KRAS is required for panitumumab efficacy in patients with metastatic colorectal cancer. J Clin Oncol. 2008;26:1626–34.
13. Vogelstein B, Kinzler KW. Cancer genes and the pathways they control. Nat Med. 2004;10:789–99.
14. Wood LD, Parsons DW, Jones S, Lin J, Sjöblom T, Leary RJ, Shen D, Boca SM, Barber T, Ptak J, Silliman N, Szabo S, Dezso Z, Ustyanksky V, Nikolskaya T, Nikolsky Y, Karchin R, Wilson PA, Kaminker JS, Zhang Z, Croshaw R, Willis J, Dawson D, Shipitsin M, Willson JK, Sukumar S, Polyak K, Park BH, Pethiyagoda CL, Pant PV, Ballinger DG, Sparks AB, Hartigan J, Smith DR, Suh E, Papadopoulos N, Buckhaults P, Markowitz SD, Parmigiani G, Kinzler KW, Velculescu VE, Vogelstein B. The genomic landscapes of human breast and colorectal cancers. Science. 2007;318:1108–13.
15. Lievre A, Bachet JB, Le Corre D, Boige V, Landi B, Emile JF, Côté JF, Tomasic G, Penna C, Ducreux M, Rougier P, Penault-Llorca F, Laurent-Puig P. KRAS mutation status is predictive of response to cetuximab therapy in colorectal cancer. Cancer Res. 2006;66:3992–5.
16. COSMIC DATABASE Catalog of Somatic Mutation, Sanger Institute. http://www.sanger.ac.uk/perl/genetics/CGP/cosmic?action=bycancer&ln=KRAS&sn=large_intestine&ss=colon&sh=adenocarcinoma&hn=carcinoma. 2012.
17. Buhrman G, Wink G, Mattos C. Transformation efficiency of RasQ61 mutants linked to structural features of the switch regions in the presence of Raf. Structure. 2007;15:1618–29.
18. Smith G, Bounds R, Wolf H, Steele RJ, Carey FA, Wolf CR. Activating K-Ras mutations outwith 'hotspot' codons in sporadic colorectal tumors—implications for personalised cancer medicine. Br J Cancer. 2010;102:693–703.
19. Loupakis F, Ruzzo A, Cremolini C, Vincenzi B, Salvatore L, Santini D, Masi G, Stasi I, Canestrari E, Rulli E, Floriani I, Bencardino K, Galluccio N, Catalano V, Tonini G, Magnani M, Fontanini G, Basolo F, Falcone A, Graziano F. KRAS codon 61, 146 and BRAF mutations predict resistance to cetuximab plus irinotecan in KRAS codon 12 and 13 wild-type metastatic colorectal cancer. Br J Cancer. 2009;101:715–21.

20. De RW, Claes B, Bernasconi D, De Schutter J, Biesmans B, Fountzilas G, Kalogeras KT, Kotoula V, Papamichael D, Laurent-Puig P, Penault-Llorca F, Rougier P, Vincenzi B, Santini D, Tonini G, Cappuzzo F, Frattini M, Molinari F, Saletti P, De Dosso S, Martini M, Bardelli A, Siena S, Sartore-Bianchi A, Tabernero J, Macarulla T, Di Fiore F, Gangloff AO, Ciardiello F, Pfeiffer P, Qvortrup C, Hansen TP, Van Cutsem E, Piessevaux H, Lambrechts D, Delorenzi M, Tejpar S. Effects of KRAS, BRAF, NRAS, and PIK3CA mutations on the efficacy of cetuximab plus chemotherapy in chemotherapy-refractory metastatic colorectal cancer: a retrospective consortium analysis. Lancet Oncol. 2010;11:753–62.
21. Phase III Trial of Panitumumab vs BSC in mCRC: genetic markers of response. AACR annual meeting; 2010.
22. McCubrey JA, Sokolosky ML, Lehmann BD, Taylor JR, Navolanic PM, Chappell WH, Abrams SL, Stadelman KM, Wong EW, Misaghian N, Horn S, Bäsecke J, Libra M, Stivala F, Ligresti G, Tafuri A, Milella M, Zarzycki M, Dzugaj A, Chiarini F, Evangelisti C, Martelli AM, Terrian DM, Franklin RA, Steelman LS. Alteration of Akt activity increases chemotherapeutic drug and hormonal resistance in breast cancer yet confers an achilles heel by sensitization to targeted therapy. Adv Enzyme Regul. 2008;48:113–35.
23. Davies H, Bignell GR, Cox C, Stephens P, Edkins S, Clegg S, Teague J, Woffendin H, Garnett MJ, Bottomley W, Davis N, Dicks E, Ewing R, Floyd Y, Gray K, Hall S, Hawes R, Hughes J, Kosmidou V, Menzies A, Mould C, Parker A, Stevens C, Watt S, Hooper S, Wilson R, Jayatilake H, Gusterson BA, Cooper C, Shipley J, Hargrave D, Pritchard-Jones K, Maitland N, Chenevix-Trench G, Riggins GJ, Bigner DD, Palmieri G, Cossu A, Flanagan A, Nicholson A, Ho JW, Leung SY, Yuen ST, Weber BL, Seigler HF, Darrow TL, Paterson H, Marais R, Marshall CJ, Wooster R, Stratton MR, Futreal PA. Mutations of the BRAF gene in human cancer. Nature. 2002;417:949–54.
24. Di Nicolantonio F, Martini M, Molinari F, Sartore-Bianchi A, Arena S, Saletti P, De Dosso S, Mazzucchelli L, Frattini M, Siena S, Bardelli A. Wild-type BRAF is required for response to panitumumab or cetuximab in metastatic colorectal cancer. J Clin Oncol. 2008;26:5705–12.
25. Rajagopalan H, Bardelli A, Lengauer C, Kinzler KW, Vogelstein B, Velculescu VE. Tumorigenesis: RAF/RAS oncogenes and mismatch-repair status. Nature. 2002;418:934.
26. Saridaki Z, Tzardi M, Papadaki C, Sfakianaki M, Pega F, Kalikaki A, Tsakalaki E, Trypaki M, Messaritakis I, Stathopoulos E, Mavroudis D, Georgoulias V, Souglakos J. Impact of KRAS, BRAF, PIK3CA mutations, PTEN, AREG, EREG expression and skin rash in >/=2 line cetuximab-based therapy of colorectal cancer patients. PLoS ONE. 2011;6:e15980.
27. Souglakos J, Philips J, Wang R, Marwah S, Silver M, Tzardi M, Silver J, Ogino S, Hooshmand S, Kwak E, Freed E, Meyerhardt JA, Saridaki Z, Georgoulias V, Finkelstein D, Fuchs CS, Kulke MH, Shivdasani RA. Prognostic and predictive value of common mutations for treatment response and survival in patients with metastatic colorectal cancer. Br J Cancer. 2009;101:465–72.
28. French AJ, Sargent DJ, Burgart LJ, Foster NR, Kabat BF, Goldberg R, Shepherd L, Windschitl HE, Thibodeau SN. Prognostic significance of defective mismatch repair and BRAF V600E in patients with colon cancer. Clin Cancer Res. 2008;14:3408–15.
29. Saridaki Z, Papadatos-Pastos D, Tzardi M, Mavroudis D, Bairaktari E, Arvanity H, Stathopoulos E, Georgoulias V, Souglakos J. BRAF mutations, microsatellite instability status and cyclin D1 expression predict metastatic colorectal patients' outcome. Br J Cancer. 2010;102:1762–8.
30. Oliveira C, Pinto M, Duval A, Brennetot C, Domingo E, Espín E, Armengol M, Yamamoto H, Hamelin R, Seruca R, Schwartz S Jr. BRAF mutations characterize colon but not gastric cancer with mismatch repair deficiency. Oncogene. 2003;22:9192–6.
31. Domingo E, Laiho P, Ollikainen M, Pinto M, Wang L, French AJ, Westra J, Frebourg T, Espín E, Armengol M, Hamelin R, Yamamoto H, Hofstra RM, Seruca R, Lindblom A, Peltomäki P, Thibodeau SN, Aaltonen LA, Schwartz S Jr. BRAF screening as a low-cost effective strategy for simplifying HNPCC genetic testing. J Med Gene. 2004;41:664–8.

32. Wang L, Cunningham JM, Winters JL, Guenther JC, French AJ, Boardman LA, Burgart LJ, McDonnell SK, Schaid DJ, Thibodeau SN. BRAF mutations in colon cancer are not likely attributable to defective DNA mismatch repair. Cancer Res. 2003;63:5209–12.
33. Tol J, Nagtegaal ID, Punt CJ. BRAF mutation in metastatic colorectal cancer. N Engl J Med. 2009;361:98–9.
34. Van CE, Köhne CH, Láng I, Folprecht G, Nowacki MP, Cascinu S, Shchepotin I, Maurel J, Cunningham D, Tejpar S, Schlichting M, Zubel A, Celik I, Rougier P, Ciardiello F. Cetuximab plus irinotecan, fluorouracil, and leucovorin as first-line treatment for metastatic colorectal cancer: updated analysis of overall survival according to tumor KRAS and BRAF mutation status. J Clin Oncol. 2011;29:2011–9.
35. Rodriguez-Viciana P, Warne PH, Dhand R, Vanhaesebroeck B, Gout I, Fry MJ, Waterfield MD, Downward J. Phosphatidylinositol-3-OH kinase as a direct target of Ras. Nature. 1994;370:527–32.
36. Huang CH, Mandelker D, Schmidt-Kittler O, Samuels Y, Velculescu VE, Kinzler KW, Vogelstein B, Gabelli SB, Amzel LM. The structure of a human p110alpha/p85alpha complex elucidates the effects of oncogenic PI3Kalpha mutations. Science. 2007;318:1744–8.
37. Samuels Y, Diaz LA Jr, Schmidt-Kittler O, Cummins JM, Delong L, Cheong I, Rago C, Huso DL, Lengauer C, Kinzler KW, Vogelstein B, Velculescu VE. Mutant PIK3CA promotes cell growth and invasion of human cancer cells. Cancer Cell. 2005;7:561–73.
38. Laurent-Puig P, Cayre A, Manceau G, Buc E, Bachet JB, Lecomte T, Rougier P, Lievre A, Landi B, Boige V, Ducreux M, Ychou M, Bibeau F, Bouché O, Reid J, Stone S, Penault-Llorca F. Analysis of PTEN, BRAF, and EGFR status in determining benefit from cetuximab therapy in wild-type KRAS metastatic colon cancer. J Clin Oncol. 2009;27:5924–30.
39. Perrone F, Lampis A, Orsenigo M, Di Bartolomeo M, Gevorgyan A, Losa M, Frattini M, Riva C, Andreola S, Bajetta E, Bertario L, Leo E, Pierotti MA, Pilotti S. PI3KCA/PTEN deregulation contributes to impaired responses to cetuximab in metastatic colorectal cancer patients. Ann Oncol. 2009;20:84–90.
40. Prenen H, De Schutter J, Jacobs B, De Roock W, Biesmans B, Claes B, Lambrechts D, Van Cutsem E, Tejpar S. PIK3CA mutations are not a major determinant of resistance to the epidermal growth factor receptor inhibitor cetuximab in metastatic colorectal cancer. Clin Cancer Res. 2009;15:3184–8.
41. Sartore-Bianchi A, Martini M, Molinari F, Veronese S, Nichelatti M, Artale S, Di Nicolantonio F, Saletti P, De Dosso S, Mazzucchelli L, Frattini M, Siena S, Bardelli A. PIK3CA mutations in colorectal cancer are associated with clinical resistance to EGFR-targeted monoclonal antibodies. Cancer Res. 2009;69:1851–7.
42. Zhao L, Vogt PK. Helical domain and kinase domain mutations in p110alpha of phosphatidylinositol 3-kinase induce gain of function by different mechanisms. Proc Natl Acad Sci U S A. 2008;105:2652–7.
43. Martini M, Vecchione L, Siena S, Tejpar S, Bardelli A. Targeted therapies: how personal should we go? Nat Rev Clin Oncol. 2012;9:87–97.
44. Jhawer M, Goel S, Wilson AJ, et al. PIK3CA mutation/PTEN expression status predicts response of colon cancer cells to the epidermal growth factor receptor inhibitor cetuximab. Cancer Res. 2008;68:1953–61.
45. Frattini M, Saletti P, Romagnani E, Martin V, Molinari F, Ghisletta M, Camponovo A, Etienne LL, Cavalli F, Mazzucchelli L. PTEN loss of expression predicts cetuximab efficacy in metastatic colorectal cancer patients. Br J Cancer. 2007;97:1139–45.
46. Loupakis F, Pollina L, Stasi I, Ruzzo A, Scartozzi M, Santini D, Masi G, Graziano F, Cremolini C, Rulli E, Canestrari E, Funel N, Schiavon G, Petrini I, Magnani M, Tonini G, Campani D, Floriani I, Cascinu S, Falcone A. PTEN expression and KRAS mutations on primary tumors and metastases in the prediction of benefit from cetuximab plus irinotecan for patients with metastatic colorectal cancer. J Clin Oncol. 2009;27:2622–9.
47. Prenen H, Tejpar S, Van CE. Impact of molecular markers on treatment selection in advanced colorectal cancer. Eur J Cancer. 2009;45(Suppl 1):70–8.

48. Jacobs B, De RW, Piessevaux H, Van Oirbeek R, Biesmans B, De Schutter J, Fieuws S, Vandesompele J, Peeters M, Van Laethem JL, Humblet Y, Pénault-Llorca F, De Hertogh G, Laurent-Puig P, Van Cutsem E, Tejpar S. Amphiregulin and epiregulin mRNA expression in primary tumors predicts outcome in metastatic colorectal cancer treated with cetuximab. J Clin Oncol. 2009;27:5068–74.
49. Khambata-Ford S, Garrett CR, Meropol NJ, Basik M, Harbison CT, Wu S, Wong TW, Huang X, Takimoto CH, Godwin AK, Tan BR, Krishnamurthi SS, Burris HA 3rd, Poplin EA, Hidalgo M, Baselga J, Clark EA, Mauro DJ. Expression of epiregulin and amphiregulin and K-ras mutation status predict disease control in metastatic colorectal cancer patients treated with cetuximab. J Clin Oncol. 2007;25:3230–7.
50. Tabernero J, Cervantes A, Rivera F, Martinelli E, Rojo F, von Heydebreck A, Macarulla T, Rodriguez-Braun E, Eugenia Vega-Villegas M, Senger S, Ramos FJ, Roselló S, Celik I, Stroh C, Baselga J, Ciardiello F. Pharmacogenomic and pharmacoproteomic studies of cetuximab in metastatic colorectal cancer: biomarker analysis of a phase I dose-escalation study. J Clin Oncol. 2010;28:1181–9.
51. Vecchione L, Saridaki Z, Tejpar S. Clinical implications and quality assurance of molecular testing for EGFR-targeting agents in colorectal cancer. Curr Colorectal Cancer Rep. 2011;8:42–50. doi:10.1007/s11888-011-0112-3.
52. Vecchione L, Jacobs B, Normanno N, Ciardiello F, Tejpar S. EGFR-targeted therapy. Exp Cell Res. 2011;317:2765–71.
53. Baker JB, Dutta D, Watson D, Maddala T, Munneke BM, Shak S, Rowinsky EK, Xu LA, Harbison CT, Clark EA, Mauro DJ, Khambata-Ford S. Tumor gene expression predicts response to cetuximab in patients with KRAS wild-type metastatic colorectal cancer. Br J Cancer. 2011;104:488–95.
54. Moroni M, Veronese S, Benvenuti S, Marrapese G, Sartore-Bianchi A, Di Nicolantonio F, Gambacorta M, Siena S, Bardelli A. Gene copy number for epidermal growth factor receptor (EGFR) and clinical response to antiEGFR treatment in colorectal cancer: a cohort study. Lancet Oncol. 2005;6:279–86.
55. Lenz HJ, Van CE, Khambata-Ford S, Mayer RJ, Gold P, Stella P, Mirtsching B, Cohn AL, Pippas AW, Azarnia N, Tsuchihashi Z, Mauro DJ, Rowinsky EK. Multicenter phase II and translational study of cetuximab in metastatic colorectal carcinoma refractory to irinotecan, oxaliplatin, and fluoropyrimidines. J Clin Oncol. 2006;24:4914–21.
56. Sartore-Bianchi A, Moroni M, Veronese S, Carnaghi C, Bajetta E, Luppi G, Sobrero A, Barone C, Cascinu S, Colucci G, Cortesi E, Nichelatti M, Gambacorta M, Siena S. Epidermal growth factor receptor gene copy number and clinical outcome of metastatic colorectal cancer treated with panitumumab. J Clin Oncol. 2007;25:3238–45.
57. Diaz LA Jr, Williams RT, Wu J, Kinde I, Hecht JR, Berlin J, Allen B, Bozic I, Reiter JG, Nowak MA, Kinzler KW, Oliner KS, Vogelstein B. The molecular evolution of acquired resistance to targeted EGFR blockade in colorectal cancers. Nature. 2012;486:537–40.
58. Misale S, Yaeger R, Hobor S, Scala E, Janakiraman M, Liska D, Valtorta E, Schiavo R, Buscarino M, Siravegna G, Bencardino K, Cercek A, Chen CT, Veronese S, Zanon C, Sartore-Bianchi A, Gambacorta M, Gallicchio M, Vakiani E, Boscaro V, Medico E, Weiser M, Siena S, Di Nicolantonio F, Solit D, Bardelli A. Emergence of KRAS mutations and acquired resistance to anti-EGFR therapy in colorectal cancer. Nature. 2012;486:532–6.
59. Yonesaka K, Zejnullahu K, Okamoto I, Satoh T, Cappuzzo F, Souglakos J, Ercan D, Rogers A, Roncalli M, Takeda M, Fujisaka Y, Philips J, Shimizu T, Maenishi O, Cho Y, Sun J, Destro A, Taira K, Takeda K, Okabe T, Swanson J, Itoh H, Takada M, Lifshits E, Okuno K, Engelman JA, Shivdasani RA, Nishio K, Fukuoka M, Varella-Garcia M, Nakagawa K, Jänne PA. Activation of ERBB2 signaling causes resistance to the EGFR-directed therapeutic antibody cetuximab. Sci Transl Med. 2011;3:99ra86.
60. Lurkin I, Stoehr R, Hurst CD, van Tilborg AA, Knowles MA, Hartmann A, Zwarthoff EC. Two multiplex assays that simultaneously identify 22 possible mutation sites in the KRAS, BRAF, NRAS and PIK3CA genes. PLoS ONE. 2010;5:e8802.

Overcoming Resistance of Melanoma to Immunotherapy with Monoclonal Antibodies Against Checkpoints Inhibitors

Peter Hersey, Stuart Gallagher and Branka Mijatov

Abstract The introduction of monoclonal antibodies against checkpoint inhibitors on T cells such as Ipilimumab and anti PD1 has been a major advance in the treatment of metastatic melanoma. Nevertheless, the majority of patients does not receive benefit from this treatment approach. The reasons for this are likely to reflect conditioning of the microenvironment of the tumour by properties of the tumour cells that either prevent infiltration by T cells or which modulate their function. Treatments that combine monoclonal antibodies with agents that inhibit melanoma cell production of suppressive cytokines and which favor infiltration of T cells into the tumour are the focus of ongoing studies.

Keywords Melanoma · Checkpoint inhibitors · Ipilimumab · PD1 · Microenvironment · Cytokines · Chemokines · T cells

Abbreviations

BTLA	B and T cell attenuator
CT	Cancer testis
CTLA4	Cytotoxic lymphocyte antigen 4
EOMES	Eomesodermin
ICOS	Inducible costimulator
IDO	Indolamine dioxygenase
MAbs	Monoclonal antibodies
NBD	Nemo binding domain
PD1	Programmed death receptor 1
TILs	Tumour infiltrating lymphocytes
Tim3	T cell immunoglobulin mucin 3

P. Hersey (✉) · S. Gallagher · B. Mijatov
Kolling Institute of Medical Research, Royal North Shore Hospital,
St Leonards, NSW 2065, Australia
e-mail: peter.hersey@sydney.edu.au

B. Bonavida (ed.), *Resistance to Immunotherapeutic Antibodies in Cancer*,
Resistance to Targeted Anti-Cancer Therapeutics 2, DOI: 10.1007/978-1-4614-7654-2_7,

Introduction

Treatment of melanoma by various forms of immunotherapy has a long history ranging from non specific active immunotherapy with bacterial products like BCG to specific vaccines made from melanoma cells or more purified antigenic proteins, peptides or DNA coding for melanoma antigens. Treatment with antibodies directly binding to melanoma antigens has also shown little promise. More success, however, has followed from innovative approaches using antibodies that target physiological checkpoints on lymphocytes that help to maintain homeostasis in the immune system. The following reviews the key studies describing the clinical results with these antibodies, there limitations and approaches to further improve their efficacy in the treatment of melanoma.

Immunotherapy of Melanoma with Monoclonal Antibodies Against Checkpoint Receptors on T Cells Takes Center Stage

Treatment of metastatic melanoma has been revolutionized by the introduction of treatment with monoclonal antibodies (MAbs) against the checkpoint inhibitors, cytotoxic lymphocyte antigen 4 (CTLA4) and programmed death receptor 1(PD1). The MAb, Ipilimumab (Yervoy), against CTLA4, was shown in two large randomized studies to improve the survival of patients with metastatic melanoma. In the first trial reported by Hodi et al. [1], treatment with Ipilimumab was compared to immunotherapy with a vaccine against the melanoma antigen gp100 and a combination of these. The Ipilimumab-treated patients had median survivals of 10 months compared to 6.4 months in the vaccine alone treated patients and 1 and 2 year survival rates of approximately 40 and 25 %, respectively. The survival at different time points was consistently about 10 % greater than the gp 100 vaccine-treated patients. In the second trial reported by Robert et al. [2], 502 previously untreated patients were randomized to receive treatment with DTIC alone or a combination of Ipi plus DTIC. Again, median overall survivals (OS) were greater in the group receiving Ipilimumab (11.2 months compared to 9.1 months in those receiving DTIC alone). Percent survivals at 1, 2 and 3 years of 47.3, 28.5 and 20.8 %, respectively, were again approximately 10 % above those in the patients treated with DTIC alone.

These studies were the first to show improvement in survival by any treatment in melanoma and helped to emphasize the importance of immune responses against melanoma in improving survival from the disease. Nevertheless, approximately 80 % of patients still died of melanoma by 3 years indicating that further initiatives are needed to improve the effectiveness of this therapy.Studies with MAbs against PD1 in phase 1 studies with the MAb BMS 936558 in 94 patients with melanoma have shown response rates of approximately 30 % [3]. Effects of anti PD1 on survival are yet to be established but appear promising. Once more, though, it is clear that the majority of patients does not receive significant benefit from this treatment. In the following sections, we review the possible reasons why these forms of immunotherapy may fail and what strategies may be used to increase their effectiveness.

Information from Studies on Immune Responses

A number of studies have examined whether there are differences in the immune responses between patients who respond to MAbs against CTLA4 compared to non responders. These studies have proven surprisingly unhelpful. Studies (in small patient subgroups) have found clinical responses to correlate with antibodies and T cells against the cancer testis (CT) antigen NY-ESO-1. In studies on 144 patients, antibodies to NY-ESO-1 were detected in 16 % of patients before treatment and in 22 % at any time during treatment. Responses were seen in 55 % of seropositive patients compared to 30 % in seronegative patients. The correlations were even stronger in the 60 % of the seropositive patients who also had detectable T cell responses to NY-ESO-1 [4]. Another correlate was an increase in inducible costimulator (ICOS) on T cells. Eight of 14 patients with bladder cancer had a greater than 2 fold increase in ICOS on blood T cells at 7 or 12 weeks during treatment with Ipilimumab. Seven of the 8 patients had benefit from the treatment whereas none of 6 patients without an increase in ICOS had any benefit [5]. Studies on the abscopal effect of radiotherapy during treatment with Ipilimumab also noted a decrease in a subpopulation of myeloid suppressor cells [6] believed to have immunosuppressive properties [7] Increased absolute lymphocyte counts (ALC) at 7 weeks have been associated with good responses at 24 weeks [8]. Activation of CD4 T cells by Ipilimumab was shown by increased HLA DR antigen expression [9].

Ribas et al. [10] found an association between responses to another anti CTLA4 MAb called Tremelimumab and the ratio of CD8 T cells to Fox P3 regulatory T cells. Huang et al. [11] were, however, unable to establish a correlation between T cell infiltration in the first 1–2 months of treatment and clinical responses. Microarray studies by Wang et al. [12] confirmed that Ipilimumab increased the expression of ICOS on CD4 T cells and drew attention to the possible significance of levels of the transcription factor Eomesodermin (EOMES) in CD8 T cells as a marker of responses following Ipilimumab treatment. EOMES is believed to regulate IFN gamma and Granzyme-B production and is down regulated by the CTLA4 pathway. Values below the median were associated with poor relapse free survivals in adjuvant studies on patients with melanoma.

Unfortunately, these studies on immune responses in patients have not resulted in robust tests to select likely responders to treatment with Ipilimumab.

Changes in the Microenvironment of Melanoma as the Key to Understanding Resistance to Immunotherapy with Checkpoint Inhibitor Antibodies

Given that studies on the immune response have provided very few insights into the resistance of patients to immunotherapy, increasing evidence points to the microenvironment around tumours as the main determinant of clinical responses to immunotherapy with MAbs against checkpoint inhibitors. It has long been known that tumour stroma is important in the outcome of immunotherapy [13] but increased attention was focused on its importance as a result of gene expression studies showing that favorable clinical responses to cytokines and melanoma vaccines were associated with a relatively small gene expression signature that included cytokines, chemokines and inflammatory mediators associated with T cells [14]. Factors that influence the tumour microenvironment include production of soluble factors from the tumour cells as described for melanoma [15] or induction of innate immune sensing by release of factors such as HMGB1 [16] from the nucleus of damaged cells or interaction of Toll like receptors on melanoma with ligands in tissues [17]. Certain tissues are rich in ligands that interact with receptors on melanoma cells such as FGF1 in the brain and hepatocyte growth factor in the liver and may influence the microenvironment indirectly by activating certain resistance pathways in melanoma [18]. Production of factors by the melanoma cells are, however, most likely to be the major influence on the microenvironment and influence infiltration of T cells or modulate their function.

Regulation of T Cell Infiltration into Melanoma Tumours

The importance of T cell infiltration into primary melanoma is shown by their powerful influence on survival. One of the most comprehensive studies on relation of tumour infiltrating lymphocytes (TILs) to prognosis was by Azimi et al. on tissue sections from 1,831 patients. Patients with marked (grade 3) T cell infiltrates had no recurrences but unfortunately only 3 % of patients had such grade 3 infiltrates whereas 35 % had no infiltrates at all [19]. The causes of low numbers of TILs are likely to be multifactorial but absence of VCAM on blood vessels around melanoma may be one such factor as described by Piali et al. [20]. Studies by Delfortrie et al. [21] showed that certain tumours release a soluble factor called VE-statin which down regulates both VCAM and ICAM on endothelial cells so preventing adhesion of T cells. Another factor may be the release of Endostatins from melanoma cells as studies in animal models showed that the absence of TILs was related to Endostatin receptor B expression on endothelial cells around the tumour and that knockout of this receptor allowed marked infiltration by TILs [22, 23] Endothelins were shown to induce CXCL1 and CXCL8 production in melanoma [24] and promote the invasive behavior of melanoma [25].

Chemokines from melanoma are known to mediate infiltration of T cells by interaction with chemokine receptors on T cells [15, 26–28]. The chemokines CCL4 (MIP 1b), CCL5 (Rantes), CXCL10 (IP10) attract both CD4 and CD8 T cells. CCL22 may attract regulatory T cells and CCL21 attracts T cells to secondary lymphoid tissue. In contrast, CXCL8 (IL-8) may inhibit T cell infiltration. CXCR3 is expressed preferentially on Th1 cells whereas CCR4 determines homing to skin and CCR9 to intestine [29, 30]. The studies of Muthuswamy et al. [30] were of much interest in that they were able to show that a mixture of poly I:C, indomethacin and interferon alpha was able to activate NF-κB and induce chemokines favoring T cell infiltration but at the same time inhibited chemokines associated with infiltration by regulatory T cells. A more indirect influence on T cell infiltration was suggested by the studies of Lesokhin et al. [31] who described a subpopulation of monocyte-derived myeloid suppressor cells (CD11b, CCR2 positive) that limited the infiltration of T cells into tumours.

Therapeutic Opportunities for Increasing T Cell Infiltration into Tumours

The following studies provide a number of possible interventions that might increase T cell infiltration into tumours. Hellebraker et al. [32] observed that ICAM expression on endothelial cells in tumours could be upregulated by treatment with HDAC inhibitors or DNA demethylases. Given the safety of these agents, it would appear feasible to test their effects with the checkpoint inhibitor antibodies. Agents that inhibit endothelin receptors are also available. A small molecular inhibitor of endothelin receptors A and B (Bosentan) was tested in a randomized trial with DTIC. There was no observed benefit with the combination but the study was not designed to study effects on T cell infiltration [33]. MAb conjugates against endothelin receptor B [34] (Genentech DEDN6526A) are also being tested in phase 1 studies in patients with melanoma and might be a useful treatment to combine with agents such as Ipilimumab. The use of agents that activate NF-κB is more problematic as NF-κB can increase production of chemokines beneficial for inducing T cell infiltration but also cytokines which inhibit immune responses such as IL-10 as well as a number of inflammatory mediators which can increase the growth of tumours such as IL-6, VEGF and TNF-alpha. Targeting NF-κB is discussed in more detail below.

One of the major developments in treatment of melanoma has been the introduction of selective BRAF inhibitors such as Vemurafenib and Dabrafenib. These agents induce clinical responses or disease stabilization in a high proportion of patients but relapse from the disease remains a limitation in their use. In view of this, there is much interest in whether combining these drugs with immunotherapy will increase the duration of responses to the BRAF inhibitors and trials combining Vemurafenib and Ipilimumab are in progress. Vemurafenib was shown not to inhibit immune responses to melanoma [35] and to increase the expression of certain melanoma antigens [36]. Tumour biopsies taken from patients at 15 days after commencement of treatment with Vemurafenib or Dabrafenib showed marked infiltration with CD8 and CD4 T cells which correlated with response of the patients to treatment [37]. Whether these results were due to modulation of cytokine/chemokine production by the melanoma cells or cell death induced by the inhibitors remain an open question. In a murine model of V600 mutated melanoma, the PLX4720 BRAF inhibitor was able to inhibit tumour growth but this was associated with reduced T cell infiltration and did not increase the effectiveness of treatment with Ipilimumab [38].

Melanoma Cells Can Condition Stroma in the Microenvironment to Modulate Immune Responses

Specific evidence for the ability of melanoma cells to change the cells in their environment and inhibit immune responses was reported by Khalili et al. [39]. Gene expression analyses of melanocytes transfected with V600 mutated BRAF and of V600 mutated melanoma lines showed upregulation of IL-1 beta and alpha which could be down regulated by Vemurafenib. Fibroblast lines from patients treated with ILI-1 where able to inhibit T cell responses against melanoma. This was associated with upregulation of PD1-L1 and PD1-L2 on their surface as well as induction of COX 2 gene expression. These studies add to those of Wilson et al. [40] and Straussman et al. [41] who showed that hepatocyte growth factor (HGF) from tumour stroma could induce resistance to the selective BRAF inhibitors. Prior studies by Gallagher et al. had also shown that melanoma cells could induce production of growth stimulatory factors for melanoma such as CXCL1 [42]. As shown by the Multiplex assay results in Fig. 1, certain melanoma lines produce high amounts of multiple cytokines and chemokines.

Given the production of these factors it is not surprising that T cells in the vicinity of melanoma have a range of phenotypes associated with exhaustion or anergy of T cells. These include expression of PD1, T cell immunoglobulin mucin 3 (Tim3) and B and T cell attenuator (BTLA) [43]. Some of the changes in T cells such as down regulation of the CD3 zeta chain have been attributed to the effects of myeloid suppressor cells which may be activated by CD4 T cells [44] and other factors [45, 46].

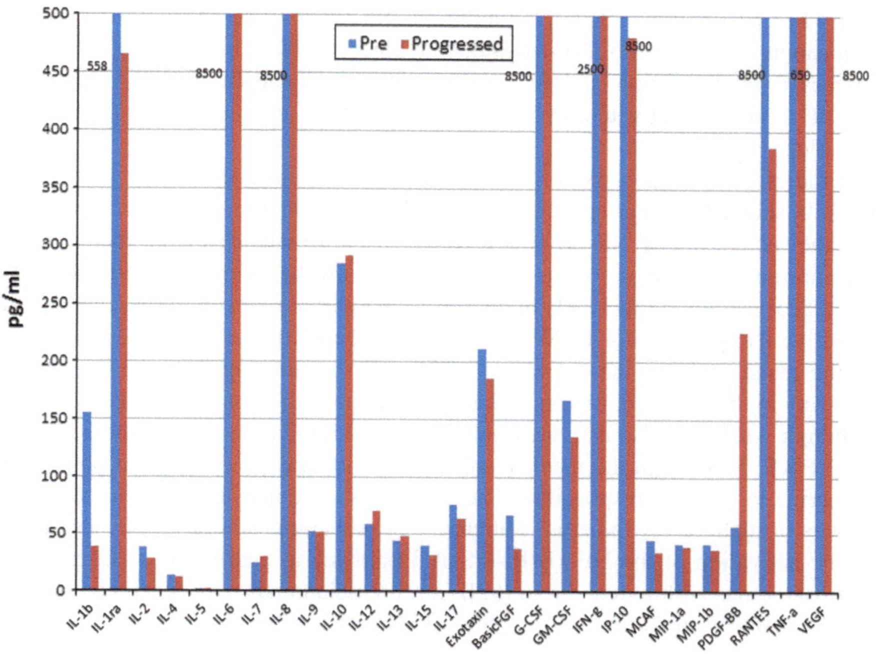

Fig. 1 Cell lines were established from a patient before treatment with Vemurafenib and after the development of resistance to the drug. Supernatants were collected from the lines after incubation in tissue culture medium for 24 h and assayed by the Biorad BIO-PLEX P 27 human cytokine Multiplex assay. (Catalogue number M500KCAFOY). The results show high levels of a range of chemokines and cytokines in both lines irrespective of their sensitivity to Vemurafenib

Activation of NF-κB as a Key Regulator of Immunomodulatory Chemokine and Cytokine Production by Melanoma

The wide array of cytokines and chemokines made by some melanoma cells has focused attention on NF-κB which is known to transcriptionally regulate a large array of such factors. NF-κB in melanoma can be activated by inflammatory mediators such as IL-1, TNF alpha, IL-6 and chemokines such as CXCL1 and CXCL8, so forming autocrine loops. In addition, NF-κB has been reported to be constitutively activated by increased activation of IKK leading to phosphorylation of IκB and release of p65/REL A complexes into the nucleus [47]. Several factors have been identified that may activate the IKK complex. These include phosphorylation by AKT [48] and increased degradation of IKK by the ubiquitin ligase beta–Trcp which is upregulated in V600 mutant BRAF melanoma [49]. In addition, p16 was shown to bind to p65 and so inhibits its activity and this restraint was lost when p16 is mutated [50]. In addition, NF-κB may be activated through the non canonical pathway by NF-κB-inducing kinase (NIK) which was reported to be increased in melanoma and to also activate the β-catenin pathway [51]. The NF-κB complex activated by this pathway results mainly in the p52/REL B complex.

Studies on cell lines established from patients failing treatment with Vemurafenib showed strong up regulation of NF-κB which raised questions as to whether activation of NF-κB was a factor in the resistance of the melanoma to Vemurafenib. Treatment of the resistant cells with the inhibitor of NF-κB, BAY 11-7082, resulted in low levels of apoptosis and partial reversal of resistance to the selective BRAF inhibitor PLX4720. Although the MEK pathway was reactivated in the resistant cells, the activation of NF-κB did not appear to be due to this pathway in that MEK inhibitors did not reduce the activation of NF-κB. Similarly, although AKT was also activated, inhibitors of AKT did not inhibit the activation of \NF-κB. Studies on the mechanism of activation are continuing but point to an autocrine loop being responsible. These findings are consistent with autocrines as drivers of malignancy in certain subgroups of melanoma similar to the description of the activation of the NF-κB/IL-6/Stat 3 pathway as a driver of malignancy in angiosarcomas with mutated p16 [52]. Certain melanomas express all components of this pathway including NF-κB, Stat3 [53] and IL-6 [54].

A logical development from these studies would be to carry out studies with inhibitors of NF-κB in patients with melanoma as discussed elsewhere [55]. Inhibition of NF-κB in patients has, however, been problematic due to lack of specificity with some agents like proteasome inhibitors (e.g. Bortezomib). Studies with more specific inhibitors of IKK, like the BMS compound 345541 [56], raise toxicity concerns due to the anti-apoptotic actions of NF-κB in the liver. Targeting NEMO/IKK interactions with cell permeable Nemo binding domain (NBD) inhibitory peptides is also under development. Inhibition of NF-κB has been examined in other inflammatory diseases such as Rheumatoid arthritis. In these states, the drugs have targeted mainly downstream targets of NF-κB such as TNF alpha (Infliximab, Etanercept, Adalimumab [57], and MAbs against IL-6 or IL-6 receptors [58]). Inhibitors of Stat3 also remain under development but upstream activators of STAT 3 such as Janus kinases (JAK) have been targeted by a number of drugs [57, 59–61]. Inhibitors of bromodomain epigenetic reader proteins are possible new inhibitors of NF-κB. One of these agents; I BET 151, was shown to protect mice from LPS-induced shock and had selective effects on different cytokines and chemokines regulated by NF-κB [62, 63]. Inhibitors of the BET proteins are believed to dissociate protein complexes containing transcription factors from nucleosomes and this may be selective for different protein complexes. The drugs are believed to have little toxicity so that future studies in patients with cancer will be of much interest.

Conclusions

The limitations in use of MAbs to checkpoint inhibitors in the treatment of melanoma discussed above apply to many forms of immunotherapy and the combination of approaches discussed for treatment with vaccines are equally relevant [64]. These include use of inhibitors of indolamine dioxygenase (IDO) that deplete tissues of tryptophan needed for T cell responses and various treatments that inhibit suppressor T cells. Myeloablative radiation has also been used to reduce myeloid suppressor macrophages. The role of signal pathway inhibitors remains under investigation but the combined use of selective BRAF and MEK inhibitors was shown in vitro to be effective in downregulating the PD-L1 ligand that inhibits T cell responses. The challenge will be to find inhibitors that do not also inhibit lymphocyte responses. Identification of agents which influence T cell infiltration into the tumour are key to the effectiveness of treatment with MAb inhibitors of immune checkpoints and several therapeutic options have been canvassed. Dysfunction of T cells in the vicinity of melanoma tumours is well documented and is most likely the result of soluble factors from melanoma that inhibit their function. Many of the factors involved appear to be regulated by the transcription factor NF-κB and more research is needed to identify agents that can be used clinically to target NF-κB-regulated cytokines and chemokines that inhibit T cell responses against the tumour. Much work is needed in the next few years to explore the effectiveness of combinations with MAbs against CTLA4 and PD1 that target the adverse microenvironment of tumours.

Conflicts of Interest
No potential conflicts of interest are disclosed.

References

1. Hodi FS, O'Day SJ, McDermott DF, Weber RW, Sosman JA, Haanen JB, Gonzalez R, Robert C, Schadekndorf D, Hassel JC, Akerley W, van den Eertwegh AJM, Lutzky J, Lorigan P, Vaubel JM, Linette GP, Hogg D, Ottensmeier CH, Lebbé C, Peschel C, Quirt I, Clark JI, Wolchok JD, Weber JS, Tian J, Yellin MJ, Nichol GM, Hoos A, Urba WJ. Improved survival with ipilimumab in patients with metastatic melanoma. N Engl J Med. 2010;363:711–23.
2. Robert C, Thomas L, Bondarenko I, O'Day S, Webe J, Garbe C, Lebbe C, Baurain JF, Testori A, Grob JJ, Davidson N, Richards J, Maio M, Hauschild A, Miller WH Jr, Gascon P, Lotem M, Harmankaya K, Ibrahim R, Francis S, Chen TT, Humphrey R, Hoos A, Wolchok JD. Ipilimumab plus dacarbazine for previously untreated metastatic melanoma. N Engl J Med. 2011;364:2517–26.
3. Topalian SL, Hodi FS, Brahmer JR, Gettinger SN, Smith DC, McDermott DF, Powderly JD, Carvajal RD, Sosman JA, Atkins MB, Leming PD, Spigel DR, Antonia SJ, Horn L, Drake CG, Pardoll DM, Chen L, Sharfman WH, Anders RA, Taube JM, McMiller TL, Xu H, Korman AJ, Jure-Kunkel M, Agrawal S, McDonald D, Kollia GD, Gupta A, Wigginton JM, Sznol M. Safety, activity, and immune correlates of anti–PD-1 antibody in cancer. N Engl J Med. 2012;366:2443–54.

4. Yuan ZR, Wang R, Solomon J, Luo X, Sun H, Zhang L, Shi Y. Identification and characterization of survival-related gene, a novel cell survival gene controlling apoptosis and tumourigenesis. Cancer Res. 2005;65:10716–24.
5. Carthon BC, Wolchok JD, Yuan J, Kamat A, Ng TDS, Sun J, Ku G, Troncoso P, Logothetis CJ, Allison JP, Sharma P. Preoperative CTLA-4 blockade: tolerability and immune monitoring in the setting of a presurgical clinical trial. Clin Cancer Res. 2010;16:2861–71.
6. Postow MA, Callahan MK, Barker CA, Yamada Y, Yuan J, Kitano S, Mu Z, Rasalan T, Adamow M, Ritter E, Sedrak C, Jungbluth AA, Chua R, Yang AS, Roman RA, Rosner S, Benson B, Allison JP, Lesokhin AM, Gnjatic S, Wolchok JD. Immunologic correlates of the abscopal effect in a patient with melanoma. N Engl J Med. 2012;366:925–31.
7. Filipazzi P, Valenti R, Huber V, Pilla L, Canese P, Iero M, Castelli C, Mariani L, Parmiani G, Rivoltini L. Identification of a new subset of myeloid suppressor cells in peripheral blood of melanoma patients with modulation by a granulocyte-macrophage colony-stimulation factor-based antitumour vaccine. J Clin Oncol. 2007;25:2546–53.
8. Ku GY, Yuan J, Page DB, Schroeder SE, Panageas KS, Carvajal RD, Chapman PB, Schwartz GK, Allison JP, Wolchok JD. Single-institution experience with ipilimumab in advanced melanoma patients in the compassionate use setting: lymphocyte count after 2 doses correlates with survival. Cancer. 2010;116:1767–75.
9. Maker AV, Phan GQ, Attia P, Yang JC, Sherry RM, Topalian SL, Kammula US, Royal RE, Haworth LR, Levy C, Kleiner D, Mavroukakis SA, Yellin M, Rosenberg SA. Tumour regression and autoimmunity in patients treated with cytotoxic T lymphocyte-associated antigen 4 blockade and interleukin 2: a phase I/II study. Ann Surg Oncol. 2005;12:1005–16.
10. Ribas A, Comin-Anduix B, Economou JS, Donahue TR, de la Rocha P, Morris LF, Jalil J, Dissette VB, Shintaku IP, Glaspy JA, Gomez-Navarro J, Cochran AJ. Intratumoural immune cell infiltrates, FoxP3, and indoleamine 2,3-dioxygenase in patients with melanoma undergoing CTLA4 blockade. Clin Cancer Res. 2009;15:390–9.
11. Huang RR, Jalil J, Economou JS, Chmielowski B, Koya RC, Mok S, Sazegar H, Seja E, Villanueva A, Gomez-Navarro J, Glaspy JA, Cochran AJ, Ribas A. CTLA4 blockade induces frequent tumour infiltration by activated lymphocytes regardless of clinical responses in humans. Clin Cancer Res. 2011;17:4101–9.
12. Wang W, Yu D, Sarnaik AA, Yu B, Hall M, Morelli D, Zhang Y, Zhao X, Weber JS. Biomarkers on melanoma patient T Cells associated with ipilimumab treatment. J Transl Med. 2012;10:146.
13. Singh S, Ross SR, Acena M, Rowley DA, Schreiber H. Stroma is critical for preventing or permitting immunological destruction of antigenic cancer cells. J Exp Med. 1992; 175:139–46.
14. Gajewski TF, Fuertes M, Spaapen R, Zheng Y, Kline J. Molecular profiling to identify relevant immune resistance mechanisms in the tumour microenvironment. Curr Opin Immunol. 2011;23:286–92.
15. Harlin H, Meng Y, Peterson AC, Zha Y, Tretiakova M, Slingluff C, McKee M, Gajewski TF. Chemokine expression in melanoma metastases associated with CD8+ T-cell recruitment. Cancer Res. 2009;69:3077–85.
16. Tang D, Billiar TA, Lotze MT. A Janus tale of two active HMGB1 redox states. Mol Med. 2012;12:00314.
17. Goto Y, Arigami T, Kitago M, Nguyen SL, Narita N, Ferrone S, Morton DL, Irie RF, Hoon DS. Activation of Toll-like receptors 2, 3, and 4 on human melanoma cells induces inflammatory factors. Mol Cancer Ther. 2008;7:3642–53.
18. Vergani E, Vallacchi V, Frigerio S, Deho P, Mondellini P, Perego P, Cassinelli G, Lanzi C, Testi MA, Rivoltini L, Bongarzone I, Rodolfo M. Identification of MET and SRC activation in melanoma cell lines showing primary resistance to PLX4032. Neoplasia. 2011;13:1132–42.
19. Azimi F, Scolyer RA, Rumcheva P, Moncrieff M, Murali R, McCarthy SW, Saw RP, Thompson JF. Tumour-infiltrating lymphocyte grade is an independent predictor of sentinel

lymph node status and survival in patients with cutaneous melanoma. J Clin Oncol. 2012;30:2678–83.
20. Piali L, Fichtel A, Terpe HJ, Imhof BA, Gisler RH. Endothelial vascular cell adhesion molecule 1 expression is suppressed by melanoma and carcinoma. J Exp Med. 1995;181:811–6.
21. Delfortrie S, Pinte S, Mattot V, Samson C, Villain G, Caetano B, Lauridant-Philippin G, Baranzelli MC, Bonneterre J, Trottein F, Faveeuw C, Soncin F. Egfl7 promotes tumour escape from immunity by repressing endothelial cell activation. Cancer Res. 2011;71:7176–86.
22. Buckanovich RJ, Facciabene A, Kim S, Benencia F, Sasaroli D, Balint K, Katsaros D, O'Brien-Jenkins A, Gimotty PA, Coukos G. Endothelin B receptor mediates the endothelial barrier to T cell homing to tumours and disables immune therapy. Nat Med. 2008;14:28–36.
23. Kandalaft LE, Facciabene A, Buckanovich RJ, Coukos G. Endothelin B receptor, a new target in cancer immune therapy. Clin Cancer Res. 2009;15:4521–8.
24. Mangahas CR, dela Cruz GV, Friedman-Jimenez G, Jamal S. Endothelin-1 induces CXCL1 and CXCL8 secretion in human melanoma cells. J Invest Dermatol. 2005;125:307–11.
25. Spinella F, Caprara V, Di Castro V, Rosano L, Cianfrocca R, Natali PG, Bagnato A. Endothelin-1 induces the transactivation of vascular endothelial growth factor receptor-3 and modulates cell migration and vasculogenic mimicry in melanoma cells. J Mol Med. 2012;11:1–11.
26. Richmond A, Yang J, Su Y. The good and the bad of chemokines/chemokine receptors in melanoma. Pigment Cell Melanoma Res. 2009;22:175–86.
27. Kershaw MH, Wang G, Westwood JA, Pachynski RK, Tiffany HL, Marincola FM, Wang E, Young HA, Murphy PM, Hwu P. Redirecting migration of T cells to chemokine secreted from tumours by genetic modification with CXCR2. Hum Gene Ther. 2002;13:1971–80.
28. Chew V, Toh HC, Abastado JP. Immune microenvironment in tumour progression: characteristics and challenges for therapy. J Oncol. 2012;608406:8.
29. Fulton AM. The chemokine receptors CXCR4 and CXCR3 in cancer. Curr Oncol Rep. 2009;11:125–31.
30. Muthuswamy R, Berk E, Junecko BF, Zeh HJ, Zureikat AH, Normolle D, Luong TM, Reinhart TA, Bartlett DL, Kalinski P. NF-κB hyperactivation in tumour tissues allows tumour-selective reprogramming of the chemokine microenvironment to enhance the recruitment of cytolytic T effector cells. Cancer Res. 2012;72:3735–43.
31. Lesokhin AM, Hohl TM, Kitano S, Cortez C, Hirschhorn-Cymerman D, Avogadri F, Rizzuto GA, Lazarus JJ, Pamer EG, Houghton AN, Merghoub T, Wolchok JD. Monocytic CCR2(+) myeloid-derived suppressor cells promote immune escape by limiting activated CD8 T-cell infiltration into the tumour microenvironment. Cancer Res. 2012;72:876–86.
32. Hellebrekers DM, Castermans K, Vire E, Dings RP, Hoebers NT, Mayo KH, Oude EMG, Molema G, Fuks F, van Engeland M, Griffioen AW. Epigenetic regulation of tumour endothelial cell anergy: silencing of intercellular adhesion molecule-1 by histone modifications. Cancer Res. 2006;66:10770–7.
33. Kefford RF, Clingan PR, Brady B, Ballmer A, Morganti A, Hersey P. A randomized, double-blind, placebo-controlled study of high-dose bosentan in patients with stage IV metastatic melanoma receiving first-line dacarbazine chemotherapy. Mol Cancer. 2010;9:69–80.
34. Asundi J, Reed C, Arca J, McCutcheon K, Ferrando R, Clark S, Luis E, Tien J, Firestein R, Polakis P. An antibody-drug conjugate targeting the endothelin B receptor for the treatment of melanoma. Clin Cancer Res. 2011;17:965–75.
35. Hong DS, Vence L, Falchook G, Radvanyi LG, Liu C, Goodman V, Legos JJ, Blackman S, Scarmadio A, Kurzrock R, Lizee G, Hwu P. BRAF(V600) inhibitor GSK2118436 targeted inhibition of mutant BRAF in cancer patients does not impair overall immune competency. Clin Cancer Res. 2012;18:2326–35.
36. Boni A, Cogdill AP, Dang P, Udayakumar D, Njauw CN, Sloss CM, Ferrone CR, Flaherty KT, Lawrence DP, Fisher DE, Tsao H, Wargo JA. Selective BRAFV600E inhibition

enhances T-cell recognition of melanoma without affecting lymphocyte function. Cancer Res. 2010;70:5213–9.
37. Wilmott JS, Long GV, Howle JR, Haydu LE, Sharma R, Thompson JF, Kefford RF, Hersey P, Scolyer RA. Selective BRAF inhibitors induce marked T cell infiltration into human metastatic melanoma. Clin Cancer Res. 2012;18:1386–94.
38. Hooijkaas A, Gadiot J, Morrow M, Stewart R, Schumacher T, Blank CU. Selective BRAF inhibition decreases tumour-resident lymphocyte frequencies in a mouse model of human melanoma. Oncoimmunology. 2012;1:609–17.
39. Khalili JS, Liu S, Rodriguez-Cruz TG, Whittington M, Wardell S, Liu C, Zhang M, Cooper ZA, Frederick DT, Li Y, Joseph RW, Bernatchez C, Ekmekcioglu S, Grimm E, Radvanyi LG, Davis RE, Davies MA, Wargo JA, Hwu P, Lizee G. Oncogenic BRAF(V600E) promotes stromal cell-mediated immunosuppression via induction of interleukin-1 in melanoma. Clin Cancer Res. 2012;18:5329–40.
40. Wilson TR, Fridlyand J, Yan Y, Penuel E, Burton L, Chan E, Peng J, Lin E, Wang Y, Sosman J, Ribas A, Li J, Moffat J, Sutherlin DP, Koeppen H, Merchant M, Neve R, Settleman J. Widespread potential for growth-factor-driven resistance to anticancer kinase inhibitors. Nature. 2012;487:505–9.
41. Straussman R, Morikawa T, Shee K, Barzily-Rokni M, Qian ZR, Du J, Davis A, Mongare MM, Gould J, Frederick DT, Cooper ZA, Chapman PB, Solit DB, Ribas A, Lo RS, Flaherty KT, Ogino S, Wargo JA, Golub TR. Tumour micro-environment elicits innate resistance to RAF inhibitors through HGF secretion. Nature. 2012;487:500–4.
42. Gallagher PG, Bao Y, Prorock A, Zigrino P, Nischt R, Politi V, Mauch C, Dragulev B, Fox JW. Gene expression profiling reveals cross-talk between melanoma and fibroblasts: implications for host-tumour interactions in metastasis. Cancer Res. 2005;65:4134–46.
43. Fourcade J, Sun Z, Pagliano O, Guillaume P, Luescher IF, Sander C, Kirkwood JM, Olive D, Kuchroo V, Zarour HM. CD8(+) T cells specific for tumour antigens can be rendered dysfunctional by the tumour microenvironment through upregulation of the inhibitory receptors BTLA and PD-1. Cancer Res. 2012;72:887–96.
44. Nagaraj S, Nelson A, Youn JI, Cheng P, Quiceno D, Gabrilovich DI. Antigen-specific CD4(+) T cells regulate function of myeloid-derived suppressor cells in cancer via retrograde MHC class II signaling. Cancer Res. 2012;72:928–38.
45. Filipazzi P, Huber V, Rivoltini L. Phenotype, function and clinical implications of myeloid-derived suppressor cells in cancer patients. Cancer Immunol Immunother. 2012;61:255–63.
46. Allavena P, Mantovani A. Immunology in the clinic review series; focus on cancer: tumour-associated macrophages: undisputed stars of the inflammatory tumour microenvironment. Clin Exp Immunol. 2012;167:195–205.
47. Richmond A, Nf-κB. Chemokine gene transcription and tumour growth. Nat Rev Immunol. 2002;2:664–74.
48. Ueda Y, Richmond A. NF-κB activation in melanoma. Pigment Cell Res. 2006;19:112–24.
49. Liu J, Suresh KKG, Yu D, Molton SA, McMahon M, Herlyn M, Thomas-Tikhonenko A, Fuchs SY. Oncogenic BRAF regulates beta-Trcp expression and NF-κB activity in human melanoma cells. Oncogene. 2007;26:1954–8.
50. Becker TM, Rizos H, de la Pena A, Leclercq IA, Woodruff S, Kefford RF, Mann GJ. Impaired inhibition of NF-κB activity by melanoma-associated p16INK4a mutations. Biochem Biophys Res Commun. 2005;332:873–9.
51. Thu YM, Su Y, Yang J, Splittgerber R, Na S, Boyd A, Mosse C, Simons C, Richmond A. NF-κB inducing kinase (NIK) modulates melanoma tumourigenesis by regulating expression of pro-survival factors through the β-catenin pathway. Oncogene. 2012;31:2580–92.
52. Yang J, Kantrow S, Sai J, Hawkins OE, Boothby M, Ayers GD, Young ED, Demicco EG, Lazar AJ, Lev D, Richmond A. Ikk4a/Arf inactivation with activation of the NF-κB/IL-6 pathway is sufficient to drive the development and growth of angiosarcoma. Cancer Res. 2012;72:4682–95.
53. Zhuang L, Lee CS, Scolyer RA, McCarthy SW, Zhang XD, Thompson JF, Hersey P. Mcl-1, Bcl-XL and Stat3 expression are associated with progression of melanoma whereas Bcl-2,

AP-2 and MITF levels decrease during progression of melanoma. Mod Pathol. 2007;20:416–26.
54. Hoejberg L, Bastholt L, Schmidt H. Interleukin-6 and melanoma. Melanoma Res. 2012;22:327–33.
55. Madonna G, Ullman CD, Gentilcore G, Palmieri G, Ascierto PA. NF-κB as potential target in the treatment of melanoma. J Transl Med. 2012;10:53–61.
56. Yang J, Amiri KI, Burke JR, Schmid JA, Richmond A. BMS-345541 targets inhibitor of κB kinase and induces apoptosis in melanoma: involvement of nuclear factor κB and mitochondria pathways. Clin Cancer Res. 2006;12:950–60.
57. Benucci M, Saviola G, Manfredi M, Sarzi-Puttini P, Atzeni F. Tumour necrosis factors blocking agents: analogies and differences. Acta Biomed. 2012;83:72–80.
58. Deal Watch. BMS acquires rights for IL-6 inhibitor. Nat Rev Drug Discov. 2010;9:10.
59. Vaddi K, Luchi M. JAK inhibition for the treatment of rheumatoid arthritis: a new era in oral DMARD therapy. Expert Opin Investig Drugs. 2012;21:961–73.
60. Braun J, Sieper J. Overview of the use of the anti-TNF agent infliximab in chronic inflammatory diseases. Expert Opin Biol Ther. 2003;3:141–68.
61. Ostermeier E, Roll P, Tony HP. Janus kinase inhibitors. Z Rheumatol. 2012;71:473–8.
62. Nicodeme E, Jeffrey KL, Schaefer U, Beinke S, Dewell S, Chung CW, Chandwani R, Marazzi I, Wilson P, Coste H, White J, Kirilovsky J, Rice CM, Lora JM, Prinjha RK, Lee K, Tarakhovsky A. Suppression of inflammation by a synthetic histone mimic. Nature. 2010;468:1119–23.
63. Seal J, Lamotte Y, Donche F, Bouillot A, Mirguet O, Gellibert F, Nicodeme E, Krysa G, Kirilovsky J, Beinke S, McCleary S, Rioja I, Bamborough P, Chung CW, Gordon L, Lewis T, Walker AL, Cutler L, Lugo D, Wilson DM, Witherington J, Lee K, Prinjha RK. Identification of a novel series of BET family bromodomain inhibitors: binding mode and profile of I-BET151 (GSK1210151A). Bioorg Med Chem Lett. 2012;22:2968–72.
64. Martinez FI, Okada H, Topalian SL, Gajewski TF, Korman AJ, Melero I. Workshop on immunotherapy combinations. Society for immunotherapy of cancer annual meeting Bethesda. J Transl Med. 2012;10:108.

Strategies to Overcome TRAIL Resistance in Cancer

Simone Fulda

Abstract For decades the therapeutic induction of cell death in cancer cells represents one of the key goals of cancer therapies. However, since cancer cells have developed multiple mechanisms to resist cell death induction, we are still far from reaching this aim. In principle, the TRAIL receptor/ligand system represents a promising approach to selectively initiate cell death pathways in cancer cells and is amendable for therapeutic targeting. Therefore, further insights into the molecular mechanisms that regulate TRAIL signal transduction and the events that control sensitivity and resistance of human cancers towards TRAIL-mediated cell death are critical to exploit this approach for the treatment of human cancers.

Keywords Apoptosis · Cancer · Cell death · Resistance · TRAIL

Abbreviations

5-FU	5-fluorouracil
AML	Acute myeloid leukemia
APAF	Apoptotic protease activating factor
cFLIP	FLICE-like inhibitory protein
DISC	Death-inducing signaling complex
FADD	Fas-associated death domain
IAP	Inhibitor of apoptosis
MAPK	Mitogen-activated protein kinase
TNF	Tumor necrosis factor
LOH	Loss of heterozygosity
NF-κB	Nuclear factor kappa-B
TNFR	TNF receptor

S. Fulda (✉)
Institute for Experimental Cancer Research in Pediatrics, Goethe-University,
Komturstr. 3a 60528 Frankfurt, Germany
e-mail: simone.fulda@kgu.de

B. Bonavida (ed.), *Resistance to Immunotherapeutic Antibodies in Cancer*,
Resistance to Targeted Anti-Cancer Therapeutics 2, DOI: 10.1007/978-1-4614-7654-2_8,

TRAIL Tumor-necrosis-factor-related apoptosis-inducing ligand
XIAP X-linked inhibitor of apoptosis protein

Introduction

One common aim of all cancer therapies is to efficiently and specifically trigger cell death in cancer cells, while exerting no or little effects on non-malignant cells. Since programmed cell death is an endogenous program that is in place in every cell of our body [1], the concept to activate this cell-intrinsic program of cell death is very attractive in order to elicit cancer cell death [2]. One strategy to trigger programmed cell death in cancer cells is the use of ligands that bind to death receptors on the cell surface [2]. Similar to natural ligands, fully humanized monoclonal antibodies directed against death receptors have been shown to initiate cell death pathways in cancer cells [3]. While the strategy to engage endogenous cell death programs in cancer cells using e.g. death receptor ligands or agonistic antibodies directed against death receptors appears very attractive for cancer therapy, one of the key challenges nowadays in oncology resides in the fact that many cancers have evolved resistance to undergo programmed cell death [4]. Therefore, the elucidation of the underlying molecular mechanisms that are responsible for cancer cell resistance to undergo programmed cell death will be critical to ensure the success of cell death-targeting strategies. This review will focus on the opportunities to target the TRAIL receptor system for cancer therapy and the key mechanisms associated with cancer cell resistance to TRAIL.

The TRAIL Receptor/Ligand System

The TRAIL receptor/ligand system belongs to the family of death receptors, which are part of the superfamily of tumor necrosis factor (TNF) receptors [5]. The TNF receptor superfamily comprises more than 20 members with a broad range of biological activities [6]. Classification as death receptor requires the existence of a death domain, a stretch of about 80 amino acids that serves as a protein–protein interaction platform and is critical to transduce the death-inducing signaling from the surface to signal transduction cascades within the cell [5]. Death receptors reside within the outer plasma membrane and contain an extracellular stretch that mediates the binding of the receptor to its cognate ligand. The TRAIL receptor/ligand system is one of the prominent death receptor systems apart from CD95/APO-1/Fas and TNF receptor 1 (TNFR1) [6]. The TRAIL receptor system is composed of both agonistic receptors such as TRAIL receptor 1 and 2 (TRAIL-R1 and TRAIL-R2) and antagonistic TRAIL receptors (TRAIL-R3 to -R5) [6]. The later receptors can bind the endogenous ligand, but are incapable to signal. Since the endogenous ligand TRAIL can bind to all these TRAIL receptors, signaling outcome is at least in part controlled by the relative expression levels of TRAIL receptors on the cell surface. It is interesting to note that many cancer cells have been reported to express the agonistic TRAIL receptors, whereas many normal cells were described to harbor relatively low expression levels of agonistic TRAIL receptors, while predominantly expressing the antagonistic TRAIL receptors [6]. While this differential expression of agonistic versus antagonistic TRAIL receptors has initially been viewed as a possible explanation for the differential sensitivity of tumor versus normal cells towards TRAIL, subsequent studies have shown that expression levels of TRAIL receptors do not fully account for the differential sensitivity of cancer versus normal cells towards TRAIL [7].

TRAIL Signaling Pathway

The TRAIL signal transduction pathway is organized according to the death receptor-mediated pathway of apoptosis (extrinsic pathway) [6]. Upon binding of TRAIL to its cognate agonistic TRAIL receptors, i.e., TRAIL-R1 or -R2, TRAIL receptors homotrimerize and initiate the recruitment of the adaptor protein in Fas-associated death domain (FADD) and the proenzyme form of the initiator caspase caspase-8 to the death domain of the TRAIL receptors [8]. This recruitment leads to the formation of the so-called death-inducing signaling complex (DISC), a multimeric platform that facilitates the dimerization and cleavage of caspase-8 [6]. Upon its cleavage, caspase-8 can proteolytically process downstream substrates including the effector caspase-3, thereby initiating activation of the caspase cascade. In addition, once activated, caspase-8 can cleave the proapoptotic Bcl-2 family protein Bid into tBid, which in turn translocates to mitochondrial membranes to trigger the release of cytochrome c and to perturb mitochondrial functions. Upon translocation of tBid to mitochondrial membranes, tBid interacts with proapoptotic Bcl-2 family proteins such as Bax and Bak, leading to a conformational change in Bax and Bak, their activation and subsequently permeabilization of the outer mitochondrial membrane [9]. As a consequence, proapoptotic proteins that reside within the intermembrane space of mitochondria, such as cytochrome c and Smac, are released from the mitochondrial outer membrane space into the cytosol [10]. Cytochrome c promotes the formation of the apoptosome complex comprising, besides cytochrome c, procaspase-9 and APAF-1, which in turn results in caspase-9 activation and apoptosis. The release of Smac into the cytosol allows Smac to antagonize Inhibitor of Apoptosis (IAP) proteins, for example XIAP [10]. This, in turn, displaces XIAP from inhibiting caspase-3 and caspase-9, thereby promoting caspase activation and apoptosis. In addition to these two key apoptosis signaling cascades, there are multiple amplification and feedback mechanisms. For example, activated caspase-3 can act back on mitochondria by cleaving components of the respiratory chain, thereby causing mitochondrial dysfunction [11]. In addition, activated caspase-3 can cleave caspase-8 via caspase-6 [12], thereby initiating a feedback amplification loop of caspase activation.

Beyond the induction of apoptosis signaling pathways, the TRAIL receptor ligand system can also engage additional signaling pathways that have been implicated in the regulation of cell survival [13]. For example, TRAIL can signal to activate the transcription factor nuclear factor kappa-B (NF-κB), as well as kinase signaling pathways including the Akt/protein kinase B and mitogen-activated protein kinase (MAPK) [13]. This implies that TRAIL can in principle signal both to cell death and to survival. Therefore, inactivation of cell death pathways can unleash the pro-survival function of TRAIL, resulting in TRAIL-mediated stimulation of proliferation and survival. In view of this involvement of TRAIL and its receptors in cell survival signaling cascades, it is not surprising that TRAIL has been implicated to foster proliferation, migration, invasion and metastasis in cancers that are resistant to TRAIL-induced cell death, for example in acute lymphoblastic leukemia [14]. Here, resistance to TRAIL was associated with TRAIL-stimulated proliferation in a NF-κB-dependent fashion [14]. In pancreatic carcinoma, the failure to undergo apoptosis upon treatment with TRAIL resulted in a shift towards TRAIL-mediated metastasis in an in vivo model [15]. These studies highlight the relevance of TRAIL-mediated cell survival pathways that can paradoxically mediate increased tumor growth upon the administration of TRAIL in cancers that resist TRAIL-induced cell death.

Mechanisms of TRAIL Resistance

A variety of different mechanisms have been identified that can mediate the resistance of cancer cells towards TRAIL. On theoretical grounds, the TRAIL signal transduction pathway can be blocked at different levels, for example at the level of TRAIL receptors, at the level of the TRAIL-inducing signaling complex or intracellularly at several distinct points. There are both primary mechanisms as well as secondary (acquired) events that can confer resistance to TRAIL-induced cell death.

TRAIL Receptors

Evasion of cancer cells to TRAIL-induced cell death can be caused by absent or reduced expression levels of agonistic TRAIL receptors at the cell surface. Both TRAIL-R1 and TRAIL-R2 localize to chromosome 8p, a region in the human genome that is frequently affected by genetic alterations, including loss of heterozygosity (LOH) [3]. In addition, mutations or deletions in TRAIL-R1 or -R2 receptors have been described in several different cancers, including osteosarcoma, non-Hodgkin's lymphoma, colorectal cancer, breast cancer, lung cancer and head and neck carcinoma [16, 17]. Besides genetic alterations, also epigenetic events, such as hypermethylation of gene promoters, can contribute to downregulation of agonistic TRAIL receptors in human cancers, for example in glioblastoma or ovarian cancer [18, 19]. Another mechanism accounting for reduced TRAIL receptor expression on the cell surface is the aberrant storage of TRAIL receptor in intracellular compartments and their defective transport to the plasma membrane. For example, TRAIL-R1 and TRAIL-R2 were found to be retained in the endoplasmic reticulum in colon carcinoma cells, resulting in defective TRAIL receptor signaling [20]. Furthermore, aberrant expression levels of TRAIL decoy receptors may interfere with TRAIL signal transduction. Since TRAIL decoy receptors such as TRAIL-R3 and TRAIL-R4 can form heterodimers with the agonistic TRAIL receptors TRAIL-R1 and TRAIL-R2, these heterodimers composed of both antagonistic and agonistic TRAIL receptors hamper effective TRAIL receptor signaling and confer resistance to TRAIL-induced apoptosis. In the case of TRAIL-R3 blockade of TRAIL signal transduction, this has been attributed to sequestration of TRAIL within lipid rafts, thereby resulting in inhibition of the formation of the TRAIL DISC [21]. By comparison, the TRAIL-R4 decoy receptor has been described to inhibit TRAIL-induced apoptosis at the level of the TRAIL DISC by blocking caspase-8 activation [21]. TRAIL-R3 expression has been described in different cancer entities, including acute myeloid leukemia (AML), colorectal carcinoma and breast carcinoma [22–25]. High expression levels of TRAIL-R3 were associated with poor prognosis, for example in AML and colorectal carcinoma [23, 24]. It is important to note that also the decoy receptors *TRAIL-R3* and *TRAIL-R4* are p53 target genes, in addition to the agonistic TRAIL receptors. This implies that treatment with DNA-damaging agents, including chemotherapeutic drugs or radio therapy, can transcriptionally upregulate TRAIL-R3 or -4 expression levels [22, 25, 26]. Furthermore, TRAIL-mediated activation of Akt has been linked to signaling via TRAIL-R4, leading to increased tumor growth and evasion of apoptosis in response to TRAIL receptor stimulation [27].

Furthermore, sensitivity of human cancers to TRAIL-induced cell death is modulated by O-glycosylation. In fact, the expression levels of O-glycosylation enzymes such as GALNT14 and fucosyltransferase-3/-6 were found to correlate with the sensitivity of cancer cells to TRAIL-induced cell death [28]. This association was also identified in primary human tumor tissues, indicating that this parameter might serve as a diagnostic option in order to identify cancers that are sensitive towards TRAIL-based therapies.

Aberrant Expression of Antiapoptotic Proteins Containing the Death Domain

In addition to death receptors, there are also several antiapoptotic proteins that contain the death domain motif, including cellular FLICE-like inhibitory protein (cFLIP) and phosphoprotein enriched in diabetes/phospoprotein enriched in astrocytes-15 kDa (PED/PEA-15) [29, 30]. Due to the presence of the death domain, cFLIP and PED/PEA-15 are recruited to the TRAIL DISC upon ligation of TRAIL receptors, where they inhibit the recruitment of caspase-8 to activated TRAIL-R1 or -R2. This results in reduced caspase-8 activation and inhibition of TRAIL-induced apoptosis. cFLIP is an antiapoptotic protein that is highly expressed in a large variety of human cancers and has been implicated in conferring resistance to both receptor- as well as chemotherapy-mediated cell death [31–33]. In pancreatic adenocarcinoma, differential expression of cFLIP in tumor versus non-malignant cells was recently reported in primary tumor specimens [32]. While cFLIP was expressed at high levels in pancreatic tumor tissue, normal pancreatic ducts showed low expression levels of cFLIP [32]. cFLIP can exist in distinct isoforms, including the long and short isoform [34]. While the long isoform of cFLIP shares high-sequence homology with caspase-8 with the exception of some critical amino acids that are substituted in $cFLIP_L$ resulting in its lack of proteolytic activity, the short isoform of cFLIP is completely devoid of the caspase homology domain and contains only the two death effector domains [34]. It is interesting to note that cFLIP has been implicated both in suppressing as well as promoting cell death, depending on the cellular context. In pancreatic cancer, downregulation of cFLIP either by genetic knockdown or exposure to some anticancer drug such as 5-fluorouracil (5-FU) resulted in enhancement of TRAIL-mediated cell death, demonstrating that both isoforms of cFLIP confer resistance to TRAIL-induced apoptosis in pancreatic cancer [32].

Regulation of Caspase-8

Alterations in caspase-8 represent another mechanism that can confer resistance to TRAIL-induced cell death. Caspase-8 is a key signaling molecule in the TRAIL pathway that plays a pivotal role in transmitting the death signal from TRAIL receptors to intracellular signaling networks. While mutations in caspase-8 have not frequently been encountered in human cancers, the *caspase-8* gene is often inactivated by epigenetic silencing [35]. Hypermethylation of a regulatory region of the *caspase-8* gene has been correlated with absent or reduced expression levels of caspase-8 in different human cancers [10, 36–40]. For example, epigenetic silencing of caspase-8 resulting in low or absent caspase-8 protein expression was found in the vast majority of neuroblastoma primary specimens as well as in neuroblastoma cell lines [40, 41]. It is interesting to note that loss of caspase-8 expression did not correlate with parameters of advanced stage of the disease, including amplification of the oncogene *MycN*, 1p36 aberrations or clinical factors of poor prognosis such as disease stage, age at diagnosis or histology [40]. While absent caspase-8 expression did not correlate with event-free or overall survival rates of neuroblastoma patients in one study [40], another study reported an association of caspase-8 hypermethylation and the risk to relapse in neuroblastoma [42]. These findings indicate that additional factors might be involved in conferring an adverse prognosis in neuroblastoma patients lacking caspase-8 expression. As far as medulloblastoma is concerned, a correlation between lack of caspase-8 expression and adverse prognosis was described [43].

In addition to wild-type caspase-8, a dominant-negative version of caspase-8, i.e., caspase-8L, was identified both in malignant as well as non-malignant cells, for example, in CD34-positive hematopoietic progenitor cells as well as in leukemia and neuroblastoma [44–47]. Mechanistically, caspase-8L acts in a dominant-negative manner by interfering with the binding of caspase-8 to activated death receptors within the death-inducing signaling complex (DISC), since caspase-8L is recruited in a similar manner as wild-type caspase-8 to activated death receptors [47].

Besides these aberrations in expression or structure of caspase-8, the function of caspase-8 can also be modified by posttranslational modifications. For example, phosphorylation of caspase-8 can interfere with its enzymatic activity. To this end, the tyrosine kinase Src was shown to phosphorylate caspase-8 on residue tyrosine 308 which lies within the linker loop of caspase-8 [48]. This phosphorylation step, in turn, results in reduced enzymatic activity of caspase-8 [48]. Integrin- as well as growth factor ligand-mediated activation of Src have been implied to mediate elevated phosphorylation of caspase-8 at this residue in human cancers [48, 49]. As a consequence, the phosphorylated form of caspase-8 is not only impaired in its apoptotic activity but also harbors an increased ability to migrate, indicating that this phosphorylation event affects both apoptotic as well as non-apoptotic functions of caspase-8.

Conclusions

The TRAIL receptor/ligand system represents an attractive therapeutic target in human cancers, as it is differentially dysregulated in cancer versus non-malignant cells which may open important perspectives for tumor-selective induction of cell death. However, since TRAIL-mediated signal transduction is frequently impaired at different levels of the signaling cascade in human cancers, it will be critical to identify the key mechanisms that confer resistance towards TRAIL receptor agonists in human cancers. A better knowledge of the molecular mechanisms that are involved in the regulation of sensitivity versus resistance towards TRAIL will lay the ground for the successful application of TRAIL receptor reagents for the treatment of human cancers.

Acknowledgments The expert secretarial assistance of C Hugenberg is greatly appreciated. This work has been partially supported by grants from the Deutsche Forschungsgemeinschaft, the Ministerium für Bildung und Forschung (01GM1104C), European Community and IAP VII P7/32.

Conflicts of Interest

No potential conflicts of interest were disclosed.

References

1. Lockshin RA, Zakeri Z. Cell death in health and disease. J Cell Mol Med. 2007;11:1214–24.
2. Fulda S, Debatin KM. Extrinsic versus intrinsic apoptosis pathways in anticancer chemotherapy. Oncogene. 2006;25:4798–811.
3. Ashkenazi A. Directing cancer cells to self-destruct with pro-apoptotic receptor agonists. Nat Rev Drug Discov. 2008;7:1001–12.
4. Fulda S. Tumor resistance to apoptosis. Int J Cancer. 2009;124:511–15.
5. Gerspach J, Wajant H, Pfizenmaier K. Death ligands designed to kill: development and application of targeted cancer therapeutics based on proapoptotic TNF family ligands. Results Probl Cell Differ. 2009;49:241–73.
6. Ashkenazi A. Targeting the extrinsic apoptosis pathway in cancer. Cytokine Growth Factor Rev. 2008;19:325–31.
7. Pennarun B, Meijer A, de Vries EG, Kleibeuker JH, Kruyt F, de Jong S. Playing the DISC: turning on TRAIL death receptor-mediated apoptosis in cancer. Biochim Biophys Acta. 2010;1805:123–40.
8. Holland PM. Targeting Apo2L/TRAIL receptors by soluble Apo2L/TRAIL. Cancer Lett. 2013;332:156–162.
9. Adams JM, Cory S. The Bcl-2 apoptotic switch in cancer development and therapy. Oncogene. 2007;26:1324–37.
10. Fulda S, Vucic D. Targeting IAP proteins for therapeutic intervention in cancer. Nat Rev Drug Discov. 2012;11:109–24.
11. Ricci JE, Munoz-Pinedo C, Fitzgerald P, Bailly-Maitre B, Perkins GA, Yadava N, Scheffler IE, Ellisman MH, Green DR. Disruption of mitochondrial function during apoptosis is mediated by caspase cleavage of the p75 subunit of complex I of the electron transport chain. Cell. 2004;117:773–86.
12. Cowling V, Downward J. Caspase-6 is the direct activator of caspase-8 in the cytochrome c-induced apoptosis pathway: absolute requirement for removal of caspase-6 prodomain. Cell Death Differ. 2002;9:1046–56.
13. Falschlehner C, Emmerich CH, Gerlach B, Walczak H. TRAIL signalling: decisions between life and death. Int J Biochem Cell Biol. 2007;39:1462–75.
14. Ehrhardt H, Fulda S, Schmid I, Hiscott J, Debatin KM, Jeremias I. TRAIL induced survival and proliferation in cancer cells resistant towards TRAIL-induced apoptosis mediated by NF-kappaB. Oncogene. 2003;22:3842–52.
15. Trauzold A, Siegmund D, Schniewind B, Sipos B, Egberts J, Zorenkov D, Emme D, Roder C, Kalthoff H, Wajant H. TRAIL promotes metastasis of human pancreatic ductal adenocarcinoma. Oncogene. 2006;25:7434–39.
16. Dechant MJ, Fellenberg J, Scheuerpflug CG, Ewerbeck V, Debatin KM. Mutation analysis of the apoptotic "death-receptors" and the adaptors TRADD and FADD/MORT-1 in osteosarcoma tumor samples and osteosarcoma cell lines. Int J Cancer. 2004;109:661–67.
17. Pai SI, Wu GS, Ozoren N, Wu L, Jen J, Sidransky D, El-Deiry WS. Rare loss-of-function mutation of a death receptor gene in head and neck cancer. Cancer Res. 1998;58:3513–18.
18. Horak P, Pils D, Haller G, Pribill I, Roessler M, Tomek S, Horvat R, Zeillinger R, Zielinski C, Krainer M. Contribution of epigenetic silencing of tumor necrosis factor-related apoptosis inducing ligand receptor 1 (DR4) to TRAIL resistance and ovarian cancer. Mol Cancer Res. 2005;3:335–43.
19. Elias A, Siegelin MD, Steinmuller A, von Deimling A, Lass U, Korn B, Mueller W. Epigenetic silencing of death receptor 4 mediates tumor necrosis factor-related apoptosis-inducing ligand resistance in gliomas. Clin Cancer Res. 2009;15:5457–65.
20. Jin Z, McDonald ER 3rd, Dicker DT, El-Deiry WS. Deficient tumor necrosis factor-related apoptosis-inducing ligand (TRAIL) death receptor transport to the cell surface in human colon cancer cells selected for resistance to TRAIL-induced apoptosis. J Biol Chem. 2004;279:35829–39.

21. Merino D, Lalaoui N, Morizot A, Schneider P, Solary E, Micheau O. Differential inhibition of TRAIL-mediated DR5-DISC formation by decoy receptors 1 and 2. Mol Cell Biol. 2006;26:7046–55.
22. Ruiz de Almodovar C, Ruiz-Ruiz C, Rodriguez A, Ortiz-Ferron G, Redondo JM, Lopez-Rivas A. Tumor necrosis factor-related apoptosis-inducing ligand (TRAIL) decoy receptor TRAIL-R3 is up-regulated by p53 in breast tumor cells through a mechanism involving an intronic p53-binding site. J Biol Chem. 2004;279:4093–101.
23. Chamuleau ME, Ossenkoppele GJ, van Rhenen A, van Dreunen L, Jirka SM, Zevenbergen A, Schuurhuis GJ, van de Loosdrecht AA. High TRAIL-R3 expression on leukemic blasts is associated with poor outcome and induces apoptosis-resistance which can be overcome by targeting TRAIL-R2. Leuk Res. 2011;35:741–49.
24. Granci V, Bibeau F, Kramar A, Boissiere-Michot F, Thezenas S, Thirion A, Gongora C, Martineau P, Del Rio M, Ychou M. Prognostic significance of TRAIL-R1 and TRAIL-R3 expression in metastatic colorectal carcinomas. Eur J Cancer. 2008;44:2312–18.
25. Sheikh MS, Huang Y, Fernandez-Salas EA, El-Deiry WS, Friess H, Amundson S, Yin J, Meltzer SJ, Holbrook NJ, Fornace AJ Jr. The antiapoptotic decoy receptor TRID/TRAIL-R3 is a p53-regulated DNA damage-inducible gene that is overexpressed in primary tumors of the gastrointestinal tract. Oncogene. 1999;18:4153–59.
26. Meng RD, McDonald ER 3rd, Sheikh MS, Fornace AJ Jr, El-Deiry WS. The TRAIL decoy receptor TRUNDD (DcR2, TRAIL-R4) is induced by adenovirus-p53 overexpression and can delay TRAIL-, p53-, and KILLER/DR5-dependent colon cancer apoptosis. Mol Ther. 2000;1:130–44.
27. Lalaoui N, Morle A, Merino D, Jacquemin G, Iessi E, Morizot A, Shirley S, Robert B, Solary E, Garrido C, Micheau O. TRAIL-R4 promotes tumor growth and resistance to apoptosis in cervical carcinoma HeLa cells through AKT. PLoS ONE. 2011;6:e19679.
28. Wagner KW, Punnoose EA, Januario T, Lawrence DA, Pitti RM, Lancaster K, Lee D, von Goetz M, Yee SF, Totpal K, Huw L, Katta V, Cavet G, Hymowitz SG, Amler L, Ashkenazi A. Death-receptor O-glycosylation controls tumor-cell sensitivity to the proapoptotic ligand Apo2L/TRAIL. Nat Med. 2007;13:1070–77.
29. Hao C, Beguinot F, Condorelli G, Trencia A, Van Meir EG, Yong VW, Parney IF, Roa WH, Petruk KC. Induction and intracellular regulation of tumor necrosis factor-related apoptosis-inducing ligand (TRAIL) mediated apotosis in human malignant glioma cells. Cancer Res. 2001;61:1162–70.
30. Krueger A, Baumann S, Krammer PH, Kirchhoff S. FLICE-inhibitory proteins: regulators of death receptor-mediated apoptosis. Mol Cell Biol. 2001;21:8247–54.
31. Fulda S, Meyer E, Debatin KM. Metabolic inhibitors sensitize for CD95 (APO-1/Fas)-induced apoptosis by down-regulating Fas-associated death domain-like interleukin 1-converting enzyme inhibitory protein expression. Cancer Res. 2000;60:3947–56.
32. Haag C, Stadel D, Zhou S, Bachem MG, Moller P, Debatin KM, Fulda S. Identification of c-FLIP(L) and c-FLIP(S) as critical regulators of death receptor-induced apoptosis in pancreatic cancer cells. Gut. 2011;60:225–37.
33. Longley DB, Wilson TR, McEwan M, Allen WL, McDermott U, Galligan L, Johnston PG. c-FLIP inhibits chemotherapy-induced colorectal cancer cell death. Oncogene. 2006;25:838–48.
34. Fulda S. Targeting c-FLICE-like inhibitory protein in cancer. Expert Opin Ther Targets. 2013;17:195–201.
35. Fulda S. Caspase-8 in cancer biology and therapy. Cancer Lett. 2009;281:128–33.
36. Friesen C, Fulda S, Debatin KM. Deficient activation of the CD95 (APO-1/Fas) system in drug-resistant cells. Leukemia. 1997;11:1833–41.
37. Fulda S, Scaffidi C, Susin SA, Krammer PH, Kroemer G, Peter ME, Debatin KM. Activation of mitochondria and release of mitochondrial apoptogenic factors by betulinic acid. J Biol Chem. 1998;273:33942–48.
38. Finlay D, Howes A, Vuori K. Critical role for caspase-8 in epidermal growth factor signaling. Cancer Res. 2009;69:5023–29.

39. Fulda S, Debatin KM. 5-Aza-2′-deoxycytidine and IFN-gamma cooperate to sensitize for TRAIL-induced apoptosis by upregulating caspase-8. Oncogene. 2006;25:5125–33.
40. Fulda S, Poremba C, Berwanger B, Hacker S, Eilers M, Christiansen H, Hero B, Debatin K-M. Loss of caspase-8 expression does not correlate with MYCN amplification, aggressive disease, or prognosis in neuroblastoma. Cancer Res. 2006;66:10016–23.
41. Teitz T, Wei T, Valentine MB, Vanin EF, Grenet J, Valentine VA, Behm FG, Look AT, Lahti JM, Kidd VJ. Caspase 8 is deleted or silenced preferentially in childhood neuroblastomas with amplification of MYCN. Nat Med. 2000;6:529–35.
42. Grau E, Martinez F, Orellana C, Canete A, Yanez Y, Oltra S, Noguera R, Hernandez M, Bermudez JD, Castel V. Hypermethylation of apoptotic genes as independent prognostic factor in neuroblastoma disease. Mol Carcinog. 2011;50:153–62.
43. Pingoud-Meier C, Lang D, Janss AJ, Rorke LB, Phillips PC, Shalaby T, Grotzer MA. Loss of caspase-8 protein expression correlates with unfavorable survival outcome in childhood medulloblastoma. Clin Cancer Res. 2003;9:6401–409.
44. Himeji D, Horiuchi T, Tsukamoto H, Hayashi K, Watanabe T, Harada M. Characterization of caspase-8L: a novel isoform of caspase-8 that behaves as an inhibitor of the caspase cascade. Blood. 2002;99:4070–78.
45. Horiuchi T, Himeji D, Tsukamoto H, Harashima S, Hashimura C, Hayashi K. Dominant expression of a novel splice variant of caspase-8 in human peripheral blood lymphocytes. Biochem Biophys Res Commun. 2000;272:877–81.
46. Miller MA, Karacay B, Zhu X, O'Dorisio MS, Sandler AD. Caspase 8L, a novel inhibitory isoform of caspase 8, is associated with undifferentiated neuroblastoma. Apoptosis. 2006;11:15–24.
47. Mohr A, Zwacka RM, Jarmy G, Buneker C, Schrezenmeier H, Dohner K, Beltinger C, Wiesneth M, Debatin KM, Stahnke K. Caspase-8L expression protects CD34 + hematopoietic progenitor cells and leukemic cells from CD95-mediated apoptosis. Oncogene. 2005;24:2421–29.
48. Cursi S, Rufini A, Stagni V, Condo I, Matafora V, Bachi A, Bonifazi AP, Coppola L, Superti-Furga G, Testi R, Barila D. Src kinase phosphorylates Caspase-8 on Tyr380: a novel mechanism of apoptosis suppression. EMBO J. 2006;25:1895–905.
49. Barbero S, Barila D, Mielgo A, Stagni V, Clair K, Stupack D. Identification of a critical tyrosine residue in caspase 8 that promotes cell migration. J Biol Chem. 2008;283:13031–34.

Unnatural Amino Acid Antibody Conjugates as Next Generation Biologics

Vaughn Smider

Abstract Trastuzumab represents a monoclonal antibody therapeutic with substantial clinical benefit, but tumors ultimately evolve resistance to its mechanism of action, often while maintaining HER2 expression and signaling dependence. Thus, "next-generation" biologics targeting HER2 but providing novel effector mechanisms of action may provide avenues to combat resistance. The ability to encode unnatural amino acids allows unique site-specific drug conjugates as well as multispecific molecules to be made and developed against HER2-dependent tumors. This broad-based technology could potentially be applied to any antibody therapeutic target.

Keywords Antibody drug conjugate · Bispecific antibody · Herceptin · Multispecific antibody · Unnatural amino acid

Abbreviations

ADC	Antibody drug conjugate
EGFR	Epidermal growth factor receptor
PCR	Polymerase chain reaction

Introduction

There are now over 30 FDA approved therapeutic antibodies on the U.S. market, with 14 antibodies approved for oncologic indications. The first of these to target solid tumors, trastuzumab (Herceptin; Roche), was approved in 1998 to treat

V. Smider (✉)
Department of Cell and Molecular Biology, The Scripps Research Institute,
La Jolla, CA 92037, USA
e-mail: vvsmider@scripps.edu

B. Bonavida (ed.), *Resistance to Immunotherapeutic Antibodies in Cancer*,
Resistance to Targeted Anti-Cancer Therapeutics 2, DOI: 10.1007/978-1-4614-7654-2_9,

HER2 overexpressing metastatic breast cancer as a first-line treatment in combination with paclitaxel, then in 2006 as adjuvant treatment of node positive HER2 overexpressing breast cancer, and in 2010 in combination with a fluoropyrimidine to treat HER2 overexpressing metastatic gastric adenocarcinoma [1]. In 2012, the monoclonal antibody pertuzumab, which binds a different epitope of HER2, was approved in combination with trastuzumab and docetaxel for HER2 overexpressing metastatic breast cancer patients who have not received prior therapy. Interestingly, the phase 2 trial of pertuzumab + trastuzumab was the first to describe complete responses in patients receiving biologic therapy in the absence of chemotherapy [2, 3].

Despite the success of trastuzumab, some patients do not respond to initial treatment, and many tumors acquire resistance within 1 year [4, 5]. Thus, either primary or acquired resistance to trastuzumab is a major problem in breast cancer. Novel "next-generation" therapeutics with unique mechanisms of action could potentially overcome these problems with antibody resistance, while maintaining specificity towards the HER2 target.

Herceptin as a Model System

Trastuzumab provides a good model system for an antibody therapeutic targeting solid tumors. Trastuzumab targets HER2 (ErbB2), which is a member of the epidermal growth factor receptor family (Fig. 1). There are four members in this family: EGFR (ErbB1), HER2 (ErbB2), ErbB3, and ErbB4, and three of them are strongly implicated in oncogenesis. EGFR is the target of the antibodies cetuximab (Erbitux; Eli Lilly) and panitumumab (Vectibix; Amgen) which are approved for metastatic colorectal (Erbitux and Vectibix) and head and neck carcinoma (Erbitux). Additionally, several antibody constructs targeting ErbB3 are currently in clinical trials [6]. This receptor family and their cell signaling pathways are clearly important in oncology.

Overall, the four ErbB family members are similar in having four extracellular domains and an intracellular tyrosine kinase domain (Fig. 1). However, the individual properties of the ErbB family members are unique: ErbB2 does not contain a ligand, and is a preferred dimerization partner for the other three ErbB members, and ErbB3 does not have an *active* kinase but can pair with ErbB2 to induce intracellular signaling through the ErbB2 kinase (Fig. 1b). The ErbB2-ErbB3 interaction is thought to be the most important signaling complex in HER2 overexpressing breast cancer [7–9]. The importance of this interaction has been highlighted by the development of pertuzumab, which blocks an epitope on domain 2 of ErbB2 that dimerizes with ErbB3 (Fig. 1c).

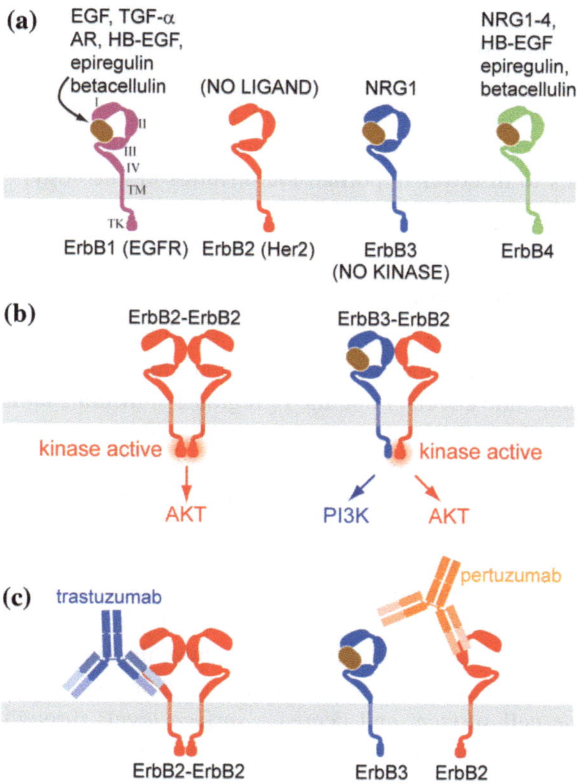

Fig. 1 The ErbB family of receptors. **a** Schematic diagram of the cell surface receptors ErbB1/EGFR (*purple*), ErbB2/HER2 (*red*), ErbB3 (*blue*), and ErbB4 (*green*), and their ligands (listed *above*). The membrane is in *grey*, and the domains are labeled I–IV, (TM) transmembrane, and (TK) tyrosine kinase. ErbB2 does not have a known ligand and is a preferential dimerization partner for the other receptors, and ErbB3 does not have an active kinase domain. **b** ErbB2/HER2 can homodimerize or heterodimerize with ErbB3 to form signaling complexes that can activate AKT (ErbB2 homodimers), or AKT and PI3K pathways (heterodimers). **c** Trastuzumab binds domain IV of HER2, and may preferentially act on HER2 dimers, whereas pertuzumab binds domain II and is thought to inhibit HER2-ErbB3 heterodimerization

Discovery of Herceptin

The mouse precursor antibody (named 4D5) to the humanized trastuzumab was discovered in 1989 through immunization of mice with NIH3T3 mouse fibroblast cells transfected with human HER2 [10]. A screen of several resulting monoclonal antibodies revealed that 4D5 could block proliferation of SK-BR-3 cells in a cell growth assay, and that 4D5 was more potent than several other antibodies including 2C4, the precursor to pertuzumab. This result is important in showing that different HER2 epitopes have different pharmacological effects on HER2 cancer cell physiology. 4D5 was subsequently "humanized" and developed as a therapeutic in preclinical models [11], then clinical trials. The revelation of the importance of the HER2-ErbB3 interaction stimulated development of pertuzumab, the humanized version of 2C4. Although it has been significantly questioned whether cultured cell lines contain the relevant physiology of in vivo tumors, the approval of both trastuzumab and pertuzumab validates the utility of cancer cell lines to discover important therapeutics in oncology.

Trastuzumab Mechanisms of Action

Trastuzumab has multiple mechanisms of action, the combination of which may mediate its therapeutic effects. First, the F_c region can mediate antibody-dependent cellular cytotoxicity (ADCC) through interaction with immune mediator cells. In xenograft models in immunodeficient mice, trastuzumab has little effect on tumor growth [12], so this immune mediated function may be considerably important. However, it is unclear whether these cell lines are endogenously "resistant" to other trastuzumab mechanisms of action like abrogating signal transduction or HER2 shedding. Trastuzumab can also inhibit intracellular signaling, including inhibiting phosphorylation of its own C-terminal kinase domain, as well as phosphorylation of ErbB3. These effects can inhibit the PI3K and AKT pathways through ErbB3 [8, 13]. Trastuzumab can also inhibit cleavage and shedding of HER2 from the cell surface, and decrease surface levels through internalization [1]. With multiple potential mechanisms of action, it is still unclear which of these is the most important, or whether the combination of multiple actions is critical for its therapeutic effect.

Trastuzumab binds proximal to the plasma membrane in domain 4 of HER2. It binds far from the heterodimerization interface in domain 2, yet still is able to substantially inhibit ErbB3 signaling. Interestingly, incubation of cells with trastuzumab leads to a substantial but transient increase in intracellular phospho-HER2 levels, suggesting that trastuzumab may increase kinase activity but in a non-productive conformation. Trastuzumab is active in tumors with overexpression of HER2 as measured by a 3+ immunohistochemical score, or by amplification of the *HER*2 gene. HER2 overexpression leads to formation of HER2-HER2 homodimers, and the optimal activity of trastuzumab may be dependent on tumors with cell surface HER2 dimers [14].

Mechanisms of Trastuzumab Resistance

Several mechanisms have been implicated in resistance to trastuzumab (Table 1). Overactivation of other pathways can compensate for inhibition of HER2 signaling. In this regard, increased expression of IGF-1R, c-MET, EphA2, or EpoR can enhance alternate signaling pathways to maintain oncogenic transformation in

Table 1 Mechanisms of trastuzumab resistance

Mechanism	Comment	Reference
Increased expression of IGF-1R	Overexpression of IGF-1R in cells abrogates trastuzumab sensitivity	[32, 33]
	High levels of IGF-1R in tumors by immunohistochemistry correlate with poor response	
Induction of MET	Her2 expressing cells upregulate MET in response to trastuzumab, which protect against trastuzumab by abrogating induction of p27	[34]
EphA2 activation	Anti-EphA2 antibody restored sensitivity to trastuzumab resistant cells	[35]
EpoR activation	Activation of EpoR inactivates PTEN and abrogates the response to trastuzumab	[36]
ErbB1 and ErbB3 ligand overexpression	Enhanced pathway activation in resistant cells leads to decreased susceptibility	[37]
Activation of TGFβ receptors	In cells TGFβ receptor activation can lead to increased ligand secretion, and a constitutively active TGFβ receptor correlated to trastuzumab resistance and poor clinical outcome in patients	[38]
Amplification of the AKT pathway	Gain of function mutations in *PIK3CA*, mutations in *AKT*, amplification of *AKT2*, loss of PTEN, loss of *INPP4*	[4, 13, 39]
p95^{HER2}	Truncated HER2 fragments maintain kinase activity but lose trastuzumab binding. Patients with cytosolic p95HER2 have a lower response rate to trastuzumab	[40, 41]
Mucin-4 overexpression	MUC4 expression masks trastuzumab binding epitopes, resulting in acquired resistance in cell lines	[42, 43]
HER2Δ16	A splicing mutation that deletes exon 16 results in transformation of cell lines and some primary tumors and shows resistance to trastuzumab	[44–46]

the presence of HER2 inhibition. Similarly, mutations that activate the AKT pathway, such as activators of PI3K, AKT, or inhibitors of PTEN can promote resistance. Alternatively, activation of pathways that result in increased secretion of ErbB growth factors may also potentiate trastuzumab resistance. Activation of TGFβ receptors can lead to increased ligand secretion that can activate EGFR or ErbB3. Changes that lead to decreased trastuzumab binding can also mediate resistance. A truncated HER2 protein termed p95^{HER2} can still mediate HER2 signaling but not trastuzumab binding, and a splicing mutation HER2Δ16 can remove the trastuzumab binding site. Overexpression of mucin-4 has been reported to mask the trastuzumab epitope, and mediates resistance. While several of these mechanisms have been uncovered in preclinical situations, it is still unclear which, if any, are predominant mechanisms in mediating trastuzumab resistance in the clinic. The majority of these mechanisms still rely on, and maintain, HER2 expression suggesting that the HER2 target itself may still be a valid target for new therapeutics aimed at overcoming trastuzumab resistance. In this regard, adding new mechanisms of action to HER2 targeted therapy is a rational way to combat resistance. While there are potential strategies using small molecules to overcome

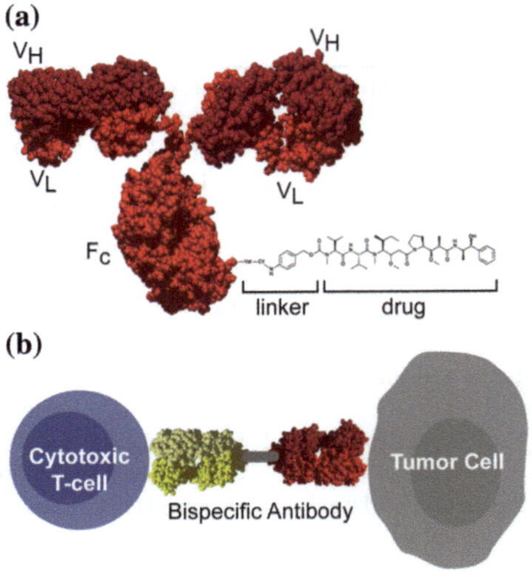

Fig. 2 Antibody drug conjugates and bispecific antibodies. **a** Schematic of an ADC showing the variable regions (V_H and V_L) and F_c, with the Fc coupled to the potent microtubule toxin auristatin through a linker. **b** A bispecific antibody binds both a T-cell (*blue*, *left*) and a target on a tumor cell (*grey*, *right*). This unique effector mechanism brings cytotoxic T-cell to the tumor and can mediate killing of multiple tumor cells per cytotoxic T-cell

trastuzumab resistance [15], here we will focus on specific strategies using novel antibody conjugates like ADCs and multispecific antibodies (Fig. 2).

Unnatural Amino Acid Background

Over the past several decades preclinical studies have demonstrated the utility of antibody-drug conjugates and bispecific antibodies in treating multiple tumor types in several in vivo models. Recently, dramatic clinical benefit has been demonstrated for brentuximab vedotin (Adcentris; Seattle Genetics), and trastuzumab-DM1 (Roche) for Hodgkin's lymphoma and HER2 overexpressing breast cancer, respectively [16–18]. These antibody-drug conjugates (ADCs) utilize potent microtubule-binding small molecules to directly induce cell death upon antibody internalization. Additionally, bispecific antibodies, such as the anti CD19-anti-CD3 "BiTE", have shown efficacy against non-Hodgkin's lymphoma [19]. Thus, new biologics that contain unique binding and effector functions could prove to be important next-generation anti-tumor therapeutics (Fig. 2).

The construction of a biologic with more than one functional moiety necessarily involves the coupling of two or more components. For an ADC, a small molecule drug is coupled to an antibody. For bispecific antibodies, two antigen binding fragments are typically genetically fused to produce the chimeric molecule. New methods for site-specific conjugation could allow both the coupling of small molecules to antibodies, as well as the coupling of antigen binding fragments to one another. Ideally, the ability to couple any combination of molecules to each other with control over the conjugation site(s) and relative orientation of the subunits would allow optimal multifunctional therapeutics to be created and tested. Furthermore, multivalent multispecific constructs beyond simple bispecific molecules are difficult to create using genetic fusion techniques. Conjugation strategies that allow the "mixing and matching" of individual components could allow targeting multiple cell surface receptors simultaneously, while also enabling novel cytotoxic effector functions.

Unnatural Amino Acids to Add Functionality to Antibodies

Over the past two decades the Schultz group has developed the technology to engineer genetically encoded unnatural amino acids into recombinant proteins [20–22]. This technology takes advantage of the natural processes involved in the central dogma of molecular biology (that DNA encodes mRNA, which through tRNA encodes protein). The mRNA coding process involves a specific tRNA coupled to its cognate amino acid (Fig. 3). Each tRNA can base pair with an individual mRNA codon during ribosomal protein synthesis. The charging of a tRNA with an amino acid is accomplished by a tRNA synthetase which is specific for each tRNA and amino acid pair. Thus, in order to ensure the fidelity of the genetic code, tRNA synthetases have evolved exceptional specificity; a tRNA synthetase does not mischarge a tRNA with the wrong amino acid, or conversely charge the wrong tRNA. The incorporation of unnatural amino acids requires (1) a 21st codon in mRNA, (2) a new tRNA not recognized by any endogenous tRNA synthetase, and (3) an engineered tRNA synthetase that specifically recognizes the new tRNA, as well as the unnatural amino acid, and can efficiently catalyze aminoacylation of the tRNA (Fig. 3). Unique positive and negative selection molecular evolution strategies have been employed to engineer tRNA synthetases that have selectivity towards the engineered tRNA as well as the unnatural amino acid. A stop codon such as TAG is utilized to specify the position of the unnatural amino acid, and the UAG in the mRNA interacts with the corresponding anticodon in the engineered tRNA. Over 50 unnatural amino acids have been encoded in recombinant proteins [20–22], with some of them comprising side chains with very useful bioorthogonal reactivity that can be used to couple to small molecules, linkers, or other proteins.

Incorporation of UAAs into the Trastuzumab Fab

Two unnatural amino acids, *p*-acetylphenylalanine and *p*-azidophenylalanine (Fig. 4), are particularly useful in generating bioconjugates through oxime ligation and click chemistry, respectively. Recently, *p*-acetylphenylalanine was successfully incorporated into several residues in the constant region of the trastuzumab Fab, with expression yields for several UAA mutants equivalent to the wild-type Fab [23, 24]. Coupling efficiency of an aminooxy-Alexa488 dye was dependent on the UAA site, but some sites could be coupled to over 90 % yield [23].

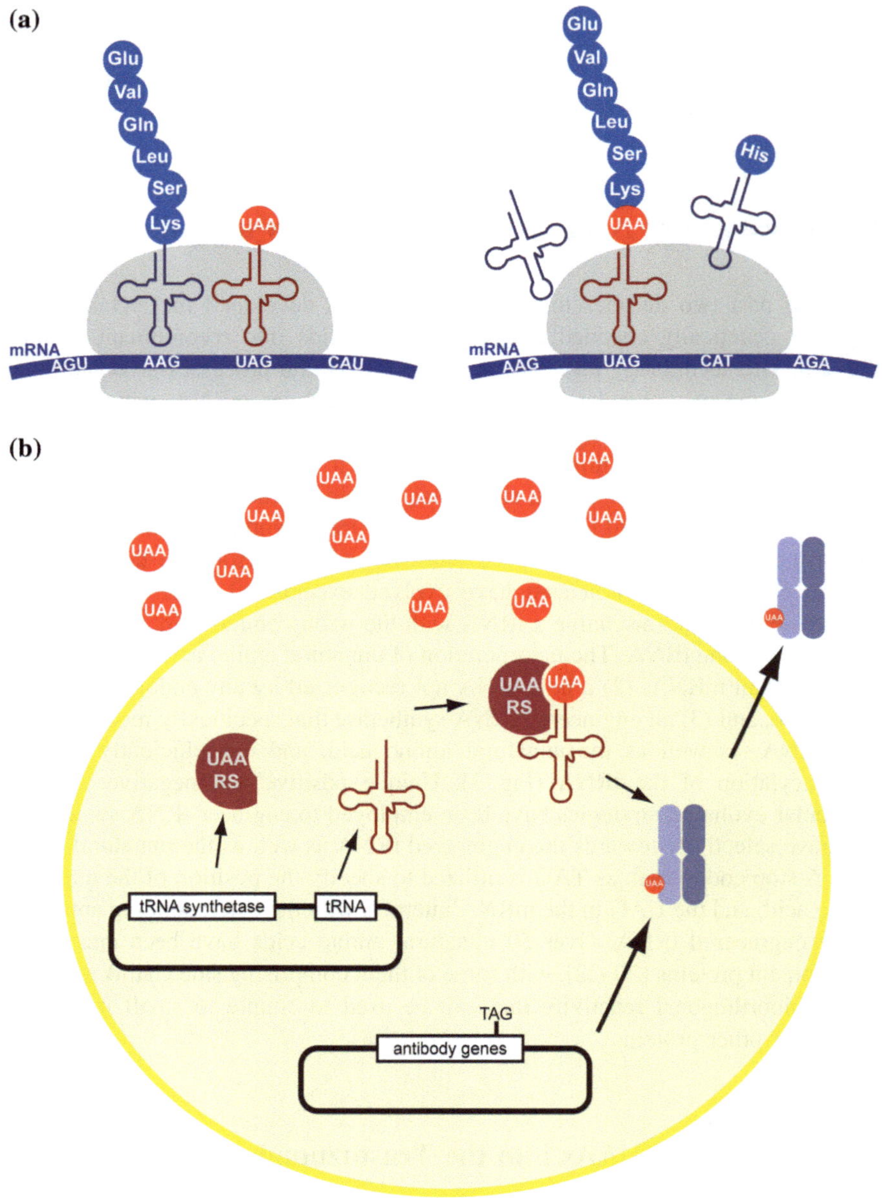

Fig. 3 Incorporation of unnatural amino acids into antibodies. **a** A tRNA that is charged with an unnatural amino acid (*red*) through an engineered tRNA synthetase is incorporated into the growing polypeptide chain. **b** Recombinantly expressed Fab fragments in *E. coli* can be engineered to incorporate an unnatural amino acid at a site of interest through the TAG amber stop codon. The antibody genes, tRNA, and tRNA synthetase are coexpressed and the unnatural amino acid is added to the media

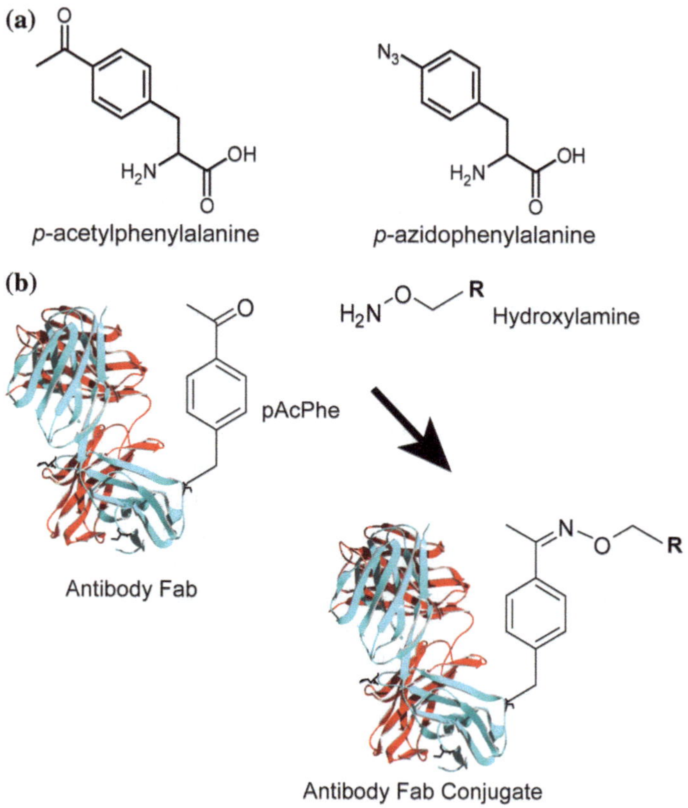

Fig. 4 Site specific coupling to unnatural amino acids. **a** Structures of *p*-acetylphenylalanine and *p*-azidophenylalanine. **b** Oxime formation between the keto side chain and a hydroxylamine to produce a site specific antibody conjugate

Homotetramers could be produced that had greater inhibitory activity than the dimeric trastuzumab IgG. Interestingly, the site of coupling impacted the activity of the tetramer in inhibiting intracellular signaling, indicating that steric factors are important in mediating binding and activity of a multimer [23].

Unnatural amino acids were used to create site-specifically linked protein–protein dimers in the form of both an antibody-toxin conjugate [24] and a bispecific antibody [25]. Short small molecule linkers were used to couple the trastuzumab Fab to the ribosomal toxin saporin at a *p*-acetylphenylalanine in the Fab and a surface cysteine in saporin. The resulting antibody-toxin conjugate could specifically kill HER2 overexpressing cell lines, with relatively little activity against HER2-negative cells. The activity was mediated by the Fab fragment, as saporin alone could not internalize and kill cancer cells. For the bispecific construct, the trastuzumab Fab was site specifically coupled to an anti-CD3 Fab, and the resulting bispecific molecule could mediate T-cell dependent killing of HER2 overexpressing cells as well as mouse xenografts. These bispecific proteins both directed different effector functions (saporin mediated toxicity, and T-cell cytotoxicity) to the same molecular target, HER2, on the tumor cells. It remains to be determined whether these molecules will be active against trastuzumab-resistant tumors in vivo, however, the unique killing mechanisms could theoretically overcome resistance mechanisms like activation of the PI3K pathway downstream of HER2 signaling.

Recently, the ADC trastuzumab-DM1 has shown biological activity in HER2 overexpressing breast tumors [16, 17]. This molecule uses the trastuzumab IgG coupled randomly at lysine residues to the maytansine microtubule binder DM1. This molecule may maintain all of the biological properties of trastuzumab, such as signaling inhibition and ADCC, but additionally carries the potent toxic payload enabling direct killing of tumor cells. Again, the resistance mechanisms (Table 1) that maintain HER2 expression could be susceptible to killing via this ADC biologic. Although trastuzumab-DM1 is quite potent, it has become clear that site specific coupling of a small molecule drug toxin improves pharmacokinetics and efficacy in preclinical models [12, 13]. Indeed, auristatin F coupled to *p*-acetylphenylalanine could be produced in high yield as trastuzumab Fab fragments or as IgG, and could mediate specific killing of HER2 overexpressing cells in vitro, or in orthotopic tumor models in vivo with complete tumor regression at a single dose of 5 mg/kg [12]. Thus, unnatural amino acids allow creation of homogenous conjugate products that may have more desireable features than current state-of-the-art coupling technologies.

Oligobodies

The ability to encode a chemical "handle" through an unnatural amino acid at a protein surface opens new opportunities in designing macromolecular complexes, which could extend into building nanotechnology structures (Fig. 5). In this vein, oligonucleotides have been coupled to a single UAA to produce molecules that can serve as templates for PCR [26], or to construct multimers through the basepairing properties of nucleic acids. These hybridization properties can allow novel bi-, tri-, or higher order hetero-multimers to be created. Such molecules self-assemble in solution at high efficiency. These new biologic structures should allow simultaneous targeting of two or more cell surface receptors, while allowing unique effector moieties to mediate novel mechanisms of action. With regards to trastuzumab resistance, targeting cell surface receptors like IGF-1R, ErbB3, or MET (Table 1) simultaneously with HER2, along with novel killing molecules like toxins or T-cell recruitment molecules may enable effective treatment of tumors that have progressed on antibody therapy.

Alternatively, it is clear that synergistic efficacy can be achieved by targeting two epitopes on the same receptor. Combination of trastuzumab which binds domain 4 and pertuzumab which binds domain 2 has shown efficacy in the clinic both as an antibody combination, as well as in conjunction with chemotherapy.

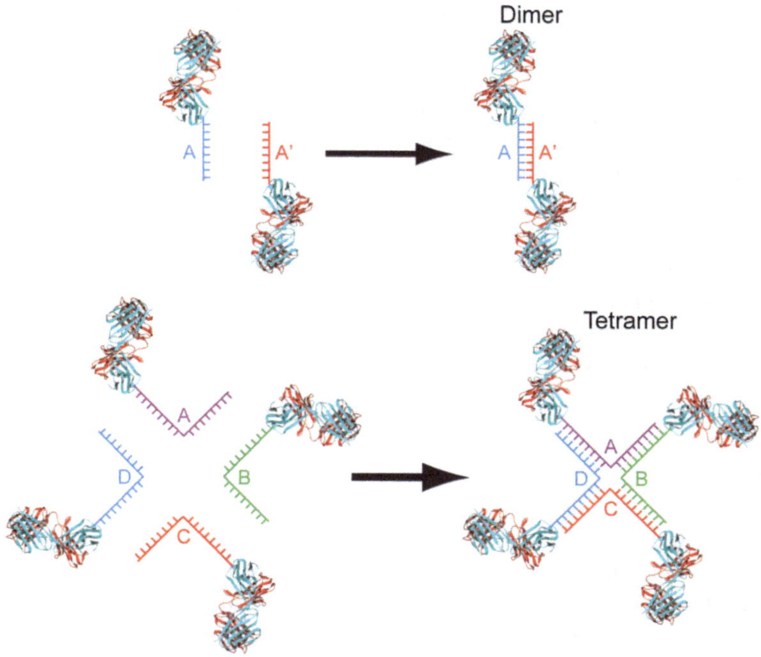

Fig. 5 Formation of "oligobodies". Complementary oligonucleotides (labeled A in *blue* and A' in *red*) are site specifically labeled to Fab fragments, then mixed to form a bispecific antibody (*top*). Alternatively, oligonucleotides are designed to allow hybridization in a cruciform structure, thus forming a tetramer (*bottom*). Oligonucleotides (DNA, RNA, PNA, or other analogs) can be designed to have other unique hybridization properties, and allow formation of a large number of molecular structures with different valencies

Multiple preclinical models have shown efficacy of combinations of antibodies against different epitopes on the same receptor [27–29]. An interesting application of unnatural amino acid technology would be to combine two or more antibody fragments targeting different epitopes on a single receptor into a single multivalent molecule.

Potential Adverse Affects

The incorporation of unnatural amino acids into therapeutics brings up potential issues of toxicity and pharmacokinetics and pharmacodynamics of this new biologic class. Any alteration of an amino acid in a "self" protein can potentially create a T-cell epitope and induce an immune response against the therapeutic. Indeed, the unnatural amino acid *p*-nitro-phenylalanine could break tolerance against TNFα in animal models when it replaced certain tyrosine or phenylalanine residues. This effect was dependent of the UAA position, and was clearly dependent on inducing a T-cell response [30]. Conversely, some positions of the UAA could not break tolerance. The immunogenic response, therefore, is likely no different than any other "natural" mutation that creates a T-cell epitope in a human protein. Each position would need to be evaluated in order to ascertain its propensity to induce an antibody response.

The construction of multivalent molecules linked by nucleic acids could have unique safety or pharmacokinetic issues. Oligonucleotides should be tested for their inability to activate Toll-like receptors, which could produce unwanted adverse immune effects. Such molecules may have a larger size and different charge than a typical IgG, and could affect biodistribution and serum or tissue half-life. None of these issues has yet been explored, and certain pharmacologic properties may need to be engineered into, or out of, each individual biomolecule.

Conclusions

With the introduction of therapeutic antibodies into the arsenal against cancer, tumors have inevitably evolved resistance mechanisms to enable disease progression. Tumors can be unresponsive to trastuzumab in the primary setting, or develop acquired resistance during the course of treatment. As trastuzumab was one of the first anticancer monoclonal antibodies in use clinically, it provides a model system for which to develop next-generation biologics that overcome resistance mechanisms. There are several potential mechanisms by which HER2 overexpressing tumors can develop resistance against trastuzumab, however, many of them leave the HER2 protein intact on the cell surface, suggesting that anti-HER2 therapies with novel mechanisms of action could be effective. Antibody-drug conjugates like trastuzumab-DM1 have shown efficacy in the clinic [16, 17], and newer site-specifically conjugated molecules have been efficacious in preclinical models [12, 31]. Methods to incorporate unnatural amino acids into antibody molecules allow for the creation of site-specific multivalent biologics, allowing novel binding and effector properties to be combined in a single molecule. Such molecules could represent a "next-generation" biologic that, if proven out clinically, may make an impact on tumors with primary or acquired resistance to more typical IgG therapeutic antibodies.

Conflicts of Interest
No potential conflicts of interest were disclosed.

References

1. Hudis CA. Trastuzumab–mechanism of action and use in clinical practice. N Engl J Med. 2007;357:39–51.
2. Baselga J, Cortés J, Kim SB, Im SA, Hegg R, Im YH, Roman L, Pedrini JL, Pienkowski T, Knott A, Clark E, Benyunes MC, Ross G, Swain SM. CLEOPATRA study group.

Pertuzumab plus Trastuzumab plus Docetaxel for metastatic breast cancer. N Engl J Med. 2012;366:109–19.
3. Baselga J, Gelmon KA, Verma S, Wardley A, Conte P, Miles D, Bianchi G, Cortes J, McNally VA, Ross GA, Fumoleau P, Gianni L. Phase II trial of Pertuzumab and Trastuzumab in patients with human epidermal growth factor receptor 2–positive metastatic breast cancer that progressed during prior Trastuzumab therapy. J Clin Oncol. 2010;28:1138–44.
4. Garrett JT, Arteaga CL. Resistance to HER2-directed antibodies and tyrosine kinase inhibitors: mechanisms and clinical implications. Cancer Biol Ther. 2011;11:793–800.
5. Wilken JA, Maihle NJ. Primary trastuzumab resistance: new tricks for an old drug. Ann N Y Acad Sci. 2010;1210:53–65.
6. Aurisicchio L, Marra E, Roscilli G, Mancini R, Ciliberto G. The promise of anti-ErbB3 monoclonal as new cancer therapeutics. Oncotarget. 2012;3:744–58.
7. Baselga J, Swain SM. Novel anticancer targets: revisiting ERBB2 and discovering ERBB3. Nat Rev Cancer. 2009;9:463–75.
8. Lee-Hoeflich ST, Crocker L, Yao E, Pham T, Munroe X, Hoeflich KP, Sliwkowski MX, Stern HM. A central role for HER3 in HER2-amplified breast cancer: implications for targeted therapy. Cancer Res. 2008;68:5878–87.
9. Menendez JA, Lupu R. Transphosphorylation of kinase-dead HER3 and breast cancer progression: a new standpoint or an old concept revisited? Breast cancer Res BCR. 2007;9:111.
10. Hudziak RM, Lewis GD, Winget M, Fendly BM, Shepard HM, Ullrich A. p185HER2 monoclonal antibody has anti-proliferative effects in vitro and sensitizes human breast tumor cells to tumor necrosis factor. Mol Cell Biol. 1989;9:1165–72.
11. Carter P, Presta L, Gorman CM, Ridgway JB, Henner D, Wong WL, Rowland AM, Kotts C, Carver ME, Shepard HM. Humanization of an anti-p185HER2 antibody for human cancer therapy. Proc Natl Acad Sci USA. 1992;89:4285–9.
12. Axup JY, Bajjuri KM, Ritland M, Hutchins BM, Kim CH, Kazane SA, Halder R, Forsyth JS, Santidrian AF, Stafin K, Lu Y, Tran H, Seller AJ, Biroc SL, Szydlik A, Pinkstaff JK, Tian F, Sinha SC, Felding-Habermann B, Smider VV, Schultz PG. Synthesis of site-specific antibody-drug conjugates using unnatural amino acids. Proc Natl Acad Sci USA. 2012;109:16101–6.
13. Junttila TT, Akita RW, Parsons K, Fields C, Lewis Phillips GD, Friedman LS, Sampath D, Sliwkowski MX. Ligand-independent HER2/HER3/PI3K complex is disrupted by trastuzumab and is effectively inhibited by the PI3K inhibitor GDC-0941. Cancer Cell. 2009;15:429–40.
14. Ghosh R, Narasanna A, Wang SE, Liu S, Chakrabarty A, Balko JM, González-Angulo AM, Mills GB, Penuel E, Winslow J, Sperinde J, Dua R, Pidaparthi S, Mukherjee A, Leitzel K, Kostler WJ, Lipton A, Bates M, Arteaga CL. Trastuzumab has preferential activity against breast cancers driven by HER2 homodimers. Cancer Res. 2011;71:1871–82.
15. Puglisi F, Minisini AM, De Angelis C, Arpino G. Overcoming treatment resistance in HER2-positive breast cancer: potential strategies. Drugs. 2012;72:1175–93.
16. Burris HA 3rd, Rugo HS, Vukelja SJ, Vogel CL, Borson RA, Limentani S, Tan-Chiu E, Krop IE, Michaelson RA, Girish S, Amler L, Zheng M, Chu YW, Klencke B, O'Shaughnessy JA. Phase II study of the antibody drug conjugate trastuzumab-DM1 for the treatment of human epidermal growth factor receptor 2 (HER2)-positive breast cancer after prior HER2-directed therapy. J Clin Oncol: Official J Am Soc Clin Oncol. 2011;29:398–405.
17. Krop IE, Beeram M, Modi S, Jones SF, Holden SN, Yu W, Girish S, Tibbitts J, Yi JH, Sliwkowski MX, Jacobson F, Lutzker SG, Burris HA. Phase I study of Trastuzumab-DM1, an HER2 antibody-drug conjugate, given every 3 weeks to patients with HER2-positive metastatic breast cancer. J Clin Oncol. 2010;28:2698–704.
18. Younes A, Bartlett NL, Leonard JP, Kennedy DA, Lynch CM, Sievers EL, Forero-Torres A. Brentuximab vedotin (SGN-35) for relapsed CD30-positive lymphomas. N Engl J Med. 2010;363:1812–21.

19. Bargou R, Leo E, Zugmaier G, Klinger M, Goebeler M, Knop S, Noppeney R, Viardot A, Hess G, Schuler M, Einsele H, Brandl C, Wolf A, Kirchinger P, Klappers P, Schmidt M, Riethmüller G, Reinhardt C, Baeuerle PA, Kufer P. Tumor regression in cancer patients by very low doses of a T cell-engaging antibody. Science. 2008;321:974–7.
20. Wang L, Xie J, Schultz PG. Expanding the genetic code. Annu Rev Biophys Biomol Struct. 2006;35:225–49.
21. Xie J, Schultz PG. Adding amino acids to the genetic repertoire. Curr Opin Chem Biol. 2005;9:548–54.
22. Young TS, Schultz PG. Beyond the canonical 20 amino acids: expanding the genetic lexicon. J Biol Chem. 2010;285:11039–44.
23. Hutchins BM, Kazane SA, Staflin K, Forsyth JS, Felding-Habermann B, Schultz PG, Smider VV. Site-specific coupling and sterically controlled formation of multimeric antibody fab fragments with unnatural amino acids. J Mol Biol. 2011;406:595–603.
24. Hutchins BM, Kazane SA, Staflin K, Forsyth JS, Felding-Habermann B, Smider VV, Schultz PG. Selective formation of covalent protein heterodimers with an unnatural amino acid. Chem Biol. 2011;18:299–303.
25. Kim CH, Axup JY, Dubrovska A, Kazane SA, Hutchins BA, Wold ED, Smider VV, Schultz PG. Synthesis of bispecific antibodies using genetically encoded unnatural amino acids. J Am Chem Soc. 2012;134:9918–21.
26. Kazane SA, Sok D, Cho EH, Uson ML, Kuhn P, Schultz PG, Smider VV. Site-specific DNA-antibody conjugates for specific and sensitive immuno-PCR. Proc Natl Acad Sci U S A. 2012;109:3731–6.
27. Spiridon CI, Ghetie MA, Uhr J, Marches R, Li JL, Shen GL, Vitetta ES. Targeting multiple Her-2 epitopes with monoclonal antibodies results in improved antigrowth activity of a human breast cancer cell line in vitro and in vivo. Clin Cancer Res. 2002;8:1720–30.
28. Vaidyanath A, Hashizume T, Nagaoka T, Takeyasu N, Satoh H, Chen L, Wang J, Kasai T, Kudoh T, Satoh A, Fu L, Seno M. Enhanced internalization of ErbB2 in SK-BR-3 cells with multivalent forms of an artificial ligand. J Cell Mol Med. 2011;15:2525–38.
29. Yamashita-Kashima Y, Iijima S, Yorozu K, Furugaki K, Kurasawa M, Ohta M, Fujimoto-Ouchi K. Pertuzumab in combination with Trastuzumab shows significantly enhanced antitumor activity in HER2-positive human gastric cancer xenograft models. Clin Cancer Res. 2011;17:5060–70.
30. Grünewald J, Hunt GS, Dong L, Niessen F, Wen BG, Tsao ML, Perera R, Kang M, Laffitte BA, Azarian S, Ruf W, Nasoff M, Lerner RA, Schultz PG, Smider VV. Mechanistic studies of the immunochemical termination of self-tolerance with unnatural amino acids. Proc Natl Acad Sci U S A. 2009;106:4337–42.
31. Junutula JR, Flagella KM, Graham RA, Parsons KL, Ha E, Raab H, Bhakta S, Nguyen T, Dugger DL, Li G, Mai E, Lewis Phillips GD, Hiraragi H, Fuji RN, Tibbitts J, Vandlen R, Spencer SD, Scheller RH, Polakis P, Sliwkowski MX. Engineered thio-trastuzumab-DM1 conjugate with an improved therapeutic index to target human epidermal growth factor receptor 2-positive breast cancer. Clin Cancer Res. 2010;16:4769–78.
32. Harris LN, You F, Schnitt SJ, Witkiewicz A, Lu X, Sgroi D, Ryan PD, Come SE, Burstein HJ, Lesnikoski BA, Kamma M, Friedman PN, Gelman R, Iglehart JD, Winer EP. Predictors of resistance to preoperative Trastuzumab and Vinorelbine for HER2-positive early breast cancer. Clin Cancer Res. 2007;13:1198–207.
33. Nahta R, Yuan LX, Zhang B, Kobayashi R, Esteva FJ. Insulin-like growth factor-I receptor/human epidermal growth factor receptor 2 heterodimerization contributes to trastuzumab resistance of breast cancer cells. Cancer Res. 2005;65:11118–28.
34. Shattuck DL, Miller JK, Carraway KL 3rd, Sweeney C. Met receptor contributes to trastuzumab resistance of Her2-overexpressing breast cancer cells. Cancer Res. 2008;68:1471–7.
35. Zhuang G, Brantley-Sieders DM, Vaught D, Yu J, Xie L, Wells S, Jackson D, Muraoka-Cook R, Arteaga C, Chen J. Elevation of receptor tyrosine kinase EphA2 mediates resistance to trastuzumab therapy. Cancer Res. 2010;70:299–308.

36. Liang K, Esteva FJ, Albarracin C, Stemke-Hale K, Lu Y, Bianchini G, Yang CY, Li Y, Li X, Chen CT, Mills GB, Hortobagyi GN, Mendelsohn J, Hung MC, Fan Z. Recombinant human erythropoietin antagonizes trastuzumab treatment of breast cancer cells via JAK2-mediated Src activation and PTEN inactivation. Cancer Cell. 2010;18:423–35.
37. Ritter CA, Perez-Torres M, Rinehart C, Guix M, Dugger T, Engelman JA, Arteaga CL. Human breast cancer cells selected for resistance to trastuzumab in vivo overexpress epidermal growth factor receptor and ErbB ligands and remain dependent on the ErbB receptor network. Clin Cancer Res. 2007;13:4909–19.
38. Wang SE, Xiang B, Guix M, Olivares MG, Parker J, Chung CH, Pandiella A, Arteaga CL. Transforming growth factor beta engages TACE and ErbB3 to activate phosphatidylinositol-3 kinase/Akt in ErbB2-overexpressing breast cancer and desensitizes cells to trastuzumab. Mol Cell Biol. 2008;28:5605–20.
39. Yakes FM, Chinratanalab W, Ritter CA, King W, Seelig S, Arteaga CL. Herceptin-induced inhibition of phosphatidylinositol-3 kinase and Akt Is required for antibody-mediated effects on p27, cyclin D1, and antitumor action. Cancer Res. 2002;62:4132–41.
40. Scaltriti M, Chandarlapaty S, Prudkin L, Aura C, Jimenez J, Angelini PD, Sánchez G, Guzman M, Parra JL, Ellis C, Gagnon R, Koehler M, Gomez H, Geyer C, Cameron D, Arribas J, Rosen N, Baselga J. Clinical benefit of lapatinib-based therapy in patients with human epidermal growth factor receptor 2-positive breast tumors coexpressing the truncated p95HER2 receptor. Clin Cancer Res. 2010;16:2688–95.
41. Scaltriti M, Rojo F, Ocaña A, Anido J, Guzman M, Cortes J, Di Cosimo S, Matias-Guiu X, Ramon y Cajal S, Arribas J, Baselga J. Expression of p95HER2, a truncated form of the HER2 receptor, and response to anti-HER2 therapies in breast cancer. J Natl Cancer Inst. 2007;99:628–638.
42. Nagy P, Friedländer E, Tanner M, Kapanen AI, Carraway KL, Isola J, Jovin TM. Decreased accessibility and lack of activation of ErbB2 in JIMT-1, a herceptin-resistant, MUC4-expressing breast cancer cell line. Cancer Res. 2005;65:473–82.
43. Price-Schiavi SA, Jepson S, Li P, Arango M, Rudland PS, Yee L, Carraway KL. Rat Muc4 (sialomucin complex) reduces binding of anti-ErbB2 antibodies to tumor cell surfaces, a potential mechanism for herceptin resistance. Int J Cancer. 2002;99:783–91.
44. Castiglioni F, Tagliabue E, Campiglio M, Pupa SM, Balsari A, Ménard S. Role of exon-16-deleted HER2 in breast carcinomas. Endocr Relat Cancer. 2006;13:221–32.
45. Kwong KY, Hung MC. A novel splice variant of HER2 with increased transformation activity. Mol Carcinog. 1998;23:62–8.
46. Mitra D, Brumlik MJ, Okamgba SU, Zhu Y, Duplessis TT, Parvani JG, Lesko SM, Brogi E, Jones FE. An oncogenic isoform of HER2 associated with locally disseminated breast cancer and trastuzumab resistance. Mol Cancer Ther. 2009;8:2152–62.

Antibody-Drug Conjugates: Can Coupling Cytotoxicity and Specificity Overcome Therapeutic Resistance?

Penelope M. Drake and David Rabuka

Abstract As their name implies, antibody-drug conjugates (ADCs) comprise a humanized or fully human IgG coupled to a cytotoxic small molecule payload. The former component provides the ADC with an antibody's exquisite selectivity for its target antigen, which is typically a cell surface molecule with a tumor-restricted expression pattern. The latter component provides the ADC with a highly potent cytotoxic payload that can efficiently kill targeted cells at low concentrations (sub nM). As relatively recent additions to the armament of anti-cancer drugs, ADCs hold great promise for disease management, particularly with respect to difficult to treat, drug-resistant tumors. Here, we provide an overview of modern approaches to cancer treatment, from first-generation systemically delivered chemotherapeutics, through the contemporary use of molecularly-targeted small molecules and biologics, to the culmination of both of these approaches—the ADC. Next, we detail the particular features of ADCs that relate to their potential for overcoming drug resistance, namely, the cytotoxic small molecule and the linker component. The latter is exceptionally well-suited to modifications that can render cytotoxic payloads poor substrates for multidrug transporter-mediated efflux from the cell. Finally, we touch on the possibility that ADCs might also serve as an effective means to treat tumors that are resistant to unmodified monoclonal antibody therapies (*e.g.*, rituximab and trastuzumab).

Keywords Antibody-drug conjugate (ADC) · Mylotarg · Adcetris · T-DM1 · Linker · Payload · Bioconjugatation

Abbreviations

ADC	Antibody-drug conjugate
MDR	Multidrug resistance
mAb	Monoclonal antibody

P. M. Drake · D. Rabuka (✉)
Redwood Bioscience, 5703 Hollis Street, Emeryville, CA 94608, USA
e-mail: drabuka@redwoodbioscience.com

B. Bonavida (ed.), *Resistance to Immunotherapeutic Antibodies in Cancer*, Resistance to Targeted Anti-Cancer Therapeutics 2, DOI: 10.1007/978-1-4614-7654-2_10,

MMAE Monomethyl auristatin E
MMAF Monomethyl auristatin F
T-DM1 Trastuzumab emtansine

Introduction

Antibody-drug conjugates (ADCs) were devised to leverage the potency of highly cytotoxic small molecules and the selective tissue targeting of antibodies to improve the therapeutic index of anti-cancer drugs by reducing side effects and improving efficacy. That these expectations are being met is evidenced by the dramatic patient response rates being observed in numerous ongoing clinical trials, and the recent FDA approval of the ADC, Adcetris, for the treatment of CD30+ Hodgkin's and anaplastic large cell lymphomas. However, challenges with the technology remain, including residual toxicity issues, component optimization (*e.g.*, drug selection and linker design), conjugation strategy, and selection/control of the drug-antibody ratio. All of these factors influence an ADC's pharmacokinetic properties, which ultimately impact its efficacy in patients. Additionally, ADCs offer the chance to circumvent drug resistance by modulating drug interactions with multidrug transporters at several levels—including mode of drug internalization into the cell, and access to modified drug/linker combinations that are not substrates for transport. Furthermore, ADCs may provide alternate means to treat tumors that are resistant to monoclonal antibody therapy. This review will provide a historical overview of ADC development, and then will focus on how current and next-generation ADCs are being used to address the challenge of multidrug resistance (MDR) in cancer.

First Generation Chemotherapeutics: Systemically Delivered Cytotoxic Drugs

Nitrogen mustards, alkylating agents that predominantly affect DNA replication, repair, and transcription, were the first clinically used chemotherapeutics. As the initial clinical trials, published in the early to mid-1940s, revealed, the drugs were efficacious against lymphomas and leukemias, but had reduced activity against solid tumors [1]. Next-generation alkylating agents soon appeared; one of them, chlorambucil, introduced in the mid-1950s, is still commonly used today to treat low-grade leukemias [2]. Over the following decades, both rational drug design and large-scale compound library screens led to the discovery of a variety of new cytotoxic drugs, including anti-folates (*e.g.*, methotrexate, introduced in the late

1940s), additional alkylating reagents (*e.g.*, cyclophosphamide, introduced in the mid-1950s), anthracyclines (*e.g.*, daunorubicin and doxorubicin, introduced in the late 1960s), platinum complexes (*e.g.*, cisplatin, introduced in the early 1970s), and taxoids (*e.g.*, paclitaxel, introduced in the late 1980s) [3].

It is interesting to note how many of these reagents, some of which have been around for more than 30 years, are still in first-line clinical use today, either alone or in combination with other drugs. For example, daunorubicin and doxorubicin are used to treat leukemias and skin cancers, respectively; cisplatin is used to treat ovarian, cervical, prostate, skin, and lung cancers; and paclitaxel is prescribed for breast, ovarian, and lung cancers [2]. The long clinical lifespan of these drugs says less about their clinical efficacy, which is modest, and more about the difficulty of finding small molecules that fit the narrow cytotoxic window required by drugs that work systemically to inhibit cell division. By definition, such agents must be only potent enough to kill the most rapidly dividing cells within an organism, but not so toxic that the entire animal (or patient) succumbs. The drugs in clinical use inhibit cellular processes such as DNA division/repair and microtubule transport, and thereby preferentially target highly proliferative tumor cells over non-transformed cells with lower division rates. Unfortunately, the drugs also demonstrate off-target effects on normal, highly proliferative tissues, such as the hematopoietic system, the lining of the gut, and hair follicles. This toxicity defines the maximum tolerated dose and thus effectively limits the amount of drug that will reach tumor cells. At the same time, drug resistance genes expressed by cancer cells serve as efflux pumps to shuttle drug molecules out of the cell, further reducing the effective dose delivered to the tumor. Together, the inherent toxicity of small molecule chemotherapeutics, coupled with drug resistance pathways that render marginal chemotherapeutic doses ineffective, highlight the need for next-generation oncology drugs to overcome these challenges.

Next-Generation Drugs: Targeted Therapeutics Customized to Tumor Subtypes

During the decades in which medicinal chemists were making first-generation chemotherapeutic drugs, the field of cancer biology was slowly but steadily discovering the signal transduction networks through which key mutations acted to perpetuate the proliferation of tumor cells. By contrast, comparatively recent advances in analytical and computing power have made it possible to generate, organize, and search huge quantities of biological information for common mutations or expression patterns. Suddenly, broad-based molecular comparisons could be made among many tumors of the same and different histological origins. These tumor profiles are now being constructed on nearly every possible biological level—from genomic and epigenetic features [4], to transcriptomic information on expression levels and alternative splicing events [5, 6], through proteomic analyses, including the status of post-translational modifications (*e.g.*, carbohydrates and phosphorylation) [7, 8]. Surprisingly, the power of bioinformatics has now turned the historical preference for hypothesis-driven research on its head, demonstrating that reams of high-quality data, when properly searched, can serve as the basis for generating testable theories related to the mechanisms underlying tumor development, propagation, and response to treatment. Furthermore, due to the unbiased nature of these inquiries, unexpected relationships can be uncovered, demonstrating novel interactions or functions.

Strikingly, as a group, these types of studies have demonstrated that not all tumors are created equal, and that distinct tumor subtypes exist even within cancers ostensibly derived from the same organ or tissue. For example, breast cancer is now recognized to be a collection of distinct neoplastic diseases with different molecular and clinical attributes. Breast tumors can be stratified into five intrinsic subtypes and a "normal-like" group according to features such as mRNA expression [9]. Interestingly, these molecularly-defined cohorts, which include luminal, basal-like, and claudin-low, are also predictive of clinical outcomes such as disease severity and treatment response [10–12]. Specifically, luminal tumors tend to be less aggressive with better survival rates, while basal-like and claudin-low lesions have generally worse prognoses [13]. These studies have also revealed that the expression of a therapeutic target such as the estrogen receptor (ER) or human epidermal growth factor receptor 2 (HER2/ErbB2) determines tumor susceptibility to drugs that interact with these molecules [14, 15]. Accordingly, tumor subtypes are now routinely determined in the clinic, and the information is used to guide treatment decisions. In addition to providing general information regarding tumor responsiveness to traditional radiation and chemotherapies, this new information regarding tumor subtype allows for the rational design of treatments that selectively shut down signaling pathways that are critical to cancer cell survival and proliferation, but are not required for most other non-transformed cells. Thus, these targeted therapies would not display the systemic cytotoxicities of traditional chemotherapeutics, but instead would be tumoricidal.

Targeted therapies have been developed using two general modalities—small molecule-based and protein-based. The flag-bearer of small molecule targeted drugs is Gleevec (imatinib), a receptor tyrosine kinase inhibitor of BCR-ABL, c-kit, and the platelet-derived growth factor receptor (PDGFR), approved in 2001 for the treatment of chronic myelogenous leukemia [16]. Gleevec had a dramatic impact on disease outcomes and patient longevity, thereby demonstrating the potential of molecularly-targeted therapeutics, and earning its originators the 2009 Lasker-DeBakey Clinical Medical Research Award for "converting a fatal cancer into a manageable chronic condition" [17]. Numerous other small molecule inhibitors targeting a range of signaling pathways have since been approved for clinical use; however, a further discussion of these agents is beyond the scope of this review.

With respect to protein-based targeted therapies, monoclonal antibodies that recognize a cancer-associated antigen are used to localize the antibody (and any cargo) preferentially to the tumor. Antibody binding then induces death of the target cell in any combination of the following ways: antibody-dependent cell-mediated cytotoxicity (ADCC), complement-dependent cytotoxicity (CDC), inhibition of growth receptor signaling networks, or through the direct or indirect induction of apoptosis. While antibody drugs can access one or more of these means of cytotoxicity, as ADCs, their efficacy is markedly enhanced by the delivery of cytotoxic small molecules directly to the cancer cell.

The first approvals of unconjugated monoclonal antibody drugs were in 1997 (rituximab) and 1998 (trastuzumab) for the treatment of non-Hodgkin's lymphoma and HER2+ breast cancer, respectively. Like Gleevec, these therapies brought significant benefits to cancer patients and forever changed the approach to drug development and patient management. Of the monoclonal antibodies currently approved by the FDA as treatments for cancer indications, seven are against leukemias/lymphomas, with four targeting the B-cell antigen CD20; of those targeting solid tumors, three were first approved for colorectal cancer, and three were first approved for breast cancer [18]. Since 1997, monoclonal antibody-based anti-cancer drugs have been approved at a rate of approximately one per year. Notably, two of these have been antibody-drug conjugates, proof-of-concept drugs that represent the first products from an expanding pipeline of ADCs in clinical trials; as such, they symbolize a marked shift in the focus of pharmaceutical companies towards this therapeutic approach.

Antibody-Drug Conjugates: Linking Potent Cytotoxics with Targeted Delivery

ADCs combine the best aspects of first-generation chemotherapeutics and contemporary targeted therapies into a single entity (Fig. 1). Accordingly, an ADC has three components: (1) an antibody that specifically recognizes an antigen with expression restricted to target tissues/cells (*e.g.*, tumors); (2) a cytotoxic small molecule; and, (3) a chemical linker joining the antibody and drug. ADCs can be viewed as sophisticated drug delivery systems that use molecular "postal codes" to send drugs to specific cellular targets. When an ADC reaches a cell expressing its cognate antigen, it binds to the antigen and is internalized via endocytosis (Fig. 2). The endocytic vesicle containing the ADC eventually fuses with a lysosome, where the ADC is degraded into its component amino acids and the drug/linker moiety. Depending on the nature of the linker—labile or stable—the cytotoxic payload is either completely liberated or remains conjugated through the linker to the modified amino acid (Fig. 2). Then, the free drug or drug derivative diffuses through the lysosomal membrane to access targets in the cytosol or nucleus, and ultimately induces cell death. The nature of this delivery system, in which ADCs are typically administered intravenously and then find their way to the tumor target(s), means that only a very small proportion (0.003–0.08 %) of the administered dose of antibody per gram of tumor will reach the cancer cells, as measured in human clinical trials [19]. Accordingly, the

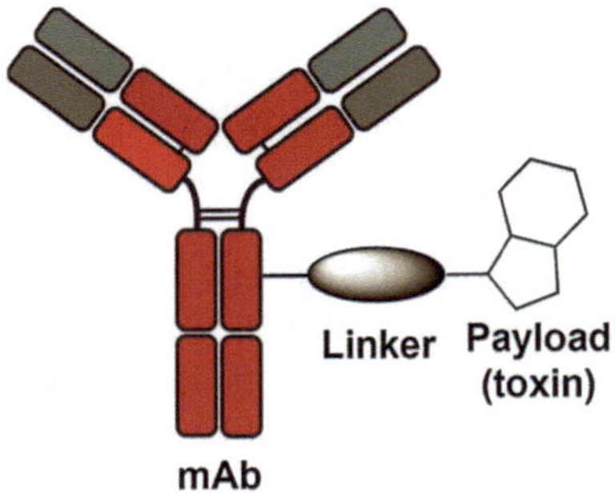

Fig. 1 An antibody-drug conjugate (ADC) incorporates the selectivity of an antibody with the potency of a small molecule cytotoxic drug. An ADC comprises the antibody, the drug, and the linker. The antibody is typically a humanized or fully human IgG that has specificity for a tumor-specific target antigen, and the drug is any of a handful of highly potent cytotoxic small molecules. The linker is the most versatile part of the molecule and is the component garnering the most attention with respect to generating modified ADCs that can overcome multidrug resistance

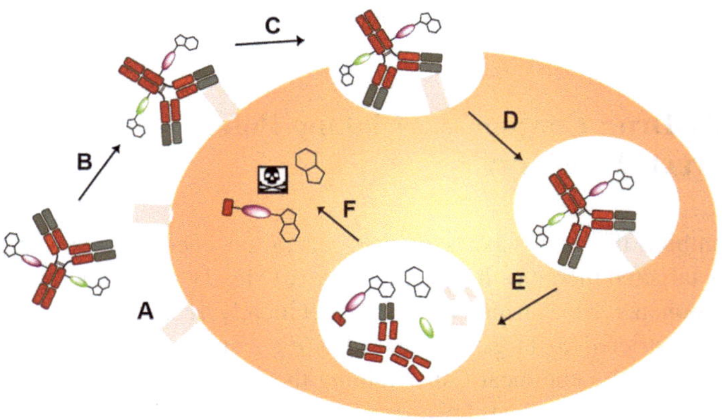

Fig. 2 The antibody-drug conjugate (ADC) enters cells via endocytosis and is degraded in the lysosome to release a membrane-permeable cytotoxic molecule. **a** An ADC comprises an antibody that recognizes a disease-specific target (*tan box*), a chemical linker, and a small molecule drug. The linker can be either chemically labile/enzymatically-cleavable (as depicted in *purple*) or stable/non-cleavable under physiological conditions (as depicted in *green*). **b** The ADC binds to its antigen on the target cell (*e.g.*, tumor) and **c** is internalized via endocytosis. **d** The endosome eventually fuses with a lysosome where **e** the ADC is degraded into its component parts. Some cleavable linkers are substrates for enzymatic degradation, *e.g.*, by lysosomal proteinases, whereas others are chemically labile at the lower pH found in the lysosome. ADCs bearing cleavable linkers break down completely into amino acids, linker derivatives, and the cytotoxic drug; however, decomposition of ADCs bearing stable/non-cleavable linkers yields the drug/linker attached to the modified amino acid. **f** Both of these drug derivatives can diffuse out of the lysosome to access molecular targets in the cytosol or nucleus, where they act to inhibit cell division and induce cell death

absolute number of drug molecules that enter each cell is low; setting a requirement for a very potent cytotoxic payload that can effectively kill target cells even at low concentrations.

The first approved ADC, gemtuzumab ozogamicin (Mylotarg), developed by Wyeth (now part of Pfizer), consisted of an anti-CD33 mAb conjugated at lysine resides to the DNA damaging drug, calicheamicin. This first-in-class drug achieved a number of its goals. Critically, it enabled the use of a highly potent cytotoxic molecule at significantly higher doses than would have been possible using the unconjugated analog. In the mouse, unconjugated calicheamicin doses were optimal at 0.5–1.5 μg/kg, whereas conjugated ADCs were tolerated at doses up to 300–400 μg calicheamicin/kg [20, 21]. As a consequence of the increased cytotoxicity of the payload, Mylotarg was efficacious against CD33+ tumors. In Phase I clinical trials, leukemia was eliminated from the blood and bone marrow of 20% of the 40 patients. It is of interest to note that patient response to Mylotarg was dependent upon tumor expression of small molecule efflux pumps (*i.e.*, multidrug transporters) as determined by the exclusion of a fluorescent dye. Mylotarg induced disease remission in 50% of patients that exhibited decreased ability to exclude the dye. However, none of the patients with leukemias that efficiently cleared the dye responded to treatment [22].

Notably, Mylotarg was very heterogeneous: about half of the antibody was unconjugated, while the other half carried various molar ratios of drug (4–8), leading to a final average of 2–3 drugs per antibody [23]. In addition, the linker component contained two cleavable bonds—a relatively unstable acid-labile hydrazone linkage and a sterically hindered disulfide. A Phase II trial showed that elderly AML patients receiving the ADC exhibited a 30% combined response rate with a median relapse-free survival of 7 months [24]. These data led to the accelerated FDA approval, in 2000, of Mylotarg for the treatment of relapsed CD33+ acute myeloid leukemia in patients over 60 years of age. However, use of the drug was immediately linked to severe liver toxicity, including veno-occlusive disease, which can be fatal [25]. Follow up clinical trials failed to demonstrate a clinical benefit in patients treated with Mylotarg as compared to patients receiving chemotherapy alone; worse, there was a greater proportion of deaths in the patient population taking Mylotarg as compared to the control population. As a result of these findings, in 2010, Pfizer voluntarily pulled the drug from the market at the request of the FDA.

Eleven years passed between the approval of the first and the second ADC. Brentuximab vedotin (Adcetris) won accelerated FDA approval in 2011 for the treatment of both Hodgkin's and anaplastic large cell lymphomas (ALCL) based upon data from Phase II trials. Adcetris, developed by Seattle Genetics, is composed of an anti-CD30 mAb conjugated at cysteine residues to the microtubule disrupter, monomethyl auristatin E (MMAE). Similar to Mylotarg, this drug product is very heterogeneous, with a drug distribution ranging from 0 to 8, with an average of 4 drugs per antibody [26]. The linker is composed of a protease labile dipeptide bond that is stable in serum but is cleaved in the lysosome upon ADC internalization and lysosomal trafficking. Phase II trials show that the overall response rate is 75% (up to 87% for ALCL) with a median duration of response of ~7 months [26]. Additional clinical trials assessing the efficacy of Adcetris are in progress, including a Phase III trial to confirm the promising initial results described here.

On the heels of Adcetris, trastuzumab emtansine (T-DM1), developed by Genentech/Roche, is poised to receive early 2013 FDA approval for the treatment of HER2+ breast cancer. T-DM1 is composed of an anti-HER2 mAb conjugated at lysine residues to another microtubule inhibitor, maytansine. Like Mylotarg and Adcetris, this product is very heterogeneous, bearing 0–8 drugs per antibody, with an average drug-antibody ratio of 3.5 [27]. The conjugate is held together by a stable thioether linker. A phase III trial has been completed, showing an objective response rate of 44% and a median progression-free survival of 9.6 months [28]. Based on these results, the FDA granted T-DM1 priority review status and is expected to approve the drug by Feb 2013.

While these pioneering ADCs demonstrate the promise of this new technology, there remains room for improvement. Among the prominent issues to address are product heterogeneity (*i.e.*, how and where drugs are conjugated to the antibody) and drug/linker design. Interestingly, the modular nature of ADCs provides an opportunity to fine tune the components for various endpoints. In this regard, some researchers have begun to investigate how the drug/linkers could be designed to thwart multidrug resistant phenotypes. Additionally, ADCs show promise as alternative therapies for tumors that are resistant to monoclonal antibody-based treatments. In the following section, we discuss ADC component parts and how these relate to both issues.

Optimizing ADCs for Improved Efficacy: Reducing Toxicity and Overcoming Resistance

Early iterations of ADCs employed commonly used clinically-approved chemotherapeutics (*e.g.*, doxorubicin, methotrexate, mitomycin, 5-fluorouracil, and the vinca alkaloids) as the drug component of the immunoconjugate [29]. These drugs, when used alone, suffered from dose-limiting toxicities and small therapeutic windows; thus, it was thought that their efficacy would improve when coupled to an antibody. This was true to some extent, however it was soon appreciated that to maximize the utility of this system more potent cytotoxic drugs were needed [30]. Thus, interest heightened around compounds with sub-nM growth inhibition activity; some of which had failed as stand-alone chemotherapeutics due to severe toxicity. Among these next-generation compounds were calicheamicin, the auristatins (including MMAE), and maytansine, all of which comprise ADCs that are either approved or are currently undergoing clinical trials. Notably, all of these small molecules are also substrates for P-glycoprotein, the most predominate of the multidrug transporters that mediate xenobiotic efflux from cells [31–33].

Interestingly, two features unique to ADCs provide opportunities to contend with multidrug transporters: the mode of internalization and the drug/linker design.

Multidrug transporters bind to their substrates in the inner leaflet of the plasma membrane (*i.e.,* before the drug has reached the cytoplasm or nucleus, the major sites of action for general cytotoxic drugs) [32, 34]. While small molecules that reach the cytoplasm can still be removed by multidrug transporters, drugs that can avoid transversing the plasma membrane may show improved efficacy in multi-drug resistant cells. ADCs take just such an evasive route to enter the cell (Fig. 2); after binding to target antigens at the cell surface, they are internalized via endosomes that ultimately fuse with lysosomes. Following ADC degradation in the lysosome, the drug component (the exact nature of which depends upon the linker, as discussed below) diffuses across the lysosomal membrane to access the cytoplasm. In this way, ADCs may deliver effective intracellular concentrations of toxin to cells that overexpress multidrug transporters. Indeed, a number of studies comparing the efficacy of free drug with the analogous ADC indicate that this approach does have merit [32, 35–40]. However, it is also clear that MDR phenotypes are still broadly protective against commonly used cytotoxics, even those delivered by ADCs [31, 41–43]. Therefore, significant efforts have focused on selecting new small molecule drugs that are poor substrates for transport [44]. These include epothilones, second- and third-generation taxanes, cryptophycins, camptothecins, duocarmycins, tomaymycin, and benzodiazapines [29, 45–50]. A different strategy uses plant- and bacterial-derived protein toxins that are too big to be P-glycoprotein substrates [51]. Importantly, a number of these pharmacophores may be applicable for use in the ADC format [47, 52, 53]. Alternately, ADC prodrug strategies could be implemented to access novel pharmacophores that circumvent mechanisms of resistance for known classes of cytotoxic compounds [36, 54].

An alternative approach for using ADCs to overcome MDR is through the rational design of the drug/linker component, such that, upon degradation in the lysosome, the liberated toxic payload is not a substrate for multidrug transporters. Much of this work is now being done in combination with optimizing other facets of conjugation, namely—the location and means of attaching the drug/linker to the antibody. The first ADCs were made using established protein conjugation chemistries that exploited the nucleophilic reactivity of lysines and cysteines [55]. Lysines, which are abundant in antibody sequences, were modified using NHS-esters and isocyanates, while cysteines, which are less common and exist as either intrachain or interchain disulfides, were modified using maleimide chemistries [56, 57]. The latter route required pre-treatment with a reducing agent to liberate the redox-sensitive cysteines from intermolecular disulfide bonds before reacting with the drug/linker component [58]. Both lysine- and cysteine-mediated conjugations yielded highly heterogeneous mixtures of products wherein each ADC molecule carried varying amounts of attached drug, referred to as variable stoichiometry, while coupling to the antibody backbone occurred at a variety of amino acid locations on the antibody [59]. Thus, the complexity lay at two levels: the drug-antibody ratio (DAR) and the attachment site. It became apparent that this complexity impacted the efficacy of the ADCs by directly affecting pharmacokinetics, predominately at the level of faster clearance for ADCs with high DARs. For example, Hamblett *et al.* [59] and McDonagh *et al.* [60] have shown that ADCs with a DAR of 8 are markedly more toxic *in vivo* and have shorter half-lives. A number of engineering approaches have been tried to reduce this heterogeneity, including the THIO-MAB conjugation strategy introduced by Genentech/Roche. This method entails the introduction of ectopic cysteine residues that are conjugated using thiol-selective chemistries to produce a homogenous ADC that is modified with a drug payload at specified positions on the protein. The efficacy of this product was strikingly improved as compared to the traditional heterogenous ADC modified at disulfide bridges. Specifically, the pharmacokinetic profiles were better with a longer serum half-life, the toxicity was reduced, and the therapeutic index was improved [61–65].

Meanwhile, other groups are endeavoring to produce homogenous ADCs using new approaches that allow for the use of bioorthogonal chemistries [66, 67]. These include the incorporation of unnatural amino acids [68, 69], and the introduction of the aldehyde tag, a five amino acid sequence that is the target of the formlyglycine generating enzyme, which converts a cysteine within the consensus sequence to a formylglycine residue bearing a reactive aldehyde group [70–72]. These protein-engineering methodologies enable site-specific antibody conjugation using reagents that do not react with the 20 canonical natural amino acids. For example, α-effect nucleophiles including substituted hydrazines and alkoxyamines will only react with carbonyls engineered into a protein backbone [73].

The linker is literally the central component of an ADC. It contains the reactive group that governs the conjugation chemistry and dictates which amino acid residues are targeted by the drug; and, it serves as a chemical spacer that physically connects the drug payload to the antibody. As such, the linker is also the most versatile aspect of the ADC. It can be modified in any number of ways to influence various drug/linker characteristics (*e.g.,* solubility [35, 36]) and ADC properties (*e.g.,* potency, pharmacokinetics, therapeutic index, and efficacy in multidrug resistant cells). Indeed, the chemical nature of the linker is as structurally significant as the payload or protein component of the ADC [30, 74]. There are essentially two broad classes of ADC linkers; those that are chemically labile or enzymatically-cleavable, and those that are chemically stabile, or non-cleavable. With respect to the former, labile/cleavable linkers are designed to keep the ADC intact when in circulation but release the drug payload upon internalization by the target cell. Early examples of labile linkers contained chemical functional groups that were to be hydrolyzed selectively in endosomes [21, 75, 76]. For example, Mylotarg contained a hydrazone that was designed to hydrolyze upon exposure to the relatively low pH of the lysosome, thus releasing calicheamicin [77]. However, this linker design met with limited success because much of the drug was released while the ADC was still in circulation; this led to a narrow therapeutic window, limiting the efficacy of the ADC.

Labile linkers containing disulfide bonds have served as more effective alternatives for ADC conjugation [37, 78, 79]. Release of these linkers is mediated through chemical interactions with the relatively high intracellular concentrations of glutathione. DM1 and DM4 are examples of potent maytansinoid derivatives that use disulfide-containing linkers. Another strategy involves the use of cleavable linkers designed to be hydrolyzed by enzymes, such as cathepsin, plasmin or glycosidases [50, 54, 80]. For example, MMAE can be conjugated via a valine-citrulline dipeptide-containing linker that provides excellent stability in plasma but is efficiently cleaved by proteases in the lysosome [56]. Interestingly, upon cleavage, the remaining linker metabolite attached to MMAE self-eliminates via a 1,6-elimination of the 4-aminobenzyl group, releasing the active form of MMAE. This linker configuration results in an improved therapeutic index for the ADC [38].

All labile/cleavable linkers allow ADCs to deliver their payloads via antigen-mediated endocytosis and bypass the powerful small molecule efflux pumps in the plasma membrane that contribute to MDR. However, once the free drug has been released from the linker it is once again susceptible to multidrug transporter-mediated efflux from the cytoplasm [32]. Non-cleavable linkers provide a potential solution to this problem. By design, stable linkers do not contain chemical functionalities that are susceptible to intracellular degradation. Therefore, after an internalized ADC is trafficked to the lysosome, the antibody moiety is proteolytically degraded into amino acids while the cytotoxic drug remains attached via the linker to an amino acid residue. Exploiting structure–activity relationships in designing covalent linker-cytotoxic drug pairs enables a chemical elaboration of the lysomally processed linker-cytotoxic drug moiety that does not impact its ability to bind to its target within the cell. Thus, the drug is still efficacious as an inhibitor of cell division. However, this elaboration does provide a chemical handle that can be modified to circumvent efflux by multidrug transporters. Specifically, with respect to P-glycoprotein, the most powerful driver of clinically significant MDR, most of the reported substrates are relatively hydrophobic, planar and weakly cationic [34]. Therefore, one strategy for overcoming MDR is to modulate the drug/linker structure, especially by reducing its overall hydrophobicity by incorporating hydrophilicity into the linker component [32, 35, 37, 81]. Both maytansinoids and auristatins are compatible with non-cleavable linkers and the *in vivo* stability of ADCs with this format is superior to that of analogous ADCs with cleavable linkers [82–84]. The best example of a non-cleavable linker ADC is Genentech's very promising anti-breast cancer drug, T-DM1, which incorporates the stable thioether bond developed by ImmunoGen. Monomethyl auristatin F (MMAF) is another example of a cytotoxic drug that is compatible with non-cleavable linkers [81, 85]. One such stable linker, developed by Seattle Genetics, that used a bromoacetamidecaproyl reactive group to achieve conjugation to the mAb was maintained in the circulation with no detectable degradation for up to 14 days [82].

Finally, ADCs may also serve as effective treatments for tumors that display innate or acquired resistance to monoclonal antibody therapies, such as rituximab and trastuzumab. Although these monoclonal antibody drugs induce dramatic responses in patients with non-Hodgkin's lymphoma and HER2+ breast cancer, respectively, disease remission is often followed by relapse within a few years [86, 87]. Although the specifics vary according to target antigen, tumor origin, and a patient's genetic background, a number of mechanisms that contribute to monoclonal antibody therapy resistance have been identified. These include complement inhibition [88, 89], the downregulation of cell surface target antigens [90], the blockade of apoptotic pathways [91], the hyperactivity of certain signaling pathways (*i.e.*, PI3K/AKT) [92, 93], and the activation of cytokine feedback loops that lead to the expansion of cancer stem cell populations [94]. A number of investigators are exploring the possibility that through the direct delivery of a potent cytotoxic drug, ADCs may be effective against these resistance mechanisms. For rituximab-resistant leukemias, a general strategy has been to use ADCs that target alternative B-cell antigens in order to bypass loss of efficacy due to the downregulation of CD20 [91]. In addition, ADCs may help to downregulate the cell surface expression of complement inhibitory proteins, such as DAF/CD55, thereby removing a blockade to monoclonal antibody efficacy. For this reason, combination ADC/monoclonal antibody therapy approaches may be useful [88]. Interestingly, the ADC, T-DM1, which uses the trastuzumab antibody as its backbone, has demonstrated efficacy against trastuzumab-resistant cell lines *in vitro* [95]. This may be, in part, because a significant component of trastuzumab resistance appears to be due to the activation of downstream signaling pathways (*e.g.*, PTEN/PI3K), whose actions can be overwhelmed by the potent microtubule inhibitory effects of T-DM1's maytansine payload [92, 93].

Conclusion

Although Mylotarg was initially approved in 2000, it has taken the field years to work out the biology and chemistries necessary to produce safe, efficacious ADCs. Now, with one FDA-approved drug and at least 20 new ADCs in clinical trials, the era of this class of molecules is just beginning. Accordingly, we do not know very much yet about how ADCs can be used and/or developed to treat diseases that are resistant to conventional drugs and monoclonal antibody therapies. However, researchers and clinicians are already addressing these pressing questions and undoubtedly over the next several years much more will be learned. The use of ADCs to overcome MDR is an area to watch with interest as it develops.

Acknowledgments The authors would like to thank Gregory Landes and Zev Gartner for a critical reading of the manuscript and helpful discussions.

Conflict of Interest

No potential conflicts of interest were disclosed

References

1. Goldenberg GJ, Moore MJ. Nitrogen Mustards. In: Teicher BA, editor. Cancer therapeutics: experimental and clinical agents. NJ: Humana Press; 1997. p. 3–22.
2. Almeida CA, Barry SA. Cancer: basic science and clinical aspects. 1st ed. NJ: Blackwell Publishing; 2010.
3. Teicher BA. Cancer therapeutics: experimental and clinical agents. NJ: Humana Press; 1997.
4. Korkola J, Gray JW. Breast cancer genomes–form and function. Curr Opin Genet Dev. 2010;20:4–14.
5. Neve RM, Chin K, Fridlyand J, Yeh J, Baehner FL, Fevr T, Clark L, Bayani N, Coppe JP, Tong F, Speed T, Spellman PT, DeVries S, Lapuk A, Wang NJ, Kuo WL, Stilwell JL, Pinkel D, Albertson DG, Waldman FM, McCormick F, Dickson RB, Johnson MD, Lippman M, Ethier S, Gazdar A, Gray JW. A collection of breast cancer cell lines for the study of functionally distinct cancer subtypes. Cancer Cell. 2006;10:515–27.
6. Lapuk A, Marr H, Jakkula L, Pedro H, Bhattacharya S, Purdom E, Hu Z, Simpson K, Pachter L, Durinck S, Wang N, Parvin B, Fontenay G, Speed T, Garbe J, Stampfer M, Bayandorian H, Dorton S, Clark TA, Schweitzer A, Wyrobek A, Feiler H, Spellman P, Conboy J, Gray JW. Exon-level microarray analyses identify alternative splicing programs in breast cancer. Mol Cancer Res. 2010;8:961–74.
7. Drake PM, Schilling B, Niles RK, Prakobphol A, Li B, Jung K, Cho W, Braten M, Inerowicz HD, Williams K, Albertolle M, Held JM, Iacovides D, Sorensen DJ, Griffith OL, Johansen E, Zawadzka AM, Cusack MP, Allen S, Gormley M, Hall SC, Witkowska HE, Gray JW, Regnier F, Gibson BW, Fisher SJ. Lectin chromatography/mass spectrometry discovery workflow identifies putative biomarkers of aggressive breast cancers. J Proteome Res. 2012;11:2508–20.
8. Boyd ZS, Wu QJ, O'Brien C, Spoerke J, Savage H, Fielder PJ, Amler L, Yan Y, Lackner MR. Proteomic analysis of breast cancer molecular subtypes and biomarkers of response to targeted kinase inhibitors using reverse-phase protein microarrays. Mol Cancer Ther. 2008;7:3695–706.
9. Perou CM, Borresen-Dale AL. Systems biology and genomics of breast cancer. Cold Spring Harb Perspect Biol. 2010;3:1–18.
10. O'Brien KM, Cole SR, Tse CK, Perou CM, Carey LA, Foulkes WD, Dressler LG, Geradts J, Millikan RC. Intrinsic breast tumor subtypes, race, and long-term survival in the Carolina breast cancer study. Clin Cancer Res. 2010;16:6100–10.
11. Espinosa E, Vara JA, Navarro IS, Gamez-Pozo A, Pinto A, Zamora P, Redondo A, Feliu J. Gene profiling in breast cancer: time to move forward. Cancer Treat Rev. 2011;37:416–21.
12. Prat A, Parker JS, Karginova O, Fan C, Livasy C, Herschkowitz JI, He X, Perou CM. Phenotypic and molecular characterization of the claudin-low intrinsic subtype of breast cancer. Breast Cancer Res. 2010;12:R68.
13. Toft DJ, Cryns VL. Minireview: basal-like breast cancer: from molecular profiles to targeted therapies. Mol Endocrinol. 2011;25:199–211.
14. Abramson V, Arteaga CL. New strategies in HER2-overexpressing breast cancer: many combinations of targeted drugs available. Clin Cancer Res. 2011;17:952–8.
15. McDermott U, Settleman J. Personalized cancer therapy with selective kinase inhibitors: an emerging paradigm in medical oncology. J Clin Oncol. 2009;27:5650–9.
16. Fischer OM, Streit S, Hart S, Ullrich A. Beyond herceptin and gleevec. Curr Opin Chem Biol. 2003;7:490–5.
17. Grindlinger B. Trio receives Lasker Foundation Clinical Award for breakthroughs in leukemia treatment. J Clin Invest. 2009;119:2863–5.
18. Reichert JM. Antibody-based therapeutics to watch in 2011. MAbs. 2011;3:76–99.
19. Erickson HK, Lambert JM. ADME of antibody-maytansinoid conjugates. Aaps J. 2012;14:799–805.

20. Zein N, Sinha AM, McGahren WJ, Ellestad GA. Calicheamicin gamma1I: an antitumor antitumor antibiotic that cleaves double-stranded DNA site specifically. Science. 1988;240:1198–201.
21. Hamann PR, Hinman LM, Hollander I, Beyer CF, Lindh D, Holcomb R, Hallett W, Tsou HR, Upeslacis J, Shochat D, Mountain A, Flowers DA, Bernstein ID. Gemtuzumab ozogamicin, a potent and selective anti-CD33 antibody-calicheamicin conjugate for treatment of acute myeloid leukemia. Bioconjug Chem. 2002;13:47–58.
22. Sievers EL, Appelbaum FR, Spielberger RT, Forman SJ, Flowers DA, Smith FO, Shannon-Dorcy K, Berger MS, Bernstein ID. Selective ablation of acute myeloid leukemia using antibody-targeted chemotherapy: a Phase I study of an anti-CD33 calicheamicin immunoconjugate. Blood. 1999;93:3678–84.
23. Wu AM, Senter PD. Arming antibodies: prospects and challenges for immunoconjugates. Nat Biotechnol. 2005;23:1137–46.
24. Schrama D, Reisfeld RA, Becker JC. Antibody targeted drugs as cancer therapeutics. Nat Rev Drug Discov. 2006;5:147–59.
25. Rajvanshi P, Shulman HM, Sievers EL, McDonald GB. Hepatic sinusoidal obstruction after gemtuzumab ozogamicin (Mylotarg) therapy. Blood. 2002;99:2310–4.
26. Furtado M, Rule S. Emerging pharmacotherapy for relapsed or refractory Hodgkin's lymphoma: focus on Brentuximab Vedotin. Clin Med Insights Oncol. 2012;6:31–9.
27. Girish S, Gupta M, Wang B, Lu D, Krop IE, Vogel CL, Burris Iii HA, LoRusso PM, Yi JH, Saad O, Tong B, Chu YW, Holden S, Joshi A. Clinical pharmacology of trastuzumab emtansine (T-DM1): an antibody-drug conjugate in development for the treatment of HER2-positive cancer. Cancer Chemother Pharmacol. 2012;69:1229–40.
28. Verma S, Miles D, Gianni L, Krop IE, Welslau M, Baselga J, Pegram M, Oh DY, Dieras V, Guardino E, Fang L, Lu MW, Olsen S, Blackwell K. Trastuzumab emtansine for HER2-positive advanced breast cancer. N Engl J Med. 2012;367:1783–91.
29. Singh Y, Palombo M, Sinko PJ. Recent trends in targeted anticancer prodrug and conjugate design. Curr Med Chem. 2008;15:1802–26.
30. Ducry L, Stump B. Antibody-drug conjugates: linking cytotoxic payloads to monoclonal antibodies. Bioconjug Chem. 2010;21:5–13.
31. Matsui H, Takeshita A, Naito K, Shinjo K, Shigeno K, Maekawa M, Yamakawa Y, Tanimoto M, Kobayashi M, Ohnishi K, Ohno R. Reduced effect of gemtuzumab ozogamicin (CMA-676) on P-glycoprotein and/or CD34-positive leukemia cells and its restoration by multidrug resistance modifiers. Leukemia. 2002;16:813–9.
32. Kovtun YV, Audette CA, Mayo MF, Jones GE, Doherty H, Maloney EK, Erickson HK, Sun X, Wilhelm S, Ab O, Lai KC, Widdison WC, Kellogg B, Johnson H, Pinkas J, Lutz RJ, Singh R, Goldmacher VS, Chari RV. Antibody-maytansinoid conjugates designed to bypass multidrug resistance. Cancer Res. 2010;70:2528–37.
33. de Claro RA, McGinn K, Kwitkowski V, Bullock J, Khandelwal A, Habtemariam B, Ouyang Y, Saber H, Lee K, Koti K, Rothmann M, Shapiro M, Borrego F, Clouse K, Chen XH, Brown J, Akinsanya L, Kane R, Kaminskas E, Farrell A, Pazdur R. U.S. food and drug administration approval summary: brentuximab vedotin for the treatment of relapsed hodgkin lymphoma or relapsed systemic anaplastic large-cell lymphoma. Clin Cancer Res. 2012;18:5845–9.
34. Higgins CF. Multiple molecular mechanisms for multidrug resistance transporters. Nature. 2007;446:749–57.
35. Zhao RY, Wilhelm SD, Audette CA, Jones GE, Leece BA, Lazar AC, Goldmacher VS, Singh R, Kovtun YV, Widdison WC, Lambert JM, Chari RV. Synthesis and evaluation of hydrophilic linkers for antibody-maytansinoid conjugates. J Med Chem. 2011;54:3606–23.
36. Zhao RY, Erickson HK, Leece BA, Reid EE, Goldmacher VS, Lambert JM, Chari RV. Synthesis and biological evaluation of antibody conjugates of phosphate prodrugs of cytotoxic DNA alkylators for the targeted treatment of cancer. J Med Chem. 2012;55:766–82.
37. Hamann PR, Hinman LM, Beyer CF, Greenberger LM, Lin C, Lindh D, Menendez AT, Wallace R, Durr FE, Upeslacis J. An anti-MUC1 antibody-calicheamicin conjugate for

treatment of solid tumors. Choice of linker and overcoming drug resistance. Bioconjug Chem. 2005;16:346–53.
38. Francisco JA, Cerveny CG, Meyer DW, Mixan BJ, Klussman K, Chace DF, Rejniak SX, Gordon KA, DeBlanc R, Toki BE, C-L L, Doronina SO, Siegall CB, Senter PD, Wahl AF. cAC10-vcMMAE, an anti-CD30-monomethyl auristatin E conjugate with potent and selective antitumor activity. Blood. 2003;102:1458–65.
39. Chari RV. Targeted cancer therapy: conferring specificity to cytotoxic drugs. Acc Chem Res. 2007;41:98–107.
40. Guillemard V, Uri Saragovi H. Prodrug chemotherapeutics bypass p-glycoprotein resistance and kill tumors in vivo with high efficacy and target-dependent selectivity. Oncogene. 2004;23:3613–21.
41. Walter RB, Raden BW, Hong TC, Flowers DA, Bernstein ID, Linenberger ML. Multidrug resistance protein attenuates gemtuzumab ozogamicin-induced cytotoxicity in acute myeloid leukemia cells. Blood. 2003;102:1466–73.
42. Walter RB, Gooley TA, van der Velden VH, Loken MR, van Dongen JJ, Flowers DA, Bernstein ID, Appelbaum FR. CD33 expression and P-glycoprotein-mediated drug efflux inversely correlate and predict clinical outcome in patients with acute myeloid leukemia treated with gemtuzumab ozogamicin monotherapy. Blood. 2007;109:4168–70.
43. Takeshita A, Shinjo K, Yamakage N, Ono T, Hirano I, Matsui H, Shigeno K, Nakamura S, Tobita T, Maekawa M, Ohnishi K, Sugimoto Y, Kiyoi H, Naoe T, Ohno R. CMC-544 (inotuzumab ozogamicin) shows less effect on multidrug resistant cells: analyses in cell lines and cells from patients with B-cell chronic lymphocytic leukaemia and lymphoma. Br J Haematol. 2009;146:34–43.
44. Nobili S, Landini I, Mazzei T, Mini E. Overcoming tumor multidrug resistance using drugs able to evade P-glycoprotein or to exploit its expression. Med Res Rev. 2012;32:1220–62.
45. Suzawa T, Nagamura S, Saito H, Ohta S, Hanai N, Yamasaki M. Synthesis of a novel duocarmycin derivative DU-257 and its application to immunoconjugate using poly(ethylene glycol)-dipeptidyl linker capable of tumor specific activation. Bioorg Med Chem. 2000;8:2175–84.
46. Jin W, Trzupek JD, Rayl TJ, Broward MA, Vielhauer GA, Weir SJ, Hwang I, Boger DL. A unique class of duocarmycin and CC-1065 analogues subject to reductive activation. J Am Chem Soc. 2007;129:15391–7.
47. Burke PJ, Senter PD, Meyer DW, Miyamoto JB, Anderson M, Toki BE, Manikumar G, Wani MC, Kroll DJ, Jeffrey SC. Design, synthesis, and biological evaluation of antibody-drug conjugates comprised of potent camptothecin analogues. Bioconjug Chem. 2009;20:1242–50.
48. Boger DL, Johnson DS. CC-1065 and the duocarmycins: unraveling the keys to a new class of naturally derived DNA alkylating agents. Proc Natl Acad Sci USA. 1995;92:3642–9.
49. Baraldi PG, Bovero A, Fruttarolo F, Preti D, Tabrizi MA, Pavani MG, Romagnoli R. DNA minor groove binders as potential antitumor and antimicrobial agents. Med Res Rev. 2004;24:475–528.
50. Jeffrey SC, Torgov MY, Andreyka JB, Boddington L, Cerveny CG, Denny WA, Gordon KA, Gustin D, Haugen J, Kline T, Nguyen MT, Senter PD. Design, synthesis, and in vitro evaluation of dipeptide-based antibody minor groove binder conjugates. J Med Chem. 2005;48:1344–58.
51. Alderson RF, Kreitman RJ, Chen T, Yeung P, Herbst R, Fox JA, Pastan I. CAT-8015: a second-generation pseudomonas exotoxin A-based immunotherapy targeting CD22-expressing hematologic malignancies. Clin Cancer Res. 2009;15:832–9.
52. Wayne AS, Kreitman RJ, Findley HW, Lew G, Delbrook C, Steinberg SM, Stetler-Stevenson M, Fitzgerald DJ, Pastan I. Anti-CD22 immunotoxin RFB4(dsFv)-PE38 (BL22) for CD22-positive hematologic malignancies of childhood: preclinical studies and phase I clinical trial. Clin Cancer Res. 2010;16:1894–903.
53. Walker MA, Dubowchik GM, Hofstead SJ, Trail PA, Firestone RA. Synthesis of an immunoconjugate of camptothecin. Bioorg Med Chem Lett. 2002;12:217–9.

54. Jeffrey SC, Andreyka JB, Bernhardt SX, Kissler KM, Kline T, Lenox JS, Moser RF, Nguyen MT, Okeley NM, Stone IJ, Zhang X, Senter PD. Development and properties of beta-glucuronide linkers for monoclonal antibody-drug conjugates. Bioconjug Chem. 2006;17:831–40.
55. Carrico IS. Chemoselective modification of proteins: hitting the target. Chem Soc Rev. 2008;37:1423–31.
56. Doronina SO, Toki BE, Torgov MY, Mendelsohn BA, Cerveny CG, Chace DF, DeBlanc RL, Gearing RP, Bovee TD, Siegall CB, Francisco JA, Wahl AF, Meyer DW, Senter PD. Development of potent monoclonal antibody auristatin conjugates for cancer therapy. Nat Biotechnol. 2003;21:778–84.
57. Lyon RP, Meyer DW, Setter JR, Senter PD. Conjugation of anticancer drugs through endogenous monoclonal antibody cysteine residues. Methods Enzymol. 2012;502:123–38.
58. Sun MMC, Beam KS, Cerveny CG, Hamblett KJ, Blackmore RS, Torgov MY, Handley FGM, Ihle NC, Senter PD, Alley SC. Reduction-alkylation strategies for the modification of specific monoclonal antibody disulfides. Bioconjug Chem. 2005;16:1282–90.
59. Hamblett KJ, Senter PD, Chace DF, Sun MMC, Lenox JS, Cerveny CG, Kissler KM, Bernhardt SX, Kopcha AK, Zabinski RF, Meyer DW, Francisco JA. Effects of drug loading on the antitumor activity of a monoclonal antibody drug conjugate. Clin Cancer Res. 2004;10:7063–70.
60. McDonagh CF, Turcott E, Westendorf L, Webster JB, Alley SC, Kim K, Andreyka J, Stone I, Hamblett KJ, Francisco JA, Carter P. Engineered antibody-drug conjugates with defined sites and stoichiometries of drug attachment. Protein Eng Des Sel. 2006;19:299–307.
61. Boswell CA, Mundo EE, Zhang C, Bumbaca D, Valle NR, Kozak KR, Fourie A, Chuh J, Koppada N, Saad O, Gill H, Shen BQ, Rubinfeld B, Tibbitts J, Kaur S, Theil FP, Fielder PJ, Khawli LA, Lin K. Impact of drug conjugation on pharmacokinetics and tissue distribution of anti-STEAP1 antibody-drug conjugates in rats. Bioconjug Chem. 2011;22:1994–2004.
62. Junutula JR, Flagella K, Graham RA, Parsons KL, Ha E, Raab H, Bhakta S, Nguyen T, Dugger DL, Li GW, Mai E, LewisPhillips GD, Hiraragi H, Fuji RN, Tibbitts J, Vandlen R, Spencer SD, Scheller RH, Polakis P, Sliwkowski MX. Engineered thio-trastuzumab-DM1 conjugate with an improved therapeutic index to target human epidermal growth factor receptor-2-positive breast cancer. Clin Cancer Res. 2010;16:4769–78.
63. Junutula JR, Raab H, Clark S, Bhakta S, Leipold DD, Weir SJ, Chen Y, Simpson M, Tsai SP, Dennis MS, Lu Y, Meng YG, Ng C, Yang J, Lee CC, Duenas E, Gorrell J, Katta V, Kim A, McDorman K, Flagella K, Venook R, Ross S, Spencer SD, Wong WL, Lowman HB, Vandlen R, Sliwkowski MX, Scheller RH, Polakis P, Mallet W. Site-specific conjugation of a cytotoxic drug to an antibody improves the therapeutic index. Nat Biotechnol. 2008;26:925–32.
64. Shen BQ, Xu K, Liu L, Raab H, Bhakta S, Kenrick M, Parsons-Reponte KL, Tien J, Yu SF, Mai E, Li D, Tibbitts J, Baudys J, Saad O, Scales SJ, McDonald PJ, Haas PE, Eigenbrot C, Nguyen T, Solis WA, Fuji RN, Flagella K, Patel D, Spencer SD, Khawli LA, Ebens A, Wong WL, Vandlen R, Kaur S, Sliwkowski MX, Scheller RH, Polakis P, Junutula JR. Conjugation site modulates the in vivo stability and therapeutic activity of antibody-drug conjugates. Nat Biotechnol. 2012;30:184–90.
65. Xu K, Liu L, Saad OM, Baudys J, Williams L, Leipold D, Shen B, Raab H, Junutula JR, Kim A, Kaur S. Characterization of intact antibody-drug conjugates from plasma/serum in vivo by affinity capture capillary liquid chromatography-mass spectrometry. Anal Biochem. 2011;412:56–66.
66. Axup JY, Bajjuri KM, Ritland M, Hutchins BM, Kim CH, Kazane SA, Halder R, Forsyth JS, Santidrian AF, Stafin K, Lu Y, Tran H, Seller AJ, Biroc SL, Szydlik A, Pinkstaff JK, Tian F, Sinha SC, Felding-Habermann B, Smider VV, Schultz PG. Synthesis of site-specific antibody-drug conjugates using unnatural amino acids. Proc Natl Acad Sci USA. 2012;109:16101–6.
67. Sletten EM, Bertozzi CR. Bioorthogonal chemistry: fishing for selectivity in a sea of functionality. Angew Chem Int Ed Engl. 2009;48:6974–98.

68. Cho H, Daniel T, Buechler YJ, Litzinger DC, Maio Z, Putnam AM, Kraynov VS, Sim BC, Bussell S, Javahishvili T, Kaphle S, Viramontes G, Ong M, Chu S, Becky GC, Lieu R, Knudsen N, Castiglioni P, Norman TC, Axelrod DW, Hoffman AR, Schultz PG, DiMarchi RD, Kimmel BE. Optimized clinical performance of growth hormone with an expanded genetic code. Proc Natl Acad Sci USA. 2011;108:9060–5.
69. Yin G, Garces ED, Yang J, Zhang J, Tran C, Steiner AR, Roos C, Bajad S, Hudak S, Penta K, Zawada J, Pollitt S, Murray CJ. Aglycosylated antibodies and antibody fragments produced in a scalable in vitro transcription-translation system. MAbs. 2012;4:217–25.
70. Rabuka D, Rush JS, de Hart GW, Wu P, Bertozzi CR. Site-specific chemical protein conjugation using genetically encoded aldehyde tags. Nat Protoc. 2012;7:1052–67.
71. Carrico IS, Carlson BL, Bertozzi CR. Introducing genetically encoded aldehydes into proteins. Nat Chem Biol. 2007;3:321–2.
72. Hudak JE, Barfield RM, de Hart GW, Grob P, Nogales E, Bertozzi CR, Rabuka D. Synthesis of heterobifunctional protein fusions using copper-free click chemistry and the aldehyde tag. Angew Chem Int Ed Engl. 2012;51:4161–5.
73. Tiefenbrunn TK, Dawson PE. Chemoselective ligation techniques: modern applications of time-honored chemistry. Biopolymers. 2010;94:95–106.
74. Stack GD, Walsh JJ. Optimising the delivery of tubulin targeting agents through antibody conjugation. Pharm Res. 2012;29:2972–84.
75. Bissery MC, Guenard D, Gueritte-Voegelein F, Lavelle F. Experimental antitumor activity of taxotere (RP 56976, NSC 628503), a taxol analogue. Cancer Res. 1991;51:4845–52.
76. DiJoseph JF, Armellino DC, Boghaert ER, Khandke K, Dougher MM, Sridharan L, Kunz A, Hamann PR, Gorovits B, Udata C, Moran JK, Popplewell AG, Stephens S, Frost P, Damle NK. Antibody-targeted chemotherapy with CMC-544: a CD22-targeted immunoconjugate of calicheamicin for the treatment of B-lymphoid malignancies. Blood. 2004;103:1807–14.
77. Boghaert ER, Khandke KM, Sridharan L, Dougher M, DiJoseph JF, Kunz A, Hamann PR, Moran J, Chaudhary I, Damle NK. Determination of pharmacokinetic values of calicheamicin-antibody conjugates in mice by plasmon resonance analysis of small (5 microl) blood samples. Cancer Chemother Pharmacol. 2008;61:1027–35.
78. Erickson HK, Widdison WC, Mayo MF, Whiteman K, Audette C, Wilhelm SD, Singh R. Tumor delivery and in vivo processing of disulfide-linked and thioether-linked antibody-maytansinoid conjugates. Bioconjug Chem. 2010;21:84–92.
79. Widdison WC, Wilhelm SD, Cavanagh EE, Whiteman KR, Leece BA, Kovtun Y, Goldmacher VS, Xie H, Steeves RM, Lutz RJ, Zhao R, Wang L, Blattler WA, Chari RV. Semisynthetic maytansine analogues for the targeted treatment of cancer. J Med Chem. 2006;49:4392–408.
80. Dubowchik GM, Firestone RA, Padilla L, Willner D, Hofstead SJ, Mosure K, Knipe JO, Lasch SJ, Trail PA. Cathepsin B-labile dipeptide linkers for lysosomal release of doxorubicin from internalizing immunoconjugates: model studies of enzymatic drug release and antigen-specific in vitro anticancer activity. Bioconjug Chem. 2002;13:855–69.
81. Doronina SO, Mendelsohn BA, Bovee TD, Cerveny CG, Alley SC, Meyer DL, Oflazoglu E, Toki BE, Sanderson RJ, Zabinski RF, Wahl AF, Senter PD. Enhanced activity of monomethylauristatin F through monoclonal antibody delivery: effects of linker technology on efficacy and toxicity. Bioconjug Chem. 2006;17:114–24.
82. Alley SC, Benjamin DR, Jeffrey SC, Okeley NM, Meyer DL, Sanderson RJ, Senter PD. Contribution of linker stability to the activities of anticancer immunoconjugates. Bioconjug Chem. 2008;19:759–65.
83. Kellogg BA, Garrett L, Kovtun Y, Lai KC, Leece B, Miller M, Payne G, Steeves R, Whiteman KR, Widdison W, Xie H, Singh R, Chari RV, Lambert JM, Lutz RJ. Disulfide-linked antibody-maytansinoid conjugates: optimization of in vivo activity by varying the steric hindrance at carbon atoms adjacent to the disulfide linkage. Bioconjug Chem. 2011;22:717–27.
84. Polson AG, Calemine-Fenaux J, Chan P, Chang W, Christensen E, Clark S, de Sauvage FJ, Eaton D, Elkins K, Elliott JM, Frantz G, Fuji RN, Gray A, Harden K, Ingle GS, Kljavin NM,

Koeppen H, Nelson C, Prabhu S, Raab H, Ross S, Slaga DS, Stephan JP, Scales SJ, Spencer SD, Vandlen R, Wranik B, Yu SF, Zheng B, Ebens A. Antibody-drug conjugates for the treatment of non-Hodgkin's lymphoma: target and linker-drug selection. Cancer Res. 2009;69:2358–64.
85. Doronina SO, Bovee TD, Meyer DW, Miyamoto JB, Anderson ME, Morris-Tilden CA, Senter PD. Novel peptide linkers for highly potent antibody-auristatin conjugate. Bioconjug Chem. 2008;19:1960–3.
86. Lan KH, Lu CH, Yu D. Mechanisms of trastuzumab resistance and their clinical implications. Ann NY Acad Sci. 2005;1059:70–5.
87. Rezvani AR, Maloney DG. Rituximab resistance. Best Pract Res Clin Haematol. 2011;24:203–16.
88. Takeshita A, Yamakage N, Shinjo K, Ono T, Hirano I, Nakamura S, Shigeno K, Tobita T, Maekawa M, Kiyoi H, Naoe T, Ohnishi K, Sugimoto Y, Ohno R. CMC-544 (inotuzumab ozogamicin), an anti-CD22 immuno-conjugate of calicheamicin, alters the levels of target molecules of malignant B-cells. Leukemia. 2009;23:1329–36.
89. Beyer I, Cao H, Persson J, Wang H, Liu Y, Yumul R, Li Z, Woodle D, Manger R, Gough M, Rocha D, Bogue J, Baldessari A, Berenson R, Carter D, Lieber A. Transient removal of cd46 is safe and increases B-cell depletion by rituximab in CD46 transgenic mice and macaques. Mol Ther. 2013;21:291–9.
90. Tsai PC, Hernandez-Ilizaliturri FJ, Bangia N, Olejniczak SH, Czuczman MS. Regulation of CD20 in rituximab-resistant cell lines and B-cell non-Hodgkin lymphoma. Clin Cancer Res. 2012;18:1039–50.
91. Gerber HP, Kung-Sutherland M, Stone I, Morris-Tilden C, Miyamoto J, McCormick R, Alley SC, Okeley N, Hayes B, Hernandez-Ilizaliturri FJ, McDonagh CF, Carter PJ, Benjamin D, Grewal IS. Potent antitumor activity of the anti-CD19 auristatin antibody drug conjugate hBU12-vcMMAE against rituximab-sensitive and -resistant lymphomas. Blood. 2009;113:4352–61.
92. Nagata Y, Lan KH, Zhou X, Tan M, Esteva FJ, Sahin AA, Klos KS, Li P, Monia BP, Nguyen NT, Hortobagyi GN, Hung MC, Yu D. PTEN activation contributes to tumor inhibition by trastuzumab, and loss of PTEN predicts trastuzumab resistance in patients. Cancer Cell. 2004;6:117–27.
93. Berns K, Horlings HM, Hennessy BT, Madiredjo M, Hijmans EM, Beelen K, Linn SC, Gonzalez-Angulo AM, Stemke-Hale K, Hauptmann M, Beijersbergen RL, Mills GB, van de Vijver MJ, Bernards R. A functional genetic approach identifies the PI3 K pathway as a major determinant of trastuzumab resistance in breast cancer. Cancer Cell. 2007;12:395–402.
94. Korkaya H, Kim GI, Davis A, Malik F, Henry NL, Ithimakin S, Quraishi AA, Tawakkol N, D'Angelo R, Paulson AK, Chung S, Luther T, Paholak HJ, Liu S, Hassan KA, Zen Q, Clouthier SG, Wicha MS. Activation of an IL6 inflammatory loop mediates trastuzumab resistance in HER2+ breast cancer by expanding the cancer stem cell population. Mol Cell. 2012;47:570–84.
95. Barok M, Tanner M, Koninki K, Isola J. Trastuzumab-DM1 causes tumour growth inhibition by mitotic catastrophe in trastuzumab-resistant breast cancer cells in vivo. Breast Cancer Res. 2011;13:R46.

Index

A
Adcetris, 184, 190
Antibodies, 50
Antibody–drug conjugates, 172, 176, 184, 187, 189–192, 194
Anti-EGFR monoclonal antibodies, 125, 126, 128–133, 136
Apoptosis, 159–162

B
Bioconjugation, 184, 191, 192
Biomarkers, 126, 133, 135–137
Bispecific antibody, 175
B-lymphoma, 74, 76–78, 80
B-Non-Hodgkin Lymphoma (B-NHL), 96–98, 103, 104, 106–108, 110, 115
Breast cancer, 28, 32

C
Cancer, 158, 159, 160–163
Cancer initiating cells, 28
CD20, 50, 53, 57, 59–61, 63, 64
Cell death, 158, 160–163
Cetuximab, 9, 13–15
Checkpoint inhibitors, 144, 146, 151
Chemokines, 146–151
Colorectal cancer, 128, 129, 136
Combinatorial therapy, 39, 42
Cytokines, 146–148, 150, 151

D
Disease recurrence, 26, 28, 32, 39, 42

F
Fc receptors, 53, 64
FcγRIIb, 51, 53–61, 63
FcR polymorphism, 77

H
Head and neck cancer, 31, 32
Herceptin, 167–169

I
Immunotherapy, 50, 51, 53–55, 57, 58, 61, 64
Ipilimumab, 144, 145, 147, 148

L
Linker, 184, 187, 189–193

M
Melanoma, 144, 146, 148–151
Microenvironment, 146, 148, 151
Modulation, 57, 59–61
Monoclonal antibodies, 2
Monoclonal antibody, 26
Multispecific antibody, 172
Mylotarg, 189, 190, 192, 194

O
Ofatumumab, 80
Osteosarcoma, 28, 32, 36

B. Bonavida (ed.), *Resistance to Immunotherapeutic Antibodies in Cancer*, Resistance to Targeted Anti-Cancer Therapeutics 2, DOI: 10.1007/978-1-4614-7654-2,

P
Pancreatic cancer, 30
Payload, 187, 189, 191–194
Programmed death receptor 1 (PD1), 144, 148, 151

R
Resistance, 2, 3, 5–8, 10, 12–15, 74, 158, 160–163
Rituximab, 3–6, 8, 74, 95, 96, 98–108, 111
Rituximab-resistance, 75, 78, 79, 83, 85, 108, 110, 111

S
Signal transduction, 108–110, 113
Signal pathways, 83, 85

T
T cells, 144–148, 151
Targeted inhibitors, 116
TNF-related apoptosis-inducing ligand (TRAIL), 159–161, 163
Trastuzumab, 3, 8, 10, 11, 15
Trastuzumab emtansine (T-DM1), 190, 193, 194
Tumor antigen, 26
Tumour resistance, 57

U
Unnatural amino acid, 172, 173, 176–178

MIX
Papier aus verantwortungsvollen Quellen
Paper from responsible sources
FSC® C105338

FSC
www.fsc.org

If you have any concerns about our products,
you can contact us on
ProductSafety@springernature.com

In case Publisher is established outside the EU,
the EU authorized representative is:
Springer Nature Customer Service Center GmbH
Europaplatz 3, 69115 Heidelberg, Germany

Printed by Libri Plureos GmbH
in Hamburg, Germany